Women's Health Communication

Women's Health Communication

High-Risk Pregnancy and Premature Birth Narratives

Jennifer G. Hall

LEXINGTON BOOKS
Lanham • Boulder • New York • London

Published by Lexington Books
An imprint of The Rowman & Littlefield Publishing Group, Inc.
4501 Forbes Boulevard, Suite 200, Lanham, Maryland 20706
www.rowman.com

Unit A, Whitacre Mews, 26–34 Stannary Street, London SE11 4AB

British Library Cataloguing in Publication Information Available

Library of Congress Control Number: 2015949554
ISBN: 978-0-7391-9586-4 (cloth : alk. paper)
eISBN: 978-0-7391-9587-1

∞™ The paper used in this publication meets the minimum requirements of American National Standard for Information Sciences—Permanence of Paper for Printed Library Materials, ANSI/NISO Z39.48-1992.

Printed in the United States of America

For my girls Anna, Sarah, Lucy, and Emily who shape my story daily. May your own stories continue to be full of wonder, amazement, love, and joy

Contents

Acknowledgments

There are several people I need to acknowledge as without their help, support, and participation, this book would have never come to be. First and foremost I need to thank the women I interviewed who so generously gave me their time and so honestly shared their stories with me. Not only did these women give me material for my book, but they also helped me to heal, gave me perspective, and showed me how important and necessary a project like this is. Second, I need to acknowledge Marifran Mattson, my former advisor and current department chair, and an incredible mentor. Without her constant guidance, encouragement, support, and friendship I would have never finished my dissertation or this book. She has constantly taught me both through her words and by example that there are many paths one can take and as long as your path is one that makes you happy and allows you to engage in work that is meaningful to you, then you are on the right path. I am always forever thankful for my mother, Theresa Gibb. Not only did she raise me to believe that I could do anything I put my mind to, but she watched the girls while I was working, listened tirelessly as I talked about the stresses and challenges of my writing, and served as my personal editor, reading and copyediting all of my chapters. And last but not least I need to acknowledge my husband who lived this story with me and gave me the time and space I needed to talk with women, write, and follow my dream.

Introduction[1]

Each year, nearly 4,000,000 babies are born in the United States (Martin et al. 2015). While a majority of these pregnancies end successfully with a full-term healthy baby, there are a myriad of complications that can occur at all stages of the reproductive process including everything from difficulty conceiving to miscarriage, still birth, and premature labor and premature delivery. What is easily thought of as a routine part of the life-cycle process can sometimes be anything but that, and this book seeks to examine some of the situations when women's pregnancies are not routine and are instead, as the title of the book suggests, more like a rollercoaster ride full of ups, downs, and terrifying turns. Specifically, the purpose of this book is to explore and share the stories of women who were diagnosed as having a high-risk pregnancy, went into premature labor, or gave birth prematurely. Unfortunately this experience is more common than one might think with one out of every eight babies born in the United States being born prematurely. The number of pregnancies classified as high risk is even higher as many women fall in the category due to their age and medical conditions such as diabetes; with careful management, they are able to carry their pregnancies to term.

I chose to focus specifically on high-risk pregnancy and premature birth for three primary reasons. The first is because of the high rate of premature birth in the United States. Over ten percent of women who give birth each year have a pregnancy and delivery experience that varies from the norm. There are almost 4,000,000 births annually, which means that roughly 40,000 of those births happen before 37 weeks. The second is because high-risk pregnancy and birth are something that I have experienced firsthand. Because of my own experience I feel qualified and capable to talk about the challenges I faced in having a high-risk pregnancy, premature labor, and having my daughters 8 weeks early. Infertility and miscarriage are not part of my story so I cannot speak to the pain of these experiences firsthand. I can try to imagine what this might be like and think I can put myself in these women's shoes, but because I have never been through these times, I do not know what it is like. In the end, the most I can do is listen to their stories and offer my sympathy as I do not truly know what it feels like to struggle to get pregnant, have a miscarriage, or lose a child.

This is not to say at all that one cannot study and write about topics and issues that he or she has not personally experienced. Countless researchers, scholars, and writers have done excellent work studying people in situations and circumstances completely different from their own. In some situations there might even be an advantage in being able to observe and draw conclusions with a more objective point of view. There is a natural human instinct to interpret the people, events, and stories we encounter from our unique lens, which is inevitably shaped by our own personal history and experiences, and if we are not careful, it is easy to judge and measure each story we hear against our own. I recently read an excellent essay by Jennifer Bute, a communication professor who built her career studying infertility and miscarriage (Bute 2011). One might assume her research interest arose from personal experience, but in fact when she started her career she had never been pregnant and had never tried to have children. She admits to struggling with the question of whether she as a women without these experiences had the "right" to study such an intimate topic. She concluded though that not being immersed in the pain and struggles of infertility and pregnancy loss allowed her to see and hear things from a more objective place and to see things that might have easily been clouded by her own pain and experience. After several years of research and writing on the topic, Bute and her husband were ready to start a family and she found herself struggling to conceive and once she did conceive she had a miscarriage. Suddenly, Bute was living the very thing that she had asked so many women about before, which raised important questions for her about how her own life and viewpoint informed her work and vice versa. She does not neatly conclude her essay with the realization that her personal experience made her work that much better, but instead ends with the fact that when we are studying something we always need to be aware of our own positionality and actively consider how it influences our way of interpreting the world.

In my own research and writing, it was imperative that as I talked with women and later tried to draw conclusions from what I had heard that I listened to what was there, what was said, and what was not said. I needed to acknowledge and even recognize differences in what women thought and how women felt from each other, and particularly from myself. I consciously had to put aside my preconceived ideas of what a woman's reactions or action would or should be based on what I knew firsthand. As much as the commonalities were important to what I was trying to learn and say about the experiences of high-risk pregnancy and premature birth, the differences were equally important. I assumed when I started (and as it turns out, rightly assumed) that there would be common trends and themes which could provide more general insight into how to help and support women. I had ideas based on my own experiences of what women might need, and finding women with similar experiences was vital to my being able to draw conclusions and develop suggestions for helping these women. When a woman had a completely different emotional reaction or used an entirely different source of information it raised the question of why, which frequently lead to important information about how individual and situational differences were either helpful or detrimental to women.

For me though, the benefits of having firsthand experience and an understanding of the multiple emotional, mental, physical, and even logistical aspects of having a premature baby were numerous. Dr. Laura Ellingson (2006) wrote about the importance of researchers incorporating their own bodies into their research and acknowledging how their own physical sensations, weakness, and strengths informs their work and understanding of what they are studying. It was my own experiences that led me to the questions that I attempted to answer in this book. Without being on bed rest, going into preterm labor multiple times, and having my children spend time in the neonatal intensive care unit (NICU), I do not think that I would have known what questions needed to be asked and where the gaps were in what we do not know and what we need to understand. Had I not experienced the isolation of being the only woman I knew who had preemie triplets, I don't think I would have known that isolation and loneliness were important issues that needed to be addressed. The difficulty I had in finding the information and stories I so desperately craved was one of the driving forces behind my undertaking this project. If I couldn't find the information that I thought would have been helpful to me, to my friends and family, and even the physicians and hospital staff, then I decided that I would take it upon myself to find the information and stories that were missing and share it.

Another huge benefit of my personal experience came as I met and spoke with women about their own pregnancies, births, and time in the NICU. It was easy for me to establish rapport and trust with the women who so graciously volunteered to let me interview them and ask what could at times be very personal questions that often had very sensitive answers. Because of my own story I was not just a curious bystander but I was a member of the in-group. I am a preemie mom, I am an NICU mom, and I am a mom of multiples. Because of that, some of the walls that women might have kept up when talking with someone who was not a member of the preemie mom tribe seemed to come down. Women knew that I could not only sympathize with them, but I truly could empathize with them. The interviews I conducted rarely felt like an interview, but instead they felt more like a genuine conversation. Every so often I will hear from a woman I interviewed to update me on how her preemie is doing or even to let me know that she has had another child. Nothing makes me smile more than to learn that someone has delivered a full-term healthy baby.

There is another reason that I chose to focus specifically on high-risk pregnancy and premature birth. Many of the stories speak to the myriad of complications and outcomes that can accompany a pregnancy. For example, many of the women I interviewed dealt with infertility and as result of fertility treatments, conceived twins, triplets, or more, resulting in a high-risk pregnancy and very often a premature birth. Other mothers shared with me their incredibly painful stories of early miscarriages, late miscarriages, and what was every parent's worst nightmare, their child or children dying after they were born due to prematurity-related complications. I share these aspects of the women's stories in the book because their stories would not be complete without including these aspects of their lives. The book, however, does not focus specifically on these issues and does not make specific observations about or recommendations for supporting, for example, a woman who has suffered a miscarriage as it was outside of the scope of this project. While miscarriage, and infertility share many aspects of high-risk pregnancy and premature birth and are connected to the reproductive process, they are still distinct experiences and I firmly believe that each of these issues deserves its own book or books. Fortunately, there are books and writers dedicated to these topics and sharing the stories of women in these situations.

This book also focuses on the stories and experiences of women and mothers. This is in no way meant to discount the experiences of the fathers whose wives or partners experience pregnancy complication and whose children are born too early. In fact, until recently there has been a paucity of research and information that looks at the unique experience of husband and fathers whose partner, wives, and children experience complications due to pregnancy-related issues and premature birth. The research that has been done shows that high-risk pregnancy and premature birth place a great deal of stress on men, that men often cope differently and have different stress reactions than women, and men and fathers also are in dire need of support to help cope with the emotional and mental challenges that come with having either a partner or child in serious harm (Garten et al. 2013; Matricardi et al. 2013). I chose to focus just on women and mothers for two primary reasons. The first is because as I have said, the experience of men is inevitably different than that of women and much like other pregnancy- and birth-related conversations, the stories and experiences of men deserve their own focused project.

The second reason is the differences between what men and women experience I wanted to address the unique things that women and mothers face.

When a woman starts to have pregnancy complications, goes into preterm labor, or her cervix starts to shorten too early, it is her body that is carrying the child or children and it is her body that is not doing what she may think it was designed to do. When a baby is born prematurely, women will often carry a sense of guilt that they somehow did something wrong or let their baby down, a feeling that is unique to the woman who was pregnant and gave birth. A few weeks after I learned I was pregnant with triplets I was feeling particularly overwhelmed. Not only did I have a million worries and concerns racing through my mind, but I also felt so much pressure to do everything I could to stay pregnant for as long as possible. Everyone was helping me as much as they possibly could, but in the end it was me who needed to stay off my feet, get enough food to adequately nourish the babies, and follow doctor's orders. Each time I learned my cervix had shortened or that I was having more frequent contractions, my first thought was always, "what did I do wrong?" It was my body's responsibility to stay pregnant, and the health and well-being of my children depended on me. Scholars and researchers have written about the physical embodiment of pregnancy and the unique experience of having one's body both physically transformed from pregnancy and of sharing one's body and resources with another being (Lupton 2012; Alcalde 2011). There is something unique about the physical experience of being pregnant and giving birth, and by focusing on women I was able to explore how the physical embodiment of pregnancy complications, premature delivery, and motherhood influenced women's reactions to their situations.

This book begins with my own story. As I mentioned previously, without my own experience, I don't believe I would have been compelled to engage in this project or write this book. As much as this book is about high-risk pregnancies and premature birth, it is equally about stories and the power they have to shape our realities. This includes the stories we tell ourselves as well as the stories we encounter, hear, and read. I share how my own experiences led me to ask the questions that drove my research and investigations that I attempt to answer in this book and how my own story informed and continues to inform my understanding and interpretation of the stories that so many women generously shared with me. Following my story, the second chapter first takes a step back and explores the power of narratives and stories in shaping our reality, drawing heavily on narrative theory. It then looks more specifically at how stories relate to the pregnancy and birthing experience.

The third chapter of the book looks at the cultural stories that are told about pregnancy and childbirth and illustrates how the expectations and beliefs about these have changed as society and culture have changed. It is important to examine the dominant stories of pregnancy and birth in order to understand how women see and think about their own experiences in relation to these cultural narratives. Even though pregnancy and birth are incredibly personal events, they are also in many ways a shared and public event that is surrounded by routines and rituals ranging from announcing the pregnancy to having a baby shower. The chapter further argues that by understanding where women's expectations and beliefs about pregnancy, birth, and motherhood come from, those whose experiences do not meet those expectations and those who support these women may be better able to handle the disappointment and may also be able to develop alternative ways to fulfill those expectations.

In the fourth chapter the book begins to look more specifically at women's stories and how women felt and reacted when their own experiences did not meet their expectations of what pregnancy and birth would be like. The feeling that one's story was wrong or should not be happening was a common thread and this chapter looks at women's experiences of living out what felt like the wrong story and also suggests ways women can come to terms with their stories and embrace their uniqueness. The fifth chapter examines the role that social comparison plays in women's storytelling as well as their understanding of and reaction to their circumstances. One of the important ways that we as humans learn about the world and evaluate how we well we are doing is by comparing ourselves to those around us. How feel we are doing in relation to the comparison target will influence how we feel about ourselves. With little firsthand knowledge of high-risk pregnancies and premature infants, many women make comparison to others in order to gain understanding and perspective on their situations. These comparisons can have both esteem-enhancing and esteem-diminishing effects, and as this chapter describes, the effects of the comparisons are not always what is expected.

The sixth chapter looks at how women sought out, used, and avoided information about high-risk pregnancy complications and premature birth. While information was essential to women making informed choices and understanding their circumstances, there are often times when too much information can lead to excessive fear, extreme anxiety, and even paralysis. At the opposite end of the spectrum, the chapter looks at information and stories that women purposely avoided and the consequences of that avoidance. The difference in the amount of information women intentionally consumed leads to an interesting tension for pregnant women and NICU moms and those who care for them as they work to find the right balance between too much and too little information. The chapter also explores women's preferred sources of information as well as how they evaluated the credibility and utility of the information they encountered

Chapter 7 focuses on media portrayals or pregnancy, birth, high-risk pregnancies, and premature birth and the influences those portrayals have on women and the stories they tell about their own pregnancy and births. As birthing moved out of the home and into the hospital, fewer and fewer girls and women had first hand experience witnessing a birth, so they have to rely on books, television, and film to see what the birth process is like. One of the challenges of relying on media to learn about pregnancy and birth to set one's expectations is that both fictional and nonfictional accounts may not provide accurate accounts and therefore women and the public in general may have false expectations or inaccurate ideas of what birth should be like or what it is like to have a premature baby.

In chapter 8, women share their stories about their high-risk pregnancies and premature births. While there are numerous reasons that a pregnancy may be classified as high risk including prior health conditions, maternal age, and being pregnant with multiples, there are many similarities among women in the struggles they faced during their pregnancies. Living with constant anxiety and enduring various medical treatments to sustain a pregnancy including surgery, medication, and bed rest can take an incredible toll. Some women have perfectly normal pregnancies and suddenly develop a life-threatening complication like preeclampsia or their water breaks and without much warning their babies are born weeks or evens month early. The emergency nature of many preterm deliveries and fears over the babies' health and at times even their survival also can take an incredible toll on women.

After going through their high-risk pregnancies and births, for women whose children were born too early, usually prior to 37 weeks, the next step in the process was a stay in the NICU. A few of the women I interviewed were able to carry their babies to term or at least close enough to 37 weeks that no NICU stay was needed, but for the vast majority of women, the NICU was a part of their story and chapter 9 describes what life in the NICU was like for women and some of the challenges they faced including logistics, emotional strain, establishing their role as a parent, and in some cases even losing a child. Whether women's children spent a few days or several months in the NICU the experience was difficult and not what they had ever expected when they imagined having a baby. In addition to sharing the stories of women's NICU experiences, the chapter also offers insights and suggestions into how the experience could be improved and how women can be better supported during this time.

In chapter 10, the focus is on what life is like for mothers after their babies are discharged from the NICU and come home. Even though a baby has matured enough and is well enough to come home, preemies often have ongoing medical issues that require medications, treatments, therapy, and multiple follow-up appointments. This chapter looks at some of the ongoing issues and stressors that women dealt with as they raised a child who was born early. The overarching theme of the women's stories was that coming home from the hospital did not mean that the challenges of a having a premature baby were over. Some family's struggles and challenges resolve more quickly than others, but almost every mother I spoke with carried with her the fear and anxiety that she had lived with, often throughout her pregnancy and then during her child's time in the NICU while she continued to be on alert and concerned with her child's health and development.

Chapter 11 brings together many of the elements discussed in the prior chapters and focuses on the wide range of emotions women experience during their high-risk pregnancies including anxiety, guilt, sadness, and envy. Many women felt unprepared for the emotional ups and downs of a high-risk pregnancy and early delivery as they had not read or heard a lot of stories about this aspect of parenting. This chapter also looks at the important role that social support plays in helping women cope and the various ways that women were able to find the support they needed.

NOTE

1. Publisher's Note: The interviews used as supplemental research in this text were all conducted with the participants' knowledge and agreement that these interviews would be used in a later publication.

Chapter 1

My Story

My story begins after I heard the three words that would forever change my life, "you have three babies in there." I had gone in for what I thought was a routine ultrasound at 18 weeks. Having an older doctor who tended to be somewhat conservative, I had not had an early ultrasound to confirm the due date so as far as we knew, I was carrying one baby. I can still remember the utter shock and panic I felt when the ultrasound technician shared the news. It was hard to grasp what she had told us, let alone believe it, but sure enough there were three half-pound infants in there with strong heartbeats. Over the next few days, as my husband and I absorbed the shock and tried to come to terms with the idea that our immediate family would soon double in size (we already had an eighteen-month-old daughter), we also were thrust into the unknown and uncertain world of a high-risk pregnancy.

To give a little back story, my husband Brian and I met while in college at Indiana University and got married four years later in 2004 when we were 24. I had just graduated with my Master's degree in communication from Purdue University and had decided to stay and continue my education so Brian found a job as a fourth grade teacher at a local elementary school and we settled into married life in Lafayette, Indiana. I was one of those women who was excited for a career, but even more so, I could not wait to be a mother. Being a perpetual planner and kind of a control freak I had strong ideas about when we should have our first baby. I was working on my doctoral degree in health communication so I wanted to be done with my course work when I had a baby, which meant that we had to wait at least a year before I got pregnant and I also wanted to have a baby in May or June because as a graduate student I had summers off from teaching. People kept telling me that you do not always get to plan things like this and I knew there was a possibility that we would not get pregnant exactly when I wanted, but I was determined to try my hardest to make it happen, so I turned to Google and began to find anything I could about conception.

Through my research I learned that it took the average couple three months to conceive and I also learned what the most fertile days in a woman's cycle were. It was shocking to learn that getting pregnant wasn't necessarily as easy as I had always believed and most women can only conceive on two or three days of her cycle and the average woman has only a 35 percent chance of getting pregnant during a given cycle. I had the information and knew when the optimum times for conception were, but the one catch to this was that I had always had a very irregular cycle, and when I was not on the pill I could go months without having a period. I knew this posed a challenge to being able to plan getting pregnant so I went to my OB. His suggestion was to give me progesterone, a medication that induces menstruation in women with irregular cycles, and then to use Clomid, a medication that helps women ovulate. At this point I started taking the progesterone pills and started to research Clomid and how it worked. The one thing that caused me some anxiety was the increased chance of conceiving twins while using this medication. My husband and I discussed it and we decided that we would take the risk as it was still a small percentage and if we had to we could handle twins.

As it turns out though, I never got the opportunity to try Clomid. After waiting somewhat impatiently for two weeks after taking the progesterone my period had still not started. I feared something was very wrong with me and I began to panic. During all of this I did not feel well, but I chalked it up to stress. For some reason on a Friday I broke down and bought a pregnancy test. It was really just wishful thinking on my part that maybe the medicine had not worked because I was pregnant. I was completely shocked and delighted then when two lines quickly appeared on the test strip. In all of my worry and concern we had gotten pregnant and I was due on April 17, which was just about perfect given that it was almost to the end of the spring semester. For all of my worry and concern, things had turned out exactly how I wanted them to.

From that point on my pregnancy was perfectly ordinary. I had some morning sickness, aches and pains, and I was tired, but nothing that was unusual or unexpected. We decided not to find out the sex of the baby because we wanted to be surprised in the delivery room. I think this bothered a lot of people as they wanted to know if they should buy blue or pink, but I reasoned that my mom had never found out as it wasn't even an option when my brothers and I were born and I also wanted to get as many neutral things as possible. I knew I wanted more than one child and I assumed we would have a mix of boys and girls so an all pink or blue nursery was just not practical.

I also thought that there could be nothing more exciting than delivering your baby and in that moment learning whether you had a new son or daughter.

It is funny the things you remember in hindsight, but after each doctor's appointment I would call my mom and relay the rate of the heartbeat, how much weight I had gained and my blood pressure. These appointments were always uneventful and I remember commenting to my mom once that the appointments were almost boring. Little did I know how thankful I should be for these routine "boring" appointments. I did not worry much about the baby's or my health and in all honesty, my largest fear after attending birthing classes at the local hospital was that I might have to share my hospital room after I delivered with another mother and baby. The hospital where I delivered did not have private rooms and I could think of nothing worse than sharing a room with a stranger and their family and visitors. Again, little did I know that there could be far worse things following a delivery than sharing your postpartum room with a stranger.

As I neared the end of my pregnancy I became less and less patient and was ready for the baby to come. My due date came and passed and I had still not gone into labor; I began to despair and started trying anything to start labor from eating spicy food to scrubbing my shower. Either my tricks worked or my time had come as I woke up around 4 am on Friday morning April 21 with contractions about eight minutes apart. To make a long story short we drove to the hospital and when I was admitted I was three centimeters dilated and experiencing intense transitional labor. I had briefly thought that I would try to have a nonmedicated birth but as the contractions kept coming I quickly opted for an epidural. At 1:45 our daughter Anna was born weighing 7 pounds 11 ounces. In many ways it was just like what I had seen on TV. They let me hold her right away and I instantly loved her and could hardly believe that this little girl was ours.

Fast forward a year and we were celebrating Anna's first birthday. Of course having a baby had been difficult at times, but we loved her so much, I wanted her to have siblings and my thinking was that if one child made us this happy, two would mean we would be even happier. I again sat down and started to figure out things like due dates and when to conceive. We had conceived so easily and quickly with Anna, but I still worried that we might not be successful. I started charting my temperature religiously and paid careful attention to any minor fluctuations. Once again my planning seemed to work and on July 8 we were visiting my parents and went out to lunch. After eating I started to feel incredibly ill and spent the rest of the day lying on the couch. I thought maybe I was pregnant so I went home the next day and took a pregnancy test and just like when I was pregnant with Anna the second line appeared on the indicator stick almost immediately. I called my OB and the nurse told me I did not need to be seen until I was at least 10 weeks so I sat back and tried to enjoy being pregnant.

From the beginning, this pregnancy was very different than the first. I had felt queasy with Anna on and off, but this time I felt sick all day long and would wake up in the night with nausea. I was so tired, but I blamed that on the fact that I was taking care of a one year old. I remember calling my mom once and asking her if she thought maybe I was pregnant with twins because I had read morning sickness was much worse with multiples because of the extra hormones. "No," she told me confidently, "if you were pregnant with twins they would have figured it out by now." That made sense to me and I just tried to cope with the pregnancy as best as I could trying everything from sucking on sour candy to wearing tight wrist bands that people sometimes wear on cruises to ward of motion sickness. Because I was so sick I only gained a pound during my first trimester, and because we were not telling anyone I was pregnant yet, it was easy to hide.

Shortly after my first trimester ended I started to feel a little better, was able to eat a little and my stomach popped out so I started to tell people I was expecting again. There was another woman in my department who was due right around the same time as me with her first baby. People were constantly telling me how much bigger I looked than her, which when you think about it is a pretty rude thing to tell a pregnant woman. I explained that you show more quickly with your second pregnancy because your body is more stretched out and really thought nothing of it. I felt the baby kick very early on, around 16 weeks and was excited about the physical evidence that Anna would soon be a big sister. We had gone home to Ohio to visit my family for a weekend and I told my mom that this little one was very active as I could already feel it kicking near my rib cage. She looked at me like I was crazy and said it must be something else because it was too early for the baby to even be up that high.

At 17 weeks I went for my monthly appointment with my OB. I stepped on the scale—definitely my least favorite part of any of my maternity appointments—and the nurse noted that I had gained 8 pounds. It seemed like a lot, but given that I had gained so little during my first trimester I figured my body was just playing catch up. When my doctor came in he asked how I was feeling and I responded jokingly, "I feel huge." I expected him to laugh but instead he looked at me nodded his head and said, "you do look huge." This is definitely not something a pregnant woman wants to hear from anyone, and especially not her doctor, but I was much larger than I should have been for being only 17 weeks pregnant.

For the rest of the appointment it became more and more obvious that something was not right. The doctor spent a lot of time with the Doppler listening to the heartbeat and noted I was measuring very far ahead of my actual gestation. He quickly suggested I go in for an ultrasound and told me that given my size we either had an incorrect due date, I had too much amniotic fluid, or he said with a laugh there might be two in there. I think this appointment was on a Thursday and when I went to schedule the ultrasound I had the option for a Friday appointment during the day which was the next day, but I wanted my husband to be there so I waited for a late afternoon appointment on Monday afternoon.

The next few days passed in a blur and I spent most of the weekend trying to figure out what could possibly be wrong. I was pretty certain my due date was not wrong, given my careful charting of my temperature, but I could be off. The idea of twins just seemed too crazy and the doctor had not seemed very serious or concerned when he said it, so I discounted that theory pretty quickly and instead became consumed with figuring out why I had too much fluid. I spent a lot of time using Google and thought that maybe something was wrong with the baby's kidneys, but also held out hope that I had just gained a lot of weight and everything would be fine. I just kept thinking that there couldn't be anything too wrong, because that is what happens to other people or that is what happens in TV shows. I was just an ordinary person with an ordinary life and I expected my pregnancy to be the same. I quickly started kicking myself for not opting for the earlier ultrasound appointment because the anticipation and unknown was killing me. Looking back I think that my willingness to wait on the ultrasound shows just how unaware I was that something could seriously be wrong. I was excited about having an ultrasound to see the baby for the first time, but I was not thinking that this would be an important diagnostic test.

I remember that I arrived for my ultrasound appointment a little early that Monday. My husband was going to pick up Anna from the sitter and bring her because I thought it would be good for her to "see" her new baby brother or sister. I remember the technician coming out and telling me she was a little ahead of schedule so if I wanted to come back and get started I could. "No thank you," I told her, "I want to wait for my husband." Normally I would have gone ahead, but something in me felt like he needed to be there and I am so glad he was.

As I lay on the ultrasound table the technician covered me with the cold goop and started to move the wand around my stomach and it seemed like a lot of blobs popped up on the screen. The blobs didn't look like anything distinct, but my first thought still was, "oh my gosh, it is twins." This is when the technician spoke and said, "Did you know there are three babies in there?" People are always interested in what my first reaction was and if I am completely honest it was utter disbelief and the feeling that she was playing a practical joke on us. I looked at my husband who looked as confused and shocked as I felt and turned to the technician and said, "can that happen? We weren't using fertility drugs." It had never once, not even for one second crossed my mind that I could possibly be pregnant with triplets. "This cannot be real," I kept thinking, "people do not just get pregnant with triplets. That does not happen." But, as I now know, apparently some people do.

The rest of that appointment passed in a blur. I know I was crying silently and my husband tried to keep Anna who was only eighteen months old occupied in the cramped room. She quickly grew restless and he took her out to walk around and all I wanted to do was jump off the table and follow him. The ultrasound took forever as the technician worked to get all of the babies' measurements. A thousand thoughts were swirling through my head; the babies would be early, how could I have four kids two and under, I would have to drop out of school, the babies might be sick or disabled, we only had one crib, we did not have a car big enough to fit everyone. Mostly, I just wanted to call my mom. She knew I had gone in for an ultrasound and had told me to call as soon as I was done. I knew she would be worried as the minutes ticked by and I also knew that she was the only one who would be able to comfort me.

After nearly two hours, the ultrasound was over. My OB came down and talked briefly to my husband and me. As I said earlier, my OB was older, more traditional, and pretty blunt. I don't think that he necessarily excelled at bedside manner, but I trusted him. When he entered the room he looked right at Brian and asked him, "What did you do?" He then warned us that the babies would come early and we needed to be prepared for a tough road ahead. I remember him telling us that he hoped we had good insurance because the babies would be in the hospital for some time. Nothing that he said was particularly reassuring, but at the same time he was being realistic and it was just the beginning of preparing us for the road ahead. Despite all of the craziness I tried to cling to the good news was that each baby was measuring almost exactly the same size, at 18 weeks and 1 day, looked perfectly healthy and my cervix was still a good length.

We had decided going in to the ultrasound that we would not find out the sex just like we had done for Anna. When the technician asked us if we wanted to know the sexes though I blurted out yes. Finding out there were triplets was surprising enough, and I needed to know if they were boys or girls so I could plan and start to gather the things we would need. Because I was only 18 weeks along and the babies were crowded the technician thought that one was a girl and she could not tell what the other two were. It took three more ultrasounds before they were finally able, about month later, to tell us that they were definitely all girls. Brian was understandably a little disappointed as we have figured there had to be a boy in there somewhere, but I was relieved. I remembered hearing once that baby girls are stronger than baby boys and that girl preemies do better than boy preemies, so we at least had that going for us.

The first thing I did as we walked out of the doctor's office was reach for my phone and call my mom. "It's triplets," I cried unable to say anything else. I know we talked more, but the details of the conversation escaped me. I drove home that evening which looking back was probably not a good idea considering that I was in shock and not thinking straight, but we had taken separate cars and we just did what we had to do. People always say that your life can change in an instant and for the first time in my life I saw that this was absolutely true. Everything that I hoped for, planned, and imagined no longer seemed possible. I don't think I slept at all that night and around 6 the next morning I called my mom back and she told me it would all be okay, that we could do this, and I had to believe her because if I didn't I could not go on.

The next step after informing family and friends that I was expecting not one but three babies was to learn as much as we could about triplets and a triplet pregnancy. I had no idea what to expect, what it would be like to carry three infants instead of one, and what sort of issues our children could be facing, so I immediately turned to the internet for any information I could find. I first looked up facts. I just needed basic facts such as what was the probability of having spontaneous (i.e. the term I quickly learned was the correct one to describe triplets conceived without the use of fertility treatments) triplets which is 1 in 8100. That number still seems fairly high to me, but, I was thinking more like one in a million, but it was still pretty uncommon. Still baffled as to how I got pregnant with triplets I also researched the factors that would make someone more likely to have twins or triplets, which include being a twin yourself, being older, and being taller—none of which describe me. Finally, and most seriously I need to know what the survival rate of triplets was. After learning that 98 percent of triplets born after 28 weeks survive, I felt much better. I honestly was not worried about the babies surviving, I was just worried what types of issues they would have. I know now that I was naïve and I could have easily delivered before 28 weeks, but I will always be grateful for my ignorance as it was just one less thing to worry about.

Although these facts were important and interesting, they were not enough, so I sought out stories of others who had multiples. I think it is important at this point to note that as worried as I was about having preemies, I was equally if not more worried about having triplets. I could not begin to even fathom how one takes care of three babies at once. My first step was to go to my neighbor Terra who had identical twin girls who were six. She kindly gave me a few books she had on raising multiples and answered all of my questions about her pregnancy, her time on bed rest, and her delivery. She was one of those amazing women who had a scheduled C-section at 38 weeks and brought home her healthy babies with her. It was reassuring to talk to her, but I also knew that carrying triplets was much different than carrying twins and I needed to find more people who were like me.

I did not know anyone personally who had triplets so unable to tap into my own social network I turned to the internet. I had used the internet to discover facts about the babies' development and potential complications, but I wanted to find actual women who had triplets and learn what they had done and how they survived. Through the magic of Google I found several forums for parents of multiples and quickly found a forum for parents of triplets and higher-order multiples on Tripletconnection.com. I was amazed at how many triplet moms there seemed to be. I obsessively read the stories of other women who had been pregnant with triplets, paying extra attention to their symptoms, how long they had carried their infants, and the details of their children's NICU stays.

At first I would read anything I could find and found myself overwhelmed by the variety of stories I encountered that included everything from triplets born at 24 weeks who did not survive to triplets born at 36 weeks who spent no time in the NICU and everything in between. I then began more tailored searches, trying to find women who seemed to most closely resemble me. I tried to find women who had spontaneous triplets, hoping the spontaneous nature of my pregnancy would in some way guarantee a better outcome. In my naïve thinking I thought that my body would not have allowed me to conceive triplets if I could not physically carry them. I also tried to determine how tall women were, how old, and what other children they had. The more similar they were to me the more I felt that their story could relate to mine and I sought to predict the outcome of my pregnancy from their stories.

As I continued to seek out information and stories, the babies and my belly continued to grow. After discovering the triplets, my OB in town scheduled me for weekly visits and also referred me to a perinatologist in Indianapolis who would also follow my case. At the first doctor's appointment after the ultrasound my OB informed me that I would be on strict bed rest at 24 weeks, which at this point was only six weeks away, and that the goal was to make it to at least 28 weeks, but ideally I would deliver at 34 weeks, with the average gestation for triplets being 32 weeks. I remember trying to formulate intelligent questions thinking that it was my obligation as a mother to be as informed as possible, but my mind was still swirling and it still didn't seem quite real. In many ways I felt like I was an actress playing a role. This could not be my life. This was something that happened to other people, this was something you saw on TV. I did ask how much I should be eating and he told me as much as I could and that it was especially important to eat a lot of protein because it helped with brain development. At this point in my life after being a vegetarian for several years I ate only chicken and this was a only a couple of times a week. It wasn't for moral reasons, it was more about trying to be healthy and I just didn't like meat that much. On that day though, I decided I would embrace meat in all of its forms and true to my word I spent the next weeks chowing down on ground beef, ham, chicken, turkey, and protein bars determined to give the babies' brains the greatest chance possible.

I tried to be as optimistic as I could, but it was hard. For not knowing anyone with triplets before I got pregnant, it now seemed like everyone I met was related to triplets, knew someone who had triplets, or had heard some incredible story of triplets. Thankfully the majority of these stories were positive, but some were alarming as the triplets had significant developmental delays or disabilities or the mother had delivered so early that the babies had spent months in the NICU. My cousin works as a special education teacher for preschoolers. While I was pregnant she had a set of triplets in her class that had been born very early and while they had all survived, they had significant delays which is why all three were in her class. I knew that negative outcomes were a distinct possibility, but hearing the accounts firsthand was too much and too scary. Reading facts was one thing, I could be objective and distant, but stories with names and faces were too real.

One thing that was hard for me was how excited some people were when they heard the news. So many people told me how lucky and blessed we were and what a miracle it was that three infants had been simultaneously conceived and were growing inside me. A favorite thing that people liked to tell me was that God does not make mistakes or that God does not give us more than we can handle. I could not disagree more! I was quite convinced at the time that this was a mistake and was sure that my husband and I were in completely over our heads and this was not something we could handle. I understand that people thought it was amazing because triplets are rare, but I couldn't help but think that they might not be so happy and positive if it was happening to them.

Faced with the optimism of others I had trouble giving an honest account of what I was experiencing. So many people have wanted to know what I thought when I first heard the news. I usually respond that we were shocked, but glad that the infants were all healthy during that first ultrasound. What I did not tell people is the scary thoughts that ran through my mind, that the infants would be sick or disabled or that I could not cope with four children. I did not tell people that I had no idea how we would afford three infants at once and I did not tell people that I secretly wished that it was all just a big medical error. I kept waiting at the next few ultrasounds for the technician to tell us that someone had miscounted and there were really only two infants in there. I could wrap my mind around twins, but not triplets. I certainly did not tell people that for the next few days after I learned the news I lay in bed each night silently crying. When my husband woke and asked me what was wrong I dared to whisper the words that had been drumming through my mind, "I don't want three infants," I told him, "I cannot do it." Even now it is hard for me to articulate this story to others as it certainly does not portray me as a joyful or even loving mother. What mother does not want her children? I had wanted so badly to get pregnant, so who was I to complain when I got more than I asked for. I was trying so hard to come to terms with the fact that I was now a mother of triplets and a mother of four children, but the story I was living and what I was thinking was not helping as there was nothing motherly about my reaction.

Before I knew it, 24 weeks had arrived and I was on bed rest. Thanks to the help of my mom, our incredibly generous family and friends, and my husband's amazing coworkers we had amassed all of the equipment, supplies and clothes we would need to bring the babies home. As I sat in a glider with my feet up I watched Brian and my mom set up the nursery and was overwhelmed by how much we had been given. My twenty-fourth week was at the beginning of December so the teachers at Brian's school had set up a Christmas tree in the teacher's lounge with ornaments that had the things we needed such as car seats, onesies, and high chairs. Our last name is Hall and the tree was topped with a sign encouraging anyone who wanted to "Deck the Halls." Not only was the idea clever, but to this day I am amazed and humbled by what they did for us. They also found us a used chest freezer and stocked it with meals so that Brian did not have to worry about cooking for over two months while I was stuck upstairs in bed and later when I was at the hospital. Not only did they provide meals, but they tried to make them as protein heavy as possible, knowing that my goal was to eat as much protein a day as I could. A moms' group I was a part of at a local church held a diaper drive for us and volunteered to bring freshly cooked meals once the girls were home from the hospital. It would be impossible to name all of the incredible things people did for us during this time, but it did help me to realize that as hard as this was going to be, we were not alone.

At first bed rest was not too bad, but within a few days I was uncomfortable and bored, but even worse than that, I was anxious. I had far too much time to think and research and contemplate everything that could go wrong. The hardest part was being so uninvolved in caring for Anna. Each day after she got home from daycare she would run to my room and climb up on the bed where we would play and read stories. Being so young she had a short attention span and wanted to get up and move so she would turn to me with the sweetest little grin and ask me to "c'mon" and beckon for me to follow her. How do you explain to a toddler than mommy can't get up to play? The guilt was overwhelming, but I knew that the best possible thing I could do for Anna was to give her siblings that were as healthy as possible and this knowledge was what kept me glued to the bed day in and day out.

When you are stuck in bed, there are only so many books you can read and so many old episodes of *Beverly Hills 90210* you can watch which meant I had a lot of time to think. One thing that struck me was how stories I had heard in the past were coming back to me. For example, one day I started thinking about the woman who had taught our childbirth class when I was pregnant with Anna telling us about how she delivered one of her daughters prematurely. She had never planned to breastfeed, but once her daughter was in the NICU she pumped her milk consistently, glad that there was something she could do for her struggling infant. I had not breastfed my first baby, but I began to think about how I would pump for my triplets, so I, like that mother, could do something for my infants. My mom also reminded me of my dad's best friend from high school. His wife got pregnant with spontaneous triplets when their older daughter was two. The triplets were about a year younger than me and she actually found a picture of a two-year-old me posing with the triplets lined up in their car seats.

Additionally I found that words and phrases from the stories I had heard or read easily slipped into the stories I told. It became second nature to tell people that I would much rather be in pain myself than watch my infants suffer or to explain that bed rest wasn't so bad because it might be the last time in a long time that I would ever get to lounge in bed, phrases I had repeatedly encountered in others' tales of high-risk pregnancies. Other's stories did more than supply a lexicon for my tales though. The general philosophies, expectations, and attitudes of others shaped the story I told as I came to understand my experience. The stories my mother, aunts, and grandmother told of labor and birth had surrounded me since I had been a child. Their ideas and beliefs strongly shaped my own. For instance, my mother had refused any pain medication during her first two labors which had been long and difficult. She often told the story of how she never cried out in pain, as she was not one to let others know she was suffering. I adopted this attitude and rarely complained about the many aches and pains I suffered, and when I did break down and complain I always tried to accompany the complaints with some sort of disclaimer of how I knew it could be worse or at least I was still pregnant. I read so many stories of women who had struggled for years with infertility or who had suffered multiple miscarriages and even though they were facing tremendous struggles with preterm labor of having very small babies in the NICU, their stories had a tone of gratitude that at least they were still pregnant or had a child. There stories also had a lot of hope in them and I tried as hard as I could to echo their sentiments.

I DON'T WANT TO HEAR THAT

Although hearing and reading stories was an important way to learn during my pregnancy, I also avoided many stories. The website for mothers of triplets I visited multiple times a day while pregnant had a forum about children with special needs, a forum that I never dared to enter. There also was a forum for bereaved parents which I never did click on; I could not let myself consider the possibility that one or more of our infants would not survive. I could comprehend a story that featured sick infants, but not a story in which I did not eventually bring three infants home. This avoidance of negative stories seemed entirely reasonable. If I wanted to stay positive I had to surround myself with positive stories.

At 27 weeks, after three weeks on bed rest, I went into the hospital when I began to experience frequent contractions. We learned that my cervix had shortened and I was put on trebutaline, a medication to halt contractions. After being released from the hospital, my cervix continued to shorten and I was put on a trebutaline pump. A needle was placed in my thigh so I could receive a continuous dosage of medication. It seemed surreal the night a nurse came to our home and taught my husband how to insert and change the needle and how to hook up a machine that would monitor my contractions from home. Additionally I was told to lay in the Trendelenberg position which involved placing bricks underneath the foot of the bed so that I was lying with my head lower than my feet in order to minimize the pressure on my cervix. It is never comfortable to have all of your blood rush to your head and it is even less comfortable to have gravity pushing three small babies into your rib cage. Until this point I believed that I would make it to 34 weeks and I would spend my long days on bed rest at home. Suddenly 34 weeks seemed like a lofty goal and I began to concentrate on one day at a time.

On January 8 when I was 29 weeks and 3 days pregnant, the trebutaline could no longer stop my contractions and I was admitted to the hospital again around 11:00 that night. At this point I was put on an IV of magnesium sulfate, more commonly referred to as mag, to slow down my contractions and halt labor. The doctors believed I might deliver any minute; it was an anxious waiting game. Once again I felt as if I was living someone else's life. As I lay on the hospital bed in pain in the middle of the night I cried. The girls could not come this early, it was too soon and we had worked too hard to keep them in. I was not ready and neither were they. Thankfully the medications were effective in controlling my labor and the infants were not born that night.

To this day I have a love/hate relationship with mag. I credit it with being a miracle drug as it stopped my labor, but it also made me feel sicker than I ever have in my entire life. The best way I can describe it is that it is like having the most horrible hangover of your entire life, but there is no hope that it will ever go away. In addition to nausea and congestion, hot flashes, double vision, and confusion are all side effects. The drug relaxes not just your uterine muscles, but all of your muscles so after a week on a continuous IV drip I had lost all of my reflexes and was unable to stand on my own. One time I paged the nurse, very concerned that I could clearly see two of my husband, but she assured me this was just a side effect of the medication. They had inserted a catheter when I was first admitted to the hospital and kept it in, so the only time I was up out of my bed was once a day I sat in a chair while they changed my bedding and every few days I was allowed to sit in a chair for a brief shower.

From this point on until the end of my pregnancy, I no longer wanted to hear or read stories of women who had carried their infants 35 weeks or of women who were able to take their infants home with them from the hospital. Instead of giving me hope, these stories made me feel as if I had somehow failed. I was doing everything I was supposed to do; I had been lying in bed for weeks, I only left the house to go to the doctor, and I drank gallons of water each day, but for some reason my body was giving out. Why were those women so much better at this than me? I distinctly remembered a nurse telling me about the last set of triplets who had been born at the hospital. They had been born at 34 weeks and the nurse referred to the mother as the "poster child" for prenatal care. Her story shot a pain through my heart. "I tried to be the poster child too," I wanted to scream. Her story was in no way a condemnation of me, but that is how I felt about it.

In addition to avoiding positive stories, I still did not want to hear stories about very premature infants—those born at 24 or 25 weeks. The stories of extremely long NICU stays with multiple complications were still too scary. Also, I did not want to hear stories about women having perfectly ordinary pregnancies and births involving one infant. I was angry and bitter about my own situation and had a hard time hearing the stories that I so desperately wanted for my own. Our hospital had a tradition that whenever a baby was born they would play a lullaby over the speaker system. Something that I would have once thought was incredibly cute and exciting just made me sad. I kept imagining people having and holding their full-term babies and it was hard because I still had no idea what the health of my girls would be like. Basically, stories were no longer helpful and in fact, were almost harmful, at least to my emotional state.

My avoidance of stories was almost as important as the stories I originally sought out. Stories I heard and read had potential to become a part of my story, but the stories I refused to hear or read could not—which in a way also shaped the story I told. During this time of narrative avoidance, I noticed that others continued to want to share stories with me, which made me wonder why people are so quick to share their stories with others believing they will be both interesting and helpful to the listener. At times I had welcomed narratives as a source of information and encouragement, but now I wanted to shut out stories. Did other women with similar experiences feel the same way? Was it possible that narratives are not always a good way to provide health information or provide comfort and support?

After three weeks in the hospital on mag I was starting to fall apart both physically and emotionally. Given that I had a catheter in for three weeks I developed a bad UTI. My skin broke out in a rash due to constantly having the contraction monitor strapped on and my stretch marks were getting so big and so stretched that some started to bleed. In addition to mag I was getting regular injections of terbutaline which causes your heart to race. My body ached and as the girls grew and their space became more and more limited, baby C wedged herself up under my ribcage and with every contraction I felt like my ribs were breaking. My heartburn was terrible, I frequently had nosebleeds and my eyes burned from the mag. On a Saturday afternoon I tried to convince myself that I could do this for two more weeks, but I was just not sure anymore. At one point I asked the nurse if I could refuse to let the doctor up the level of my mag anymore. She explained that you could refuse any treatment and I told my husband and mom that when the doctor came in on rounds Monday morning I would ask him to stop upping the mag. I would agree to stay on the level I was currently on, but I just could not take what was beginning to feel like torture anymore. As it turns out though, I never got to have that conversation.

On Sunday, January 27, 2008, when I was 32 weeks and one day pregnant, the medication could no longer stop my labor. All that day I felt just off. I was throwing up regularly and I could feel the contractions where normally I was contracting all of the time, but never could feel anything. It was a busy day at the hospital so the doctor on call just kept telling the nurses to give me another shot or some pain medication. At approximately 7:00 that night, the doctor on call came to check on me as the contractions grew more and more painful and she discovered that my water had broken and baby A's foot was stuck in the birth canal. Thankfully Brian was there at the hospital with me, because I was rushed to an emergency C-section, and at 8:09 pm, baby A entered the world and was quickly followed by her sisters, baby B and baby C. I laid on the operating table and as I listened to hear each baby cry, I prayed they all would be okay. They had been born almost two months early and were so small, weighing just 3lbs 8 oz, 3 lbs 14 oz, and 3 lbs 4 oz. They briefly showed me the first two babies, Sarah and Lucy, but Emily came out not breathing so she was quickly whisked away.

Following the surgery, I was wheeled to recovery and Brian went to the NICU to see how the girls were doing. I would like to say that I was consumed with worry and concern, but the reality is that the drugs I was on were making me incredibly tired and even though I tried to stay awake, I quickly feel asleep. My husband woke me up when he returned with pictures of the girls that I viewed on the small screen on the back of our digital camera. I was happy to see them and hear that none of them had to be ventilated, but I was also racked with guilt. I was already failing in my role as an NICU mom, unable to even stay awake to make sure they were ok. I also started to itch all over, a reaction to the pain medication which required yet another medication be administered. I tried to focus on the girls, but for the first time in months I was only responsible for my own body, and my own discomforts were overwhelming me.

I don't remember a lot from the rest of the night, but there are two things I will never forget and am extremely thankful for. Once I was released from recovery, instead of wheeling me straight to my postpartum room they wheeled me through the NICU so I could see the girls. I had not expected to get to see them until the next morning so this was an unexpected gift. I was able to see that they were doing well and breathing on their own with just a little supplemental oxygen delivered through a nasal cannula. I even got to hold Emily for a minute. She was the smallest of the girls and I cradled her tiny head not even filling up my entire palm. She was here though and so were her sisters. One of the nurses had made tiny pink bows and fastened them to the girls head with a small dab of petroleum jelly and I am not sure why, but that image sticks in my mind. It made them seem more real in way, and even if I could not swaddle them in girly pink blankets and they were not wearing any clothes, they still looked like baby girls. They had come earlier than I wanted, but for now they were ok.

The next morning I awoke in tremendous pain, but was so relived to no longer be on mag. My legs were weak from my weeks on bed rest so it took the nurse and my husband to get me up and into a wheelchair so I could go down to the NICU. Both of our parents were there, but due to a limit in the number of the visitors allowed in at a time my parents came in first with us followed by my husband's parents. It was all so different than when I had Anna and everyone was able to come into the room and pass her around. Now we had to spend five minutes scrubbing our hands and arms before we were even able to go where the babies were, which was incredibly difficult to do when you are sitting in a wheelchair. The NICU was incredibly crowded that day so they were unable to put the three girls next to each other so Brian wheeled me from isolette to isolette so I could see them all. All were wearing just diapers and were asleep. Tubes were coming out of their noses and I quickly learned that this is how they were being fed until their suck reflex was strong enough. I might have held one or two of them, but I mostly remember the nurses telling me it was okay to put my hand in the isolete and touch them and so I opened one of the circular doors on the side and stuck my hand into the incredibly warm incubator and touched two of my daughters for the first time. Another gift was that even though I was wheeled to a double room, the nurse informed me that I would not be getting a roommate. Brian was thrilled for the extra hospital bed to sleep on instead of a plastic recliner, and I was relieved that I would not potentially share a room with another mom and her newborn while my girls were in the NICU down the hall.

My first moments with my daughters quickly ended as the heat of NICU overtook me and I began to vomit. My parents wheeled me back to my room and for the first time I felt the strangeness of leaving my daughters behind. The feelings of guilt also struck. I felt that I should be in the NICU at their bedside, but I felt so terrible and sick that all I wanted to do was go back to my bed and lay down. As my stay in the postpartum unit continued I was struck by how different things were this time around. One of the things that I had pictured over and over in my mind was Anna meeting her new sibling. I imagined her running into the room proudly sporting a shirt with the words I'm the Big Sister emblazoned across the front, eager to give me a hug and kiss me and see the baby. We would then take pictures of her holding the baby that I would treasure forever. Anna did come to visit me wearing an "I'm the big sister of triplets" shirt I had found online, but was only allowed to peer through the window at her sisters. Given that I had already been in the hospital for three weeks, there was nothing new or exciting for her about the visits postdelivery. She was not even two; I don't think she had any clue that the babies had been born. We of course told her, but honestly, how much can a twenty-one month old grasp? When Anna was born I welcomed a steady stream of visitors. This time I was reluctant to have many people outside of our families visit as I was not feeling well and while they could go into the NICU they were not allowed to hold or even touch the girls. I know this sounds terrible, but I felt like asking friends to come and see the girls was basically like saying, "hey, why don't you come stare at my babies sleeping in a box."

Three days after delivery I was discharged from the hospital. I had read a lot about how other women had felt during this moment as they left the hospital empty handed and I tried to brace myself for an onslaught of tears. Instead of feeling grief as I left the hospital though, I felt relief. After being there three and a half weeks and never once being outside it felt so good to breathe fresh air. Of course I found it strange to be leaving without the girls, but I had known ever since I found out they were triplets that they would spend some time in the NICU, so the moment did not overwhelm me. My mom actually drove me home as my husband had a million errands to run including filling my prescriptions and buying a breast pump. As I said before, the weeks on bed rest and the weeks on mag had taken a serious toll on my body. My mom had to hold me up as I walked to the couch in the living room and I needed help to get up from the couch to walk to the bathroom that was probably only 25 feet away. My husband and I fell asleep on the couch that afternoon and unbeknownst to us my mom went to pick up Anna from daycare. I can so vividly remember waking up when I heard the front door opening and Anna and my mom walked in. My little girl took one look at me and started dancing as she yelled excitedly, "my mommy, my mommy!" That poor girl must have thought I was never coming home again.

The next 30 days continued to be stressful, exhausting, and a constant juggling act. A few days after I had been discharged it felt like the world was conspiring against us. It has been an unusually cold winter so far and then we got a major snowstorm making it difficult for relatives who were coming to visit to travel and even getting to and from the hospital to visit was treacherous. There was one day when I was not able to make it to the hospital due to the bad weather and I sat and cried, imagining my girls lying all alone feeling neglected. A few mornings after I had been discharged, Anna woke up coughing with a fever and a quick trip to the pediatrician confirmed that she had RSV and she came home with prescriptions for an antibiotic and breathing treatments. Now we had a sick little girl at home that would not go to anyone but us or my mom and we were constantly exposing ourselves to RSV, the infection that we knew could be so harmful and even deadly to premature infants whose lungs were not yet developed. We were still able to go into the NICU but in addition to carefully scrubbing in we also had to wear gowns and masks which made the whole visitation not only hot and uncomfortable, but also made it seem even more surreal.

I was also pumping around the clock but was never able to get very much of a milk supply and after 20 minutes of pumping I would be lucky to have 3 ounces. I kept at it though as they kept telling me how good the milk would be for babies. I woke up in the middle of the night to pump drenched in sweat, a side effect from the hormones. A few days after getting home my legs started tingling and swelling and I thought I was having an allergic reaction to the pain medication. It was not an allergic reaction, but instead, my legs were swelling as side effect of being so malnourished during the last part of the pregnancy. After all of the discomforts and indignities I had suffered through the entire pregnancy, for some reason my swollen tree-trunk legs and Fred Flinstone feet bothered me more than anything, and one night I burst into tears as I tried to shove my gigantic feet into socks and cried to Brian that I hated having ogre legs.

After that first week, things began to run a little more smoothly as we got into a somewhat of a routine. We kept Anna in daycare so that my mom and I could go over to the NICU during the day and sit and hold the babies and feed them when they were able to drink from a bottle. We would go home for dinner and then my mom would watch Anna while Brian and I went back to visit them at night for an hour or so. For the most part the girls did really well. They had bradycardia and apnea spells but they always quickly bounced back after you reminded them to breath. They were all jaundiced and spent about three days under the lights. Eating was a bigger challenge as their sucking reflex was not very strong and they had severe reflux. At one point they were tube fed through an NG tube in the nose over a period of one hour and then had to lay flat for an hour after the feeding and 30 minutes before the next feeding leaving a very short window of time when they could be held and moved which was frustrating. Eventually they started to regain the weight they had lost after birth, but it took Emily, the smallest baby, the longest to start gaining and her weight hovered below 3 pounds for several days.

I started to feel better physically after the first two weeks and was finally able to walk from the parking garage to the NICU without using a wheelchair. I also began to gain my voice and was more confident in asking questions to the nurses and doctors so I could understand what was happening. As the girls got bigger we were also able to do more things that we had taken for granted with Anna. When their umbilical cords came off we were finally able to give them a bath which seems like such a small thing, but when your baby spends almost all day in a plastic incubator you crave normalcy and nothing is more normal than carefully submerging a tiny squirmy newborn in a bathtub. After they no longer had to be under the lights for jaundice the nurses began to dress them in clothes. The first clothes they wore were those that had been donated by families who had previously been in the NICU, but once we got the go ahead on clothes we started to do some shopping. To this day when I see preemie clothes at the store I find it hard to believe that the girls were ever that small and in fact they were so small that the preemie clothes were far too big. When the girls had finally grown out of the preemie size and had moved into "newborn" we saved a few of our favorite outfits and donated the rest of the clothes to the NICU, something that made me smile as I thought of all of the tiny girls who would one day get to use them and even more of the parents who would be so happy to see their baby in an outfit and not just in a diaper under the lights.

It was a great day the night my husband and I walked into the NICU and Lucy, the biggest of the triplets, was no longer in her isolette, but was lying just in a regular hospital crib. Even though she was still hooked up to the monitors and had an NG tube in her nose, for the first time I felt like I could just pick her up and hold her like a regular baby without needing a nurse to assist me. This was a huge thing because up until that point it never quite felt like the girls were really ours, because their care lay solely in the hands of the doctors and nurses. Sure we got to do things like change their diapers and hold them, but it was all under the direction of the hospital staff. On that day I walked in, picked her up and when we were ready to leave I laid her down and got her situated which was so easy now that I did not have to maneuver around the walls of the isolette.

One of the things that I quickly learned about being in the NICU is that you have a lot of time to just sit and think which can be a dangerous thing. From the beginning our goal had been 34 weeks and everyone around me had assured me that I could do it and when things started to get tough I went online and found encouragement there as women wrote about the importance of fighting for your baby and keeping them in for just one more day. Even though I had never asked my doctor to stop upping the mag, I felt that in my mind I had partially given up the fight and my body must have recognized my sense of defeat and that is why I delivered the girls two weeks earlier than I wanted to. Even though the girls were doing well by all accounts, I also knew that there was no way to predict the future and that they might very well face struggles down the road and I felt so consumed with guilt that my body had let them down. I had to quit going online to check in at the triplets' message boards because it seemed like everyone on there had carried their babies longer and each story of a 33 or 34 weekers seemed like an accusation and one more example of how I failed my girls. I fully recognize now how irrational these thoughts were, but at the time I felt terrible. As it grew closer to the time for them to come home the worries became overwhelming. How could we possibly take care of these girls and Anna. For one thing, it took each of the girls almost thirty minutes to finish just a 2-oz bottle. They were eating every three hours around the clock and I did not see how we would have time to do anything else. On top of that how would we afford their very expensive high-calories formula and hold them and take care of them and make sure they would all get what they needed. As I said, the quiet afternoons in the NICU could be brutal for someone whose mind could not stop racing.

While sitting there, I also learned a lot about the other babies in the unit. Our NICU was a large open room so there was not much privacy. When nursing or pumping, nurses would pull up portable screens, but these makeshift walls were hardly soundproof which meant that you knew a lot of what was going on with the babies around you. It was heartbreaking, sitting there day after day and see tiny little babies who never seemed to have a visitor. Many of the moms in the unit were teenagers who barely looked old enough to drive a car, let alone care for a premature infant. Many of the families struggled financially and I would overhear the social worker talking with them providing them with meal vouchers and gas cards so that they would be able to come and visit their baby in the hospital. It made me so sad to see how hard some of these families and babies lives were and would be, but it also helped me to put my own situation in perspective. My husband and I were and are by no means wealthy, and given that I had stopped teaching and no longer received my monthly stipend, our finances were very tight, but we thankfully had family who would help us if we needed anything and we had some savings. I knew that we would always have the resources and time to do whatever the girls would need in order to give them the best possible shot at a happy and successful life. I figured that if these girls had to be born to someone, at least it was us who had the abilities to care for them financially, emotionally, and physically.

During that time I also spent a lot of time talking with the nurses and appreciated all that they did for their tiny patients and their families. The nurses were very encouraging and spent a lot of time teaching us how to care for our girls and even more importantly helped us to feel confident and comfortable in caring for them. There were a few nurses who we got especially close to including one of the night nurses whose daughter was in my husband's fifth grade class. It is actually a funny story because in the fall she had gone on a field trip with my husband's class and at some point she told my husband she was a nurse on the L&D floor. We had not told a lot of people I was pregnant yet, and did not know it was triplets but he told her that day and said that maybe she would see us when I delivered. She told him she hoped not because she was an NICU nurse and would only see us if something went wrong. As it turns out we saw a lot of her. She was actually there the night of the delivery and it was so comforting to have a familiar face there and feel like someone who cared about us on a personal level was caring for the girls. Her oldest daughter's name was Emily so she always said she had a special bond with our Emily. I loved talking to her when we visited at night and she was on duty. The NICU which always seemed a little calmer to me than the hectic day as there were fewer visitors and doctors coming through and it felt like we had the time to really talk and I could ask her as many questions as I wanted. To this day we still keep in touch and I love keeping her updated on the girls' progress and successes.

I also formed a relationship with another one of the NICU moms. Her son was born at 34 weeks gestation a few days after the girls. As I said before, there were not a lot of families or moms who spent the days in the NICU like we did and some of the moms who did were either in and out of the NICU quickly or were young or did not speak English, but this mom was around my age, also had an older child, and spent her days in the NICU with her son who had been born at 34 weeks. It was so nice to have someone to talk to and break up the monotony of the day and our children had similar issues which were learning to eat and being able to regulate their own body temperatures. Her little boy got to go home before the girls and I wondered if we would ever see them again, but thanks to the wonders of social media we connected on Facebook and remain friends to this day.

Beyond that though, the girls' time in the NICU was very isolating. I will be forever thankful that my mom was there with me because had I spent the days in the NICU alone I think I might have gone crazy. I did not have a lot of visitors come to the hospital and by the time I got home from spending the day at the NICU I was exhausted, needed to pump again, and had an almost two-year-old to take care of so I had little time and energy to connect with friends. I would send periodic updates through mass emails and send some pictures of the girls, this was before I was on Facebook, so I would get some responses from that, but even this seemed to take too much emotional and mental effort. I cried a lot during that time, not even over the girls really, but just small things. I remember one afternoon my husband had taken some pictures of the girls to work to show people and for some reason I had asked him to bring them home that afternoon. He forgot and when I found out I burst into tears. Why, I do not know, but I remember just crying and not being able to stop.

After what at the time seemed like forever, but was only 30 days the girls were discharged from the NICU. There had been talk of one or more of them going home for the past week so until the doctor signed the discharge papers I was not fully convinced that they would really be coming. That morning was a whirlwind in the NICU as they had an eye examination and then the nurses started to fill out the paper work and get them ready to go. I listened carefully to all of the instructions as far as sleeping on an incline to help with reflux, preparing their formula, giving them iron drops, and making sure their temperatures stayed up. We packed up the toys and things that their beds had accumulated over the four weeks and dressed them in the outfits I had bought them for going home. They were still so small, all around five pounds, but compared to how they had started they seemed big to us. As we walked out the NICU doors for the last time it was another surreal moment. There were times that seemed like this day would never come. While I was pregnant I had feared that their NICU stay might last for months and when they did come home they would be facing significant health issues.

My story and our family's story does not end the day they were discharged from the hospital and in many ways it was only just beginning. The day we brought them home from the NICU was both exhilarating and terrifying. It was completely real now and my husband and I were now solely responsible for our daughters' health, development, and well-being. I remember standing at the front door at the hospital with one of our favorite nurses, the three car seats on the floor and girls covered with thick blankets my cousin had crocheted to ward off the frigid February air. The first time we snapped all three car seats into the back of our new minivan was crazy. This was our life now and good or bad, we just had to take it day by day.

That first year was an adventure to say the least. There were moments of pure joy when the girls learned to smile, rolled over, and when we first heard their intoxicating belly laughs. There were also moments of pure hell when exhaustion became overwhelming, the girls screamed inconsolably as they battled colic, and when our home felt like a prison. For three months straight the girls would start screaming around 7:00 and not stop until 11 or 12 that night. The only thing that would partially console them was to drive so my husband got into the habit of driving down one of the back countries road to the next town over where there was a Dairy Queen that we affectionately dubbed the "far away" Dairy Queen as opposed to the one just a few miles to our house. So almost nightly my husband set off with three screaming girls who quickly quieted and stayed that way while he went through the drive thru at Dairy Queen and ordered sundaes and Blizzards to go. When he got back home the girls would stay quiet for a few minutes until they woke up and started screaming again, but at least I had a large sweet treat to console me. It is a small miracle that we both didn't gain 15 pounds that year, but I think we needed those extra calories just to make it through the days.

My husband would then go to bed because he took the middle of the night shift and I would sit with three inconsolable babies and cry as I imagined getting in my van and just driving away from all of them. It was a difficult year and I struggled with overwhelming feelings of guilt as I knew I was not enjoying my new daughters like I had my first and I continued to blame myself for their early birth convinced that I had done something wrong or given up too soon. There were still moments when I woke up and wished this had all been a giant mistake. I was so happy that the girls were healthy and growing, but it was just so hard and each day began to feel just like the last as I woke up to feed babies, prepare bottles, pump, hold crying babies, change diapers, and do it all over again.

My mom had rented her apartment in town for four months and her time with us was coming to end. It had been invaluable having her there in the days to help with the girls, entertain Anna, and mostly just to keep me company. Because she was there I was able to get out some in the day, but as the day of her departure drew closer I began to panic. Not only was I constantly crying, but I was angry and snapping at everyone. One of the most tedious chores of my day was making up the twenty-one bottles we would need. Some were completely formula and some were breast milk I had pumped, and those had to have formula added in to boost the calorie content. One morning as I had everything set up at the kitchen table which was my work station, Anna wandered over to check out what I was doing and knocked a few of the bottles over. It was an innocent mistake, but I lost it and started screaming at her and crying, furious that I would have to go mix up some new formula. I think this was the point where my mom realized that something more than just exhaustion and stress was going on and started to push me to go talk to my doctor to see if I had postpartum depression.

I really resisted this at first for two major reasons. The first was that I knew that my OB could not change the circumstances of my life. He could not change that I had triplets, that I had to leave school, or that I had four young children to take care of. The second reason is that I was so afraid that I would go and tell him what I was feeling and thinking and he would just brush it off and tell me it was normal to feel this way after pregnancy and there was nothing he could do for me. In many ways that fear of having someone dismiss the pain I was feeling was the biggest thing that kept me from seeking help. It finally got to the point that my mom insisted that I call the doctor because she would not be able to leave until she knew that I was going to be ok so I reluctantly made the call and the nurse got me in the next day. As I drove myself to the visit I listened to the radio and cried and rehearsed what I would tell the doctor and braced myself for his reaction.

As it turns out though, I had nothing to fear. After filling out a quick assessment sheet and answering a few questions from the doctor to ensure that I was not thinking about hurting myself or my children he quickly confirmed that I had postpartum depression and recommended a low-dose antidepressant to help even out my feelings. Ironically, his patient right after me was a mother who also had spontaneous triplets who were now twelve years old. He asked her to come into the room and talk to me and she gave me some advice and mostly reassured me that things would get better in time. It is funny sometimes how things work out like that. Call it coincidence, fate, or God, but someone or something was looking out for me. It took a few days to adjust to the medication, but just two days later I was feeling like a new person. I was still stressed, exhausted, and overwhelmed, but for the first time in a long time I felt like I could cope. I did not start crying anytime I was alone and my reactions to events were much more appropriate for the situation. In time I was able to rise above the murkiness of depression and come to accept this new and crazy life.

As time marched on we slowly began to get into a new routine and schedule. The girls' colic finally went away and by six months they were sleeping through the night so we at least got rest at night. My husband was home for the summer with us so we had two adults to manage the herd as we called them. The girls seemed to be developing normally when we noticed that Emily's head was tilted to one side. My brain quickly jumped to cerebral palsy (CP) and after calling our pediatrician, I waited anxiously for her appointment, spending the time in between researching everything I could find on CP. Instead of CP though her doctor diagnosed her with torticollis, a fairly common condition where due to positioning in utero the neck is twisted so the head tilts to one side and the chin tilts to the other. We breathed a sigh of relief, got the referral for early intervention, and went home feeling like we had dodged another bullet.

Emily started to have weekly PT (physical therapy) sessions and we stretched her neck daily in an attempt to loosen the tight muscles in her shoulder and neck. You could tell the stretching was agonizing for her and she cringed as soon as you touched her tight shoulder, but this was the only treatment. As time went on, her condition did not seem to be getting any better and she started to have episodes about every one to two weeks where she would turn gray, get very limp, and start to vomit. These episodes lasted for a few hours until she would eventually fall asleep and when she woke up she would be fine. Our pediatrician had no idea what was going on and prescribed valium to help relax her during these episodes. When Emily was around ten months old the physical therapist was looking through pictures in a photo album with Emily and noticed that her severe head tilt was on different sides in different pictures. If Emily really had torticollis caused by positioning, there was no way her head should be switching like that.

This discovery lead to another six months of doctors' appointments and tests as we tried to figure out what was wrong. Not only was her head tilted and she was continuing to have her episodes of weakness and vomiting, but her development was lagging behind her sisters. They always tell you that you should never compare kids and all kids develop at their own pace, but it is next to impossible not to compare when your child has two siblings born within a minute of her. Our pediatrician who was becoming increasingly concerned referred us to a developmental pediatrician at the children's hospital in Indianapolis. I can still remember sitting in the waiting room filling out extensive paperwork, trying desperately to remember how old she was when she hit a variety of milestones such as reaching for objects and sitting up. I honestly had no idea, I could barely keep the days of the week straight, let alone remember who had done what and when. I called my mom, crying, who had a much better memory for things like that and she gave me the info I needed, but once again I felt like I had failed as a mother. I should have written it all down and I should have known.

Following a CAT scan, MRI, and a visit with a pediatric neurologist, we found out that Emily had decreased white matter in her brain and a rare condition called Benign Paroxymal Torticollis. As far as the decreased white matter was concerned, we quickly found out that this is one of those diagnoses that doesn't really mean anything because they have no way of knowing if it will cause any issues or delays. It was possible that time would reveal additional issues as far as cognition and physical ability were concerned, but there was no way of knowing at the time what this meant for her. Benign Paroxymal Torticollis is a migraine variant that causes clenched neck muscles, veritgo, nausea, and pain and it is something that children grow out of with time though they are at an increased risk for getting migraines later in life. There was no way to treat it other than to give her some medicine during the episodes to decrease the nausea so we just continued with therapy and treated her when the episodes occurred.

As Emily's episodes became less and less frequent and she was in less pain she began to catch up with her sisters. She finally took her first steps when she was seventeen months old and pretty much everyone we know celebrated with us. In addition to Emily's health issues, all three girls were very delayed in their speech. Emily started weekly speech therapy at eighteen months, and at two Sarah and Lucy joined her. We started to teach them sign language and even though they could say almost no words they loved to sign and soon could sign over seventy-five words including rhinoceros and cookie. Now I fully understand that there is little practical use to knowing the sign for rhinoceros, but not only was it incredibly cute, but it was so reassuring to see that the girls could learn and could comprehend, it was just a matter of them not being able to form spoken words yet. Between Emily's PT and the girls' speech, we had at least two therapy appointments and sometimes three weekly. Fortunately, early intervention service in our state came to the house for sessions so I did not have to load up and drag around everyone multiple times a week. I actually enjoyed these appointments because it meant that another adult was in my house for an hour and I had someone to talk to.

By the time the girls were three it seemed like they had pretty much caught up with their peers and I seldom worried about the effects their prematurity had on them. For so long I had heard and read that most preemies catch up by age two and for us that was not the case. There were times when I wondered if all three ever would, but luckily I was just impatient, and in their own time the girls all did. During those first three years they did get sick a lot as their immune systems still were not that strong. The nurses at the pediatrician's office knew me by name and we got so close to our pediatrician, Dr. Anne, who we love, that we were actually invited to her wedding. Other than this though, there were no major complications. Little Emily, who we were so worried about, began to thrive and though she still got dizzy sometimes and had a little trouble with her balance she had no problem keeping up and sometimes even surpassing her sisters.

A huge moment for me came the night of the girls' preschool graduation. Every year their teacher puts together a slide show with pictures of all of the kids and sets it to music. Anna had graduated two years before and I had smiled through the entire thing, happy and excited that our oldest would be starting kindergarten. As soon as the video started and a picture of the three girls together in an NICU bed came up on the screen I completely lost it and sat through the entire video with tears streaming down my face. I am not an overly sentimental person when it comes to milestones like that and I was not sad that the girls were getting older, because the older they got the more self-sufficient they were. My tears came with the powerful realization of just how far they and our family had come. Here they were standing proudly on stage, singing, smiling, and thriving in ways that I had once feared would never be possible. When so many things could have gone wrong, we were so lucky that so much went right.

I wish now that I had been able to talk with other mothers with preemies or multiples who had also dealt with postpartum depression as the only stories

I seemed to find about motherhood were those where mothers sat in their infants, rooms at night wanting nothing more than to just stare at their beautiful infants or mothers who were so thankful that they had a child or children who had survived. The internet has exploded in many ways since the girls were born and there seems to be more public sharing of stories of postpartum depression and difficulties in mothering in general, but at the time it felt like a shameful secret. Had I had more exposure to stories like mine, I perhaps would not have spent so long seeing myself as the evil mother in our story, and instead a normal woman who was dealing with surging hormones and a complete upheaval of my life.

As with all stories, the story I tell of having triplets is a way to reflect on what has happened and to make connections among events. My story has changed and continues to evolve in light of my own experience as well as additional stories that I hear and read. Now that my triplets are here and healthy I have begun to read some of the stories that I had avoided. I found and read the blog of a mother whose triplets were born at 25 weeks. Her three sons survived, but two are profoundly deaf and two have cerebral palsy. I have also listened to the stories of those who lost one or more of their infants. These stories both sadden and inspire me. The stories of extremely premature and sick infants also have changed my story in the sense that I realize how fortunate we were that I was able to carry the girls to 32 weeks, they are healthy, and they are home with us. I look at the struggles of other parents with triplets and I am better able to put our own challenges into perspective. Although the story of my pregnancy with triplets still contains elements of fear and pain, it also contains elements of awe and wonder at this incredible experience that has changed our lives forever.

At the time, I considered these other stories as a source of information and often hope, but as time went on I also realized that these stories were influencing and shaping the story I was telling. It was during my high-risk pregnancy that I experienced firsthand the power of the narratives we tell and how active the process of narrative sense-making is. There were varying stories I could tell about being pregnant with spontaneous triplets, some of which were negative and filled with fear, anxiety, and at times even sadness. I never wanted triplets and I felt that life as I knew it had ended (and in a bad way). I had to make a conscious decision and extend effort to tell a story that was more positive than what I was feeling. In some ways I believed that if I told myself and others a happier story, then reality would follow suit.

My experience also prompted me to consider the role of stories in my pre-term labor and birth experience and specifically the role that others' stories played in shaping the story I told. I saw how others' stories shaped my expectations of and influenced my decisions about a high-risk pregnancy. This led me to question how other women who have experienced high-risk pregnancies used the narratives around them as they created their stories. As I began to do more research and talk to more women, I did not anticipate how the experience of talking with so many mothers and sharing our stories together would alter my story and drastically change my understanding of what had happened to me as well as my daily life raising four young girls. I started this project to learn about others and in the process learned more about myself.

During the data collection process I was immersed in the world of high-risk pregnancies. Prior to the first interview I was incredibly nervous. I had a list of questions, but what if the women didn't talk much, what if my questions did not draw out the information I wanted, and what if the whole encounter was just awkward and uncomfortable. As I waited before the first interview, which began at a local restaurant, anxiously looking at each female customer who walked through the door, trying to determine if she matched the description the participant had given me, I felt like I was on a blind date. Thankfully my first participant was outgoing and friendly and five minutes into our conversation my nervousness subsided. After each interview, I was amazed by how smoothly the conversation had gone and how much information and ground we covered. Although I went home exhausted, I always had a smile.

One of the things I discovered as I spoke with women and went over my interview notes was that the stories we hear and read that are like our own normalize our experiences. Sitting with a fellow mother of triplets and chatting about the difficulties of feeding three infants at once felt so natural. We could relate to each others' experiences and understand them; the conversation flowed easily. For this first time since I had learned I was pregnant with triplets I felt less alone. For example, I met someone else who had been on magnesium sulfate and we could laugh at our horrible memories. Even more importantly I heard stories about other mothers who had not been happy to learn they were pregnant with multiples and of mothers who struggled to feel connected and joyful when their tiny infants were resting in the NICU.

Another thing I discovered was that women integrate others' stories into their own stories as they engage in sense-making and decision-making. With each interview I heard a new story and gained new insight and perspective into what it means to be the mother of a premature infant, or in many cases infants. Inevitably, I compared my story to the stories I heard. In the beginning it was difficult to not become obsessed with determining which women had better outcomes and which women had worse outcomes as I constantly tried to assess how well I had done gestating my daughters. I felt twinges of regret when I interviewed a mother of triplets who delivered at 35 weeks and went home shaking and incredibly thankful after interviewing a mother whose triplets were born at 23 weeks and passed away soon after.

As the interviews continued though, I began to focus less on how these women's stories compared to my story and instead saw the similarities across their stories and mine. Ultimately, whether women had quadruplets or a singleton, the primary concern was the health and well-being of their infants. As I listened to women describe their sense of failure and having done something wrong when their children were born early I wanted so badly to be able to say something to help assuage their guilt. It was obvious to me that they had done everything they could to keep their infants healthy and for some reason their bodies decided to go into early labor, but women routinely blamed themselves. Eventually these conversations led to some self-reflection on my part. It seemed ridiculous to me for women to blame themselves for the outcomes of their pregnancies, yet I still blamed myself for my daughters' earlier-than-desired arrival. Throughout my pregnancy and after my daughters were born, I spent a lot of time and energy trying to avoid stories of women whose pregnancies were more successful than mine because being exposed to those stories made me feel like a failure. Slowly though, I overcame the urge to avoid these stories and was able to appreciate the information they contained. By trying to avoid exposure to stories different than my own, I was limiting myself and my understanding of my experience.

Many of the women I talked with humbled and inspired me in the ways they coped with far more difficult situations than my own. Several of the women I interviewed had lost one of their infants either during the pregnancy or after birth. They told these stories with tears, but also with acceptance and an incredible gratitude for their children who were living and healthy. These women also reached out in different ways to help others who were in situations like their own. One woman, who lost her three triplets when they were born at 23 weeks, became an NICU nurse, and was one of my daughters' nurses. Another woman, who lost her daughter when she was thirteen months old started a foundation and is working to provide information, education, and support to fellow micropreemie parents. They served as excellent reminder that what I learned from this project should be put to use and that I want to find a way to help mothers facing situations like my own.

Through this experience I also learned from the stories of mothers whose children have long-term health issues. Even though my daughters are completely healthy and with the help of early intervention were able to overcome their minor delays, these mothers and I share elements of shock at the outcomes of our pregnancies. Few women expected to have premature infants, multiples, or a child with disabilities. Our expectations were not met and therefore we experienced regret, disappointment, and envy as we observed others who appeared as if their lives were meeting all of their expectations.

One of the women I met told me that she cried every day for the first six months after her second daughter was born with Downs Syndrome. She just could not understand why this had happened and why her daughter's life would be so different than she had imagined. She shared with me that while she was in the hospital recovering from the birth a family friend told her that her world had just gotten much larger. She did not understand the comment at the time, as she felt like the world was closing in on her. As time passed though and she met other families with children with Downs Syndrome and had conversations with strangers in the aisles of the grocery store, she began to understand. Through her daughter she began to meet people and hear stories that were inspiring, hopeful, and even happy. People she never would have talked to before stopped her to chat, offer advice, or ask a question. As she shared her story and her daughter's story she began to make unique connections and forge unique relationships. My world too has grown immensely since my daughters were born. The sight of me pushing a grocery cart full of four blond girls made many people stop and look, and often come over to talk with me and ask a few questions. I have met countless people who have a connection to multiples as well as numerous people who have been touched by prematurity. Having triplets also makes for a great conversation starter when meeting someone and it has opened the door for many engaging conversations.

As I started writing this book, I often found myself transported back in time to the first months after we learned I was carrying triplets and the first months and the sometimes overwhelming task of raising them. I think of the story I created in my mind of what the future would be like, and it never included conducting research, meeting women from across the country, or completing my dissertation. When I learned I was pregnant with triplets, I had no access to stories of women with higher-order-multiples who were able to work and pursue a life outside that of being a mother to many small children. My primary story of a woman with four children came from my own mother who devoted her entire life to me and my three brothers, often at the expense of her own dreams and goals. I wanted to be a great mom like her, but I also wanted more and I worried that all of my years of school would be wasted.

Thankfully, with the support and at times urging of family and friends a few months after the birth of my daughters, I slowly began to work on my dissertation and resumed a light teaching load. Through the interviews for this project, I met many women who continued to work, attend school, and remain active members of their communities. I wish I had known their stories when I first heard the news I was pregnant with triplets because their stories would have allowed me to at least conceive of a brighter future. Access to these stories would have shown me different alternatives to what a life with preemies and multiples could be like. I still would have been shocked, scared, and upset, but at least there could have been a glimmer of hope and possibility.

Another aspect of stories I came to understand during this process is the relative fluidity of our stories. On a good day, when my house is clean, my girls are pleasant, and I am crossing things off of my to-do list, I will tell a story that is humorous and reassure myself and the listener that life isn't too crazy and this is not so bad. On days when I had taken all four girls to the doctor, filled five prescriptions for antibiotics, sat through a speech therapy session watching my daughters struggle to speak, and almost lost one daughter at Target, I would have told you that it is incredibly difficult, and frustrating, and I am tired. On another day I may watch an episode of *Private Practice* and watch the fictional story of a couple making the difficult decision to stop interventions on their son born at 25 weeks and no matter what kind of day I am having I remind myself of how fortunate we are. All of these stories are ultimately true, as each day my perspective changes and I sometimes encounter new stories that help me to realize and consider life in new ways.

Chapter 2

Pregnancy and Narratives

Michelle had always wanted twins and specifically red-headed twins, so when she learned she was pregnant with twins she was thrilled. Michelle is slightly different than most of the women I interviewed for the book, not because of the outcome of her pregnancy or any complications she experienced, but because her twins are now 30-year-olds. The other women I interviewed were still raising their children and the majority of women had given birth in the past five years. Despite the time that had passed between her pregnancy and when we spoke, her memories and stories of that time felt as if it was recent history for her. Overall her pregnancy went fairly well. At the time she was working as an Engineer inspecting bridges around the state of Ohio which meant that she was on her feet a lot. She eventually had to take a leave from work after fainting at one of her job sites. From there she tried to take it easy and her twins, a boy and a girl were born five weeks early on April Fool's day. Her twins were small, but well enough to come home from the hospital with her after a few days. She remembers those first months as incredibly difficult as she was a first-time mother and had to learn how to take care of two infants who seemed like they were constantly needing something whether it was a bottle or a diaper change. She also remembers feeling incredibly blessed as her twins were so healthy and doing so well. Even though her twins were now adults she and I had almost a two hour conversation, a powerful illustration of just how central and enduring our stories of pregnancy and birth can be.

As I mentioned in the introduction while this book is about high-risk pregnancies and premature birth, it also about stories, the power they have to shape realities, and the different elements that influence the stories we tell. When you think about it, as a species, human beings are addicted to stories. From almost the time we are born we are surrounded by stories found in books, on TV, in nursery rhymes, and from the people who love and care for us. It is from stories that we learn important lessons about what is wrong and right, we learn about others and how they live and experience the world, and in the process we often learn more about ourselves. In teaching us about others, stories can also teach us to have compassion as we are able to put ourselves into others' shoes. Often it is stories that help us to discover what we want to do and be. When we talk to others and share our experiences and lives, it is usually by telling stories about what has happened to us or what we have seen or heard. Judith Jameson, a famous choreographer was once quoted as saying, "Just living is a telling a story. You're put on this earth to tell that story, to share those stories." It is this basic fact of the human experience, the calling to live and tell our stories that compelled me to write this book. I not only wanted to share my own story, but I also wanted to share the stories of the countless women I have met and talked to who so openly shared their own stories with me. Not only are their stories interesting, sometimes shocking, and often heartbreaking, but they also provide unique insight into the experience of a having a premature baby. I write this book too with the hope that sharing these stories will help those who travel down similar paths as they can find others who have felt, feared, said, and wished for many of the same things. Sometimes recognizing oneself in another's story can be a powerful experience as it lets us know that we are not odd, that we are not alone, and that our own stories are valid.

As someone who has studied communication since I was a freshman in college, when thinking about stories and the power they have in shaping our lived experiences I immediately think of Walter Fisher (1984) who introduced the world to his narrative paradigm by claiming we are all storytelling creatures. He proposed that instead of humans essentially being rational as was the prevailing belief, humans are *homo narrans* or essentially storytellers, and we come to know and understand our world through the narratives we read, hear, and tell. According to Fisher, narratives are central to everything that humans think and say and therefore are an integral part of all human experiences. With an innate ability to be a storyteller, each of us is responsible for crafting and choosing the stories we tell. It is the facts, details, and characters we include or omit that determine what type of story we tell. Although every story is unique, stories are informed, influenced, and shaped by other stories an individual has heard, seen, or read so there is a constant interplay between the stories one tells and the stories one consumes.

THE POWER OF A STORY

The act of creating and telling a story about pregnancy and childbirth is a common and important task for all women who experience pregnancy.

Stories about one's pregnancy and delivery provide a way for women to reflect on and make sense of their experience and they assist women as they transform into the role of mother (Brubaker and Wright 2006 Kruger 2003; Brubaker and Wright 2006). Going through a pregnancy and having a child is a pivotal and complex event in a woman's life and the story she tells helps her to integrate that experience into the framework of her life (Callister 2004). Pregnancy and birth narratives can also be cathartic and healing if the birth was traumatic or was not what women expected (Beck 2006). Affonso (1977) wrote about the "missing pieces" of women's birth experiences which were the parts of their labors and deliveries that women felt should have been there but were not. By telling her story, a woman can come to terms with her disappointments in her birth experience and construct a story that provides a coherent account of the birth. Through telling and sharing her story, a woman is also able to put traumatic events into perspective (Callister 2004). Sharing pregnancy and delivery stories also can create a connection between the teller and the listener, providing a common link among women from all generations who have experienced pregnancy, labor, and birth. Peterson (1987) wrote about the important functions pregnancy stories serve within family units. The primary function is to create a sense of connection among members and strengthen family bonds and identity. Additionally, the sharing of stories serves as a way to set expectations, offer advice, and help women and fathers embrace their parenting role.

No matter the purpose of these narratives, stories about pregnancy and childbirth are abundant and easy to access, as many women freely and eagerly share stories about their pregnancies and deliveries. All one has to do is turn on the TV to The Learning Channel or the Discovery Health channel and an entire afternoon can be absorbed by watching programs such as *A Baby Story*, *Deliver Me*, and *House of Babies*, which document women's pregnancies and birth experiences. Viewers can learn how couples prepared for their infants, what symptoms mothers experienced during pregnancy, how labor started, and they can watch as each infant comes into the world whether it is a drug-free water birth or an emergency cesarean section. Cameras are invited into some of the most personal and intimate moments of these women's lives which are then shared in a very public way. Public interest in these stories is high, and these programs are incredibly popular. When The Learning Channel introduced *A Baby Story* in 1998, it quickly became one of its highest-rated programs and has continued to be a staple of its daily programming (Champagne 1999).

Although only a small number of women have the opportunity to share their stories on TV, numerous women use the internet to post and share their stories on social media, blogs, in chat rooms, and on public message boards. A Google search of pregnancy stories returns more than 436,000 hits, many of which are sites where women are invited to write about their pregnancy and birth experiences. Sites such as babycenter.com and The Bump provide numerous forums where women can post their own stories, read other's stories, and even comment on and engage in conversations about those stories. Social media has opened up a new avenue for telling and sharing pregnancy stories and women as women can regularly share their pregnancy-related news with friends and followers with pictures and status updates. Websites such as STFU Parents have even been created with the sole purpose of mocking what many label as the constant oversharing of pregnancy and labor-related details. Entries on STFU poke fun of everything from describing bodily secretions in graphic detail to posting photos of one's placenta or completely unedited photos of the birth itself.

Women wanting to share their stories do not have to turn to a public forum though. Instead, they may share their stories in more intimate ways with friends, acquaintances, and even those they meet in brief encounters. During my first pregnancy, I was amazed at how the sight of a pregnant belly made others so eager to talk and reminisce about their own experiences while pregnant and share other stories they had heard about pregnant women. I could rarely go through a checkout line at the grocery store without another woman sharing some piece of her own story. At times these stories were told as a means of providing advice although at other times their stories were simply something interesting to share. I, too, sought out stories from those I knew such as my mother and aunts, curious as to what their experiences were, wondering if my experience would be similar. As Peterson described, the sharing of pregnancy stories with the women in my family was not only interesting, but it also reminded me of the shared experiences of multiple generations of the women I loved and made me in some ways feel even more a part of them. I also perused the internet and watched my fair share of TV shows constantly wanting to know more about what pregnancy and childbirth was like for others and what potential scenarios I could be facing.

Even though the tendency to tell and share one's story about pregnancy and birth seems to be an almost ubiquitous experience that does not need much prompting, women also are strongly encouraged to document and recount their stories as evidenced by the multiple pregnancy journals, pregnancy calendars, and baby books on the market. These products prompt women to record everything from their first thoughts upon learning they were pregnant to the date they first felt the infant moving. Many women take monthly pictures of themselves to record their growth and infants' ultrasound pictures are proudly displayed in picture frames made exclusively for this purpose. Women get maternity photos taken to professionally capture what they looked like during pregnancy and those who really want to remember the shape of their pregnant bodies will even have a cast of their belly made that they can decorate and display. In their writings on pregnancy and birth stories, Callister and others explain that one of the functions of pregnancy and birth narratives is that they help women to understand their own strengths and power. After giving birth, many women feel an immense sense of pride for their ability to create and bear a child and by recording and documenting their pregnancies women can easily recall the power and sense of accomplishment they felt (Callister 2004; Callister and Khalaf 2010).

So it is clear that these types of stories play a prominent role in our culture and in many women's lives, but what does this abundance of pregnancy and childbirth narratives mean? It illustrates not only that women have a story to tell about their pregnancy and delivery, but also many women have a desire to share their stories with others. Additionally, girls and women are frequently exposed to and confronted with multiple and sometimes conflicting or competing narratives about pregnancy, birth and motherhood which they must sift through when they are pregnant. Navigating pregnancy can be difficult and stressful as women must make decisions about their prenatal care, medical procedures, and childbirth as well as negotiate their changing identities and relationships (Besser and Priel 2003). During this time she also makes sense of the multiple narratives she encounters as she makes sense of her own experience. She decides both consciously and unconsciously how her story will follow and differ from the stories she hears and reads as she integrates these stories into her own story. Even when there are uncontrollable and unpredictable elements, as there so often are, a woman still has power over how she will react to and incorporate those elements into her story. This process can become even more challenging when a woman experiences complications with her pregnancy and specifically complications that can cause premature labor and/or birth.

The idea of pregnancy and birth and women's ability to procreate has long fascinated people. Researchers, Bondas and Eriksson (2001) conducted a phenomenological study to explore the lived experience of pregnancy. In speaking with women they found three dominant themes in the stories women told about being pregnant; a desire for the perfect baby, an altered mode of physical and emotional being, and striving for family communion. In the first theme, women's stories illustrated women's desire to have a perfect baby. They adjusted their own habits to ensure the best health for their child including altering eating and sleeping habits. Not only do women want to have the perfect baby in terms of health, but they also feel personally responsible for ensuring that perfection as it is their body that is nourishing, breathing, and housing the unborn child. Women's physical activity, what they eat, what they drink, and even their emotional state can impact the health and long-term well-being of their baby. Carrying a child also means living in an altered mode of being which was the second theme of women's stories. Women experienced physical discomforts such as fatigue and nausea as well as emotional changes such as mood swings and extreme worries about the baby and childbirth. In the third theme, women's stories expressed hopes and concerns about how the new baby would fit into the family and how the addition would alter family dynamics. As the pregnancy progressed and women were able to feel the baby move or see the baby on an ultrasound, the women felt more connected to the baby and a growing sense of expectations of the infant's place in the family. This study demonstrates that even in a "typical" or "uncomplicated" pregnancy, women encounter a wide array of physical and emotional challenges as the act of being pregnant and giving birth is so life altering and so physically consuming.

In thinking about narratives and their power, a good place to start is with the five presuppositions of Fisher's narrative paradigm. For the average person who does not spend their life studying communication and literature, a discussion of the paradigm and narrative theory may seem more like an academic exercise, but Fisher's paradigm is an incredibly practical way to look at and explain how narratives function not just as a means of communication, but as a way of organizing and understanding the world. While humans have been telling stories and using them since the first spoken language was developed, Fisher was one of the first philosophers and scholars to articulate how narratives function. The first presupposition of his paradigm is that humans' mode of decision-making is good reasons rather than logical arguments. Second, good reasons vary from situation to situation meaning that what merits a good reason and makes sense to a person is always contextual. Third, the formulation of good reasons is ruled by the situation. This is similar to the second presupposition but speaks more to the actual generation of those reasons, which are generated through the creation and telling of stories.

The fourth presupposition is that rationality is judged by narrative fidelity and probability. In layman's terms, the narrative paradigm suggests that humans make decisions and judge situations not by applying pure logic to them but based on their feelings about what is good, right and moral. These feelings frequently come from one's assessment of the stories he or she is told or tells oneself, and in order to be a rational story it must have fidelity, which simply means the story is coherent, the plot hangs together, and the probability that the story is actually true or could happen. The final presupposition is that one must choose among the many existing stories available to him or her to live a good life. It is this element of choice that really struck me as I considered the impact of the narratives women tell and hear about pregnancy and birth. Individuals must not only have the power to choose how they will craft their stories, but also must choose which existing stories or parts of existing stories they will listen to, accept, admire, strive toward, and incorporate into the stories they tell.

The idea is that multiple competing stories exist and individuals must choose which stories to tell and which stories to adhere to as they live their lives. In the narrative paradigm, stories are not just something to hear and read, but they are central to the way individuals live. When thinking about the capacity of narratives to assist women in making sense of their pregnancies and making health decisions, it must be remembered that a woman's story exists among countless other stories. Although each woman's story is unique, her story is shaped by the stories that surround her. As Fisher explained, the meaning and value of a story is always a matter of how it relates to and compares with other stories. Cottle (2002) explains that any encounter with another narrative constitutes an exchange or an interaction as we always respond to a narrative either by commenting on the words of the Other or by applying the Other's narratives to our own. Frequently the response to hearing another narrative is to respond with our own story and in doing so we can either affirm or negate another's tale. Additionally, as we reflect on the stories we hear, we allow those stories to alter our own stories and worldview. Cottle states, "we tend to hear another's story with our own stories, our lenses, as it were, shaping and refining the content and tone of what we are encountering" (p. 535).

Fisher's initial work on narrative and his presuppositions laid the foundation for further narrative inquiry. Studying and understanding narratives is important because they are fundamental to the way humans communicate. Although Fisher did not believe that narrative is the sole means for human discourse, he argued it is the most efficacious for conveying nontechnical information. Accordingly, "narration captures the experience of the world" (Fisher 1984, 6). He also explained, ". . .all human communication can be seen fundamentally as stories, as interpretations of the world occurring in time and shaped by history, culture, and character" (Fisher 1989, 57). Rather than relying solely on intellectual capacity, narratives appeal to and stimulate multiple senses and emotions. Individuals hearing narratives can be moved by imagery, plotlines, or identification with characters. In terms of pregnancy and birth most people will have a very different reaction to and engage differently to a list of facts as compared to stories and examples. Additionally, individuals are born with the innate ability to judge narratives, which means that all humans have the capacity to make decisions based on narratives, not only those educated in rational argument. Therefore, narratives are accessible to and can be used by anyone.

Because narratives are accessible, they offer a great way to learn about and understand the world. The narrative form is familiar and therefore, the information is easy to process. Adval and Wyer (1998) argued that narrative information is easier to comprehend than a list of facts or details because we most often think in terms of narratives. They found that people who made decisions based on narrative information used a more holistic approach in making their judgments as they were able to consider more aspects of a situation. When becoming absorbed in a narrative, we are transported to another world (Green and Brock 2000). This occurs when one is immersed in a favorite movie or is in the middle of reading a great novel. In this absorbed state we are so engrossed in the tale that we are less likely to find flaws in the story or generate counterarguments to the ideas being presented. This allows for greater influence from the narrative information we receive. It is important to understand then how we integrate the narratives around us to understand and make sense of the world.

Since the introduction of the narrative paradigm, communication scholars have investigated the functions and roles of narratives in the human experience. Because narrative is central to the way people think and speak (W. Fisher 1984; W. Fisher 1985), it predominates illness, disease, and health experiences including how people make sense of those experiences (Hyden 1997). Recognizing this centrality to human experience, health communication scholars have studied multiple aspects of health-related narratives. The narrative turn in social science research arose out of the recognition of the ability of individual and collective narratives to reveal much about the lived experience. The narrative turn recognizes both the centrality of narratives to human life as well as the innate agency of all storytellers (Gubrium and Holstein 2009). Narrative research has explored a wide variety of areas including narrative-based medicine and doctor-patient interaction (Chatwin 2006; Eggly 2002; Vegni, Visioli, and Moja 2005; Vanderford, Jenks, and Sharf 1997; Wheatley et al. 2008). Another line of study has focused on how individuals tell their story, and how individuals use stories in health-related situations. In exploring how individuals use narratives in health-related situations, Sharf and Vanderford (2002) identified five functions of health-related storytelling including transforming identities and social roles, asserting control, solidifying health communities, sense-making, and decision-making. By considering these functions, it becomes clear that narratives are an integral part of how individuals experience and cope with their health.

Health communication scholars began to study individual's sense-making in health situations because any disruption to one's health can be so life altering and difficult to understand. Individuals craft narratives that help them understand the disease and illness experience. Through narratives, individuals are able to piece together the multiple aspects of their illness or health-related experience and make connections among seemingly random events (Frank 1995). This can pose a significant challenge as individuals must, "construct a story that can turn mere existence and stigmatization into a meaningful social and moral life that is self-validating" (Bochner 2001, 140). Narratives are an excellent tool because the "sense-making goes beyond simply recounting the events and involves drawing conclusions about the experience and its impact, significance, and/or effect" (128). Sharf and Vanderford (2002) explained that narrative sense-making is especially powerful because it occurs after events have taken place which means that "storytellers can interpret events, ascribe meanings, justify actions, and make links in retrospect that are less likely to be discerned when the narrator experiences events in real time" (p. 17). Creating and telling a story about a health experience or illness is a way for individuals to take the many events, characters, and emotions they encounter and make sense of them. It is easier to make sense of everything surrounding a health experience because, "once a complex event is put into a story format, it is simplified. The mind doesn't need to work as hard to bring structure and meaning to it" (Pennebaker and Seagal 1999, 1250).

As individuals narrate health-related events, they cast themselves and other involved people in particular roles such as the victim, the hero, or the protagonist. The creation of these roles contributes to their understanding of what has happened and how different events have contributed to the current health situation and the casting of these roles also plays a role in how one feels about and reacts to a health situation. In telling the story of how she spent her pregnancy dealing with an incompetent cervix, a woman may cast herself as the victim as she certainly was at the mercy of her body. On the other hand, the same woman could cast herself as the protagonist in the story focusing on all that she does to help prevent premature birth. Even though her stories have the same events and plotlines, the way she thinks of herself can have a huge impact on how she thinks about what happened to her and her emotional coping.

Women who have experienced preterm labor or delivery can use their narratives to make sense of a situation that was likely far different from their expectations of a typical or normal pregnancy and delivery. During a difficult pregnancy, women's stories continuously evolve as time passes because they have more events to link together and reflect upon. Their stories might vary from day to day as each day's events shape their perspectives. A day with relatively few symptoms might prompt a more hopeful tale whereas a day including a hospital visit might produce a tale full of stress and concern. Previous research has focused on the stories women create about their typical and high-risk pregnancies and how their stories assist them in coping with and understanding their situations (Bondas and Eriksson 2001; Sassi Matthias and Babrow 2007). For example, Bondas and Erikson interviewed forty women who were hospitalized in a Danish hospital due to high blood pressure and found that women's stories focused on the health of their unborn child and their role as a mother and protector of the baby, even prior to its birth. The research illustrates how instrumental these stories are in the pregnancy experience.

One reason that sense-making stories are necessary for pregnant women is because pregnancy is so fraught with uncertainty regarding everything from the health of the unborn baby, the delivery, to the impact the child will have on the mother and the family. When there are complications or a child is born too early, the level of uncertainty rises exponentially. It is through communication with oneself and others that women are able to reduce this uncertainty or at a minimum find a way to cope with the uncertainty surrounding their situations (Sassi Matthias and Babrow 2007). Through stories, women can also attempt to make sense or explain what happened and work to construct a story that helps them to come to terms with and accept their situations. Telling and retelling their stories are one of the ways that women can heal or recover from a traumatic pregnancy or birthing experience.

For example, many women who experience preterm labor are put on bed rest at home or are admitted to the hospital for more restrictive bed rest. In these circumstances, women must create a new narrative about their pregnancies and negotiate a new existence as their abilities to care for themselves and their families are very limited. Durham (1999) studied women who had been ordered to be on bed rest at home to manage their preterm labor. He studied how the women negotiated and came to terms with their activity restriction through their stories. In the initial stages of bed rest, women felt shocked by the drastic change in their lifestyle but applied a strict adherence to their bed rest regimen in order to give their infants the best chance possible. As a woman's time on bed rest continued though, women found themselves negotiating with themselves and others more and more about how they managed their bed rest. As it became more difficult to rely on others, women became more relaxed in their bed-rest regimen, a fact that caused the women to create justifications for their additional movement. For example, women would pick up dirty laundry on the way to the bathroom since they were already up and moving. The stories the women told themselves and others assisted in their negotiation and understanding of their bed rest.

When an infant is born prematurely or with any kind of complications, the opportunity and need to tell a new narrative is created. While parents may have had a preconceived idea of what it would be like to have a new baby, they are now in a situation that calls for a new and often vastly different story about parenting a premature infant, an experience that generally varies greatly from that of parenting a healthy full-term infant. It is important to remember though that no story is created in isolation, so inevitably the story that a woman tells of having a premature baby will be told in contrast to the story she was expecting. These differences between the actual story and the story that women thought they would be telling can often lead to women having several missing pieces in their stories, or at least what feel like missing pieces to the women such as holding their newborns, introducing the baby to family, or breastfeeding. These missing pieces mark their story as different, and therefore it can be difficult to connect with other women whose birth stories are so incredibly different.

In looking at high-risk pregnancy and premature birth the stories are inevitably different. Without having a direct experience with these types of situations, one may assume that the stories will all closely resemble tragedies filled with loss, pain, and disability. Even though there are certainly sad and frightening elements to a high-risk pregnancy and premature birth, the stories are not all tragedies and for as many sad and terrible things that happen there are often just as many positive and encouraging events. It is important that we have access to and hear and read a variety of stories as they provide insight and allow us to see what it is really like to have a premature infant. After his daughter, Elizabeth Ellen was born at 25 weeks, journalist Timothy Smith was inspired to share Elizabeth's story and collect and share the stories of other very premature infants who have thrived despite their early arrival into the world. He acknowledges that his book contains the stories of infants with positive outcomes, something that not all micro-preemies have, but he intentionally selected these stories in the hopes that readers would "pick up a little balance on a very controversial subject and learn that many premature infants aren't forever doomed to a poor quality of life" (Smith 1999, xxii). This does not mean the stories in his book are completely happy tales as the stories all have sections that are sad, scary, and each tale details the ups and downs of the proverbial NICU rollercoaster. In fact, one of the overarching themes of the stories Smith presents is the continual progress and setbacks these young infants and their parents endure. Parents must sit back, relatively helpless, as medical teams do their best to help infants whose underdeveloped bodies and organs are not strong enough for the outside world. Through their stories we learn of the intense emotional toll having premature infants takes on parents and we also see how parents learn to live with their new reality, if not even embrace it.

For example, Lora and Kevin Volpe's daughter Andrea was born at 26 weeks after Lora suffered from a placental abruption. For Lora, her daughter's time in the NICU was extremely difficult for her emotionally. Even when Andrea was having a good day, Lora still felt overwhelmed. She explained the overwhelming emotions this way, "even though she [Andrea] was doing all right at the moment. . .somebody in the next incubator was dying, or they were doing some emergency surgery. It just affected you." (89). The constant ups and downs of the NICU and seeing such sick infants have been shown to lead to constant stress and worry. It is elements like this that stories of life in the NICU can help to illuminate what the struggle is like and the stories that parents themselves tell can help them make sense of what's happening and to work through their various emotions.

In addition to helping people make sense of difficult health situations, narratives also assist individuals in making health care decisions by providing reasons and justifications for the decisions as well as helping individuals consider their options. Individuals construct explanatory narratives in which they are able to explain and come to accept their decisions (Bravata, Rastegar, and Horowitz 2002). Narratives frequently play a role in decision-making processes, as these imagined or hypothetical stories can become instrumental in making decisions about one's health, care, and treatment. For example, a woman experiencing a high-risk pregnancy may have to make a decision about whether or not to be admitted to the hospital for monitoring. In making this decision she could imagine what would happen if she chose to stay at home and what could happen if she chose to be admitted to the hospital. These stories can then help her choose the option that she thinks will cause her the least amount of regret and have the best possible outcome. A key factor in this process is the information an individual has available to construct a potential story. In a health situation like this where one does not have any personal experience to draw from and has a low level of knowledge, an individual may need the assistance of a medical professional or stories from other women with similar experiences to provide details as far as what may happen in different scenarios. Even though individuals are constructing their own imagined story, that story is constructed from outside information. Individuals consider the stories that others tell as they make choices about their health, as other's stories can provide valuable information with regard to expectations about and potential outcomes of a medical decision.

In their review of the effects of narratives on decision-making, Winterbottom et al. (2008) found that narratives can have more of an effect on decision-making than purely statistical information or lists of information. This effect appeared to arise from affective arousal rather than from logical processing of the information. Their review also considered the differences in effects for first-person and third-person narratives in literature designed to help with medical decision-making. First-person narratives such as testimonials tended to have greater effects than third-person accounts. When processing pregnancy and parenting-related information, it stands to reason then that the stories a women encounters told from a first-person point of view will have a strong impact on her choices, possibly even more than facts given to her by her doctors or from stories that she reads in books or online.

When thinking about the narratives that influence individual decision-making, it is important to acknowledge that most likely the stories come from a variety of places and people. In her account of having hip replacement surgery, Sharf (2005) recalled how a friend's story of a negative experience with a physician helped her to make the decision to fire her surgeon and find a physician she was more comfortable with. Other stories come from TV, books, the internet, and even random strangers. People will both actively seek out stories, will be told stories by others or passively see them on TV, and they will also recall stories they have heard in the past and in this way, individuals listen to others' stories and incorporate them into their own stories in order to make choices about how to manage their illness or disease. The decision-making process often involves multiple parties, particularly the patient, the patient's family, and the medical team. A jointly constructed narrative can help the involved parties develop a mutually acceptable care plan (Sharf and Vanderford 2002). In these situations, the involved parties actively work to create a narrative by sharing their own stories and deciding what the basic plot of the shared story will be. I was curious when I embarked on this project about who participated in the story creation process of women as they were going through their difficult pregnancies and early births as well as when they later looked back on these events as well as what stories were the most powerful in shaping and molding the stories women told themselves and others.

This book started as a research project where I sought to find out how women who experienced a high-risk pregnancy and/or gave birth early used the stories they told to make sense of their situations, negotiate their identities, make decisions, and come to terms with their experiences and situations. I was also curious about the collaborative nature of storytelling and story construction and wanted to further explore the ways that existing stories influenced and shaped the stories women tell about being pregnant, giving birth, and parenting newborns. In searching for the answers to these questions I interviewed over ninety-five women who had a high-risk pregnancy or gave birth prematurely. These women had a variety of pregnancy-complications including being pregnant with quadruplets, triplets, and twins, having pregnancy induced conditions such as preeclampsia, placenta previa, an incompetent cervix, HELPP syndrome (a variant of preeclampsia) and PROM (premature rupture of membranes) while others had preexisting conditions such as diabetes that made their pregnancies high risk. Other women delivered early due to their children having intrauterine growth restriction (IUGR) or being in some types of fetal distress, while other women simply went into labor too early. Many women had planned to get pregnant, some were not planning a pregnancy and were surprised with the news they were expecting, and many women had used some type of fertility assistance to conceive. Some women were first-time mothers and many had older children. The women I interviewed delivered anywhere from 18 to 38 weeks and their children spent anywhere between 0 and 235 days in the NICU. The time that had passed since having their preemies was three months to twenty-seven years.

These were women I knew personally, knew my friends or family, I had met through multiples groups, or who responded to requests for interviews I posted online in different forums and on different webpages for parents of multiples and preemie parents. It was an incredibly varied group with very different experiences and stories which made this project very rich and informative. This diverse group was also a good representation of who is at a risk for having a high-risk pregnancy or deliver prematurely, which is any woman who is pregnant. It can be scary to think that anyone can have a preemie, but the reality is that this is very true. Although many women have typical, healthy pregnancies with no complications, the fact is that one in eight babies will be born too early. Pregnancy complications and premature birth are not some rare occurrence, but instead happen far more often than they should.

I conducted interviews in person, over the phone, and via Skype, and the interview lasted anywhere from 30 minutes to two hours. My husband once asked me how I could possibly talk to strangers for so long and I just laughed. He obviously did not understand women's love of talking about their pregnancies, and he also did not understand the connection that many preemie moms feel. The conversations generally began by asking each participant to share her story of her experience with preterm labor or birth starting with how she learned she was pregnant and when she learned that her pregnancy was considered high-risk or when she began to experience complications. From this story, the conversation moved to sources of information she used and other stories she may have encountered during her pregnancy. I also asked women to describe any stories she had avoided or stories she had heard or read that she did not want to pursue or that were upsetting to her. To close the interview, I asked each women to share any additional information that she thought would be relevant to the study. The course of each interview varied widely as is common with a conversation. At times the subject of the interview would veer to other topics such as raising multiples or dealing with other family members. These tangents often lead to additional information that was relevant to the study, such as women discussing how they struggled to deal with relatives who were not understanding of their stories and their situations.

In writing this book I hope to provide insight into how women work to create the stories they tell about their pregnancy, birth, and motherhood experiences. I say work because even if it is not conscious, we all make deliberate choices when we tell our stories about how we cast ourselves and others, what details we share and omit, the tone, the words, the timeline of events. Our stories change and evolve over time as we grow to understand more things, make more connections, and sometimes change our minds about the significance and meaning of certain events. Because their stories are not composed in a bubble, it is important to examine how other stories influence and shape the stories women tell. The story I tell of having preemies is much different now that I have had time to watch my daughters grow, have met other women with preemies and heard their stories, and have experienced other major life events. It is my hope in writing this book that more women have the opportunity to tell and share their stories and that more people have the opportunity to read and learn from those stories.

Chapter 3

Pregnancy as a Cultural Phenomenon

After seven years of fertility treatments, Ashley was finally pregnant and not just with one baby, but with twins, a boy and girl. After having such a difficult time conceiving, Ashley was looking forward to her pregnancy and anticipated having what she described as the "picture perfect" pregnancy and delivery. For her, her ideas of what her pregnancy would be like never included weeks on bed rest, delivering her twins at 29 weeks, and then spending the first eleven weeks of their lives with them in the NICU. Her path to becoming pregnant and then having a baby was nothing like she had expected and this was something she had to come to terms with when events took unexpected turns. Despite how difficult her pregnancy and birth were, her son and daughter are now happy and healthy three-year-olds. Even though the beginning of her story was full of trauma and drama, she is thankful that it at least has a happy ending.

After my triplets were born I spent a lot of time trying to understand what had happened, why it had happened the way it did, and all of the varied emotions I felt. So much of my story and experience was painful because it did not match my expectations or beliefs as to what my pregnancy should have been like. Like Ashley, I had to come to terms with the parts of my story that fell short of what I had wanted and how I thought things should be. When talking with women with similar experiences, the most commonly repeated phrases were, "this was wrong" and "this was not the way it was supposed to happen." Of course the circumstances of many of these women's pregnancies, deliveries, and first days of their children's lives were terrible in so many ways, so their complaints and feelings made sense, but the more we talked the more I realized that the feelings of the pregnancy and childbirth being wrong went deeper than just being concerned about medical issues. When complications started to arise, when babies were born too soon, or when mothers were unable to cuddle their babies and count their fingers and toes, there was a deep sense of being robbed of the experiences and moments that in many ways define motherhood and pregnancy. Over and over women talked about how their situations and circumstances look nothing like what they had imagined or expected, and I could relate all too well to these sentiments. William Shakespeare once wrote that "expectation is the root of all heartache" and in my case I could certainly see how this was true. In order to understand the root of so many women's pain, I began to look more closely at where these expectations came from.

As I started to look more into why women have the ideas they do of what a pregnancy should look like, it struck me that so many of our beliefs and expectations of pregnancy and child-birth should be like in the United States, incredibly modern and culturally defined. Even today you will find drastically different experiences of being pregnant, childbirth, and the postpartum period around the world. In her fascinating book, *Childbirth Across Cultures: Ideas and Practices of Pregnancy, Childbirth and the Postpartum,* Helaine Selin presents a collection of essays detailing the pregnancy and birth experiences of women across the globe. In most developing countries, women still give birth at home assisted by female relatives and friends both out of custom, and out of necessity as there are no local hospitals or physicians available. For example, in the Hmong culture women deliver at home and are expected to bear the pain of childbirth without complaining. Following the birth, the mother and child have a 30-day period of confinement where they do not leave the home and do nothing more than lie together and eat. This promotes the recovery of the mother and successful breastfeeding of the baby. For the first three days, the mother and baby lay on a bed of straw in front of the fireplace and after the third day the straw which is considered contaminated with blood and birth fluids is burned (Liamputtong 2009).

Ugandan women are also expected to bear the pains of pregnancy and delivery without complaint as they face what is known as the women's battle (childbirth). In the Ugandan culture, a woman's value and social standing is related to her ability to maintain a healthy pregnancy and to birth her children with as little assistance as possible. Women who have complications and need to be seen at a medical clinic are considered to have failed at winning the battle and are less respected and seen as less powerful women (Kyomuhendo 2009). A successful home birth in considered to be a source of pride in honor. In Trinidad and Tobago, a small Caribbean and Island nation, hospitals and obstetricians are readily available, but the majority of hospitals have strict policies that prohibit fathers from being in the delivery room. In some cases fathers are allowed, but in order to be given permission they have to meet a long list of requirements and at any time, medical personnel have the right to remove them from the delivery room. These policies lead many women to opt for home births so that men may be present ("Fathers in the Caribbean Have to Fight to See the Birth of Their Kids" 2014).

Even in more developed countries with advanced medical systems like the United States, the customs and norms still differ. In Japan, a large percentage of women still adhere to the traditional practice of Satogaeri which is the Japanese word meaning going home. Pregnant women return to their parents' home about a month prior to the delivery and return to their home after the delivery for three to four months so they can be taken care of and their mothers can help with the baby. Husbands come to visit their wives and children, but remain in their own home, making this a unique time shared between just women and their babies (Yanagisawa 2009). In China where the one-child policy means that the majority of women only give birth once, there are vast differences between pregnancy and childbirth in the rural villages and the city. Women in the cities have fully embraced the medicalized view of pregnancy and childbirth and many opt to deliver via C-section as it is considered easier and more convenient, and is also a status symbol as surgical birth is more expensive (Harvey and Buckley 2009). In rural villages where medical care is less readily available women given birth at home and are attended either by a local midwife or family and close friends.

The point of noting how birth rituals and experience vary around the world is to illustrate how women's conceptions and expectations of how different rituals and experiences during the pregnancy and birth processes will occur are bounded by the culture in which one lives. In the United States, there have been researchers and feminist scholars who have argued that dominant narratives regarding pregnancy, childbirth, and motherhood exist and serve to shape not only women's narratives, but also their expectations and understanding of these unique life experiences. Evans and O'Brien (2005) assert that pregnancy and childbearing has "shifted from being part of women's private domain to being increasingly part of the public realm" (p. 66). Bondas and Eriksson (2001) argued that "evolving societal myths and rituals and technological and scientific development surround pregnancy" (824). Root and Browner (2001) go even further in arguing that the medical and social environment has created a set of moral acts or obligations that pregnant women must perform and failure to comply with prenatal norms such as taking prenatal vitamins and failing to avoiding certain foods such as sushi or tuna is equivalent to being a bad mother.

One of the dominant narratives in the United States, and arguably the most dominant narrative, comes from the medical community and concerns the medicalized view of pregnancy and childbirth (Maher 2003). The medical view promotes the idea that pregnancy and childbirth are pathological conditions that are inherently dangerous (Kline 2007). This line of thinking brings about the idea that pregnancy is something that is a medical condition, as opposed to a natural state, that needs to be monitored and controlled. An underlying assumption of the model, is that the medical community will be successful in bringing about the birth of a healthy infant. When a pregnancy is labeled high risk or a woman begins to experience complications, her pregnancy is pushed into a realm of even more surveillance and control, something that can threaten her identity as a mother and her autonomy as she must rely on others and especially medical personnel to keep herself and her unborn child healthy. Within this model, is the idea that if a woman follows the advice of her medical team and takes the necessary medical precautions, she will be able to keep her infant healthy and safe. What happens then if something goes wrong and an infant is delivered too early, or medical interventions are not successful in stopping labor? How does this woman's story fit into the broader societal narrative of pregnancy and birth?

If we look at how the experience of pregnancy has changed through time in the United States, one of the most drastic changes outside of the physical care available has been the evolution from a personal and private experience to a public phenomenon where women proudly display their baby bumps on the cover of fashion magazines, share the intimate details of their pregnancies and deliveries through social media, and can easily turn on the TV and watch women in labor, giving birth, and bringing their babies home from the hospital. Modern pregnancy and childbirth is surrounded by a number of rituals and customs from registering for gifts, and throwing baby showers, to framing the first ultrasound picture and selecting the perfect photo for the birth announcements. Although these rituals can seem essential and for many women are defining parts of their experience, many of these rituals are relatively new and were not something that even their grandmothers would have considered. What many women now take for granted as the way things are done or should be are relatively new traditions and standards of care.

A BRIEF HISTORY OF PREGNANCY AND CHILDBIRTH IN AMERICA

As I studied more and more and read about the history of pregnancy and birth in the United States, it was fascinating to think of how different the experience of pregnancy and childbirth was 200, 100, and even just 50 years ago. Prior to the early 1800s, pregnancy and birth were considered to be exclusively in the female's realm. Women labored and gave birth at home attended by family and friends who had no formal training, but had given birth themselves and had often assisted other friends and family members during previous births giving them at least a basic understanding of the process. There were a few midwives at the time, but they were not formally trained and because medicine itself was rudimentary they had no medications or knowledge of surgery to treat common problems such as hemorrhaging or high blood pressure. In many ways, childbirth was a social event and women attending the birth would often drink and share stories to pass the time as the pregnant woman labored. Childbirth was incredibly dangerous for both mother and child, and maternal and infant death rates were very high. Even if the baby survived the birth, there was a very high chance of an infant becoming ill and dying before reaching its first birthday. It is estimated that up until 1915, the infant mortality rate was as high as 40 percent (Singh and Dyck 2010; Wegman 2001). Men were never present during the labor and birth as it was considered inappropriate, so fathers left the home and waited for the news that their new son or daughter was born. Even male doctors were excluded from the birthing process making childbirth an exclusively female event (Cassidy 2006).

In the early 1800s, medicine as a profession began to expand and more formal training of medical professionals became commonplace. Knowledge of the human body also increased which led to a shift in thinking of pregnancy as a natural state of women to a pathological condition that needed to be treated and managed. Women were still giving birth at home as hospitals were just starting to be established, but in addition to be attended by midwives more women were also being seen by doctors, especially the upper class. Husbands still were not present during the labor and birth, but male physicians were allowed into the delivery room in emergency situations when they were needed. More formal training also became available for midwives leading to a professionalization of the field although there was still a strong belief that pregnancy and childbirth were a natural part of womanhood and medical interventions were at a minimum.

One of the major changes that came about in the ways that American women experienced birth came about in 1847 when Dr. William Morton became the first physician to use anesthesia during a delivery at Massachusetts General Hospital in Boston. His patient was a woman with a severely deformed pelvis due to rickets. This was a common illness at the time and when women with rickets became pregnant the delivery often required intense and painful manipulation of the baby so that it could navigate through the deformed birth canal. Knowing how horrific and painful this experience could be, Morton used ether during the delivery and was able to lessen the pain. This initial successful use of ether paved the way for continued investigation into how medical interventions could lessen the pain of labor and childbirth. Hospital births were still rare, but it became common to administer ether during these deliveries. It was noted that women who were sedated often had trouble pushing and the newborns often struggled with their breathing as the ether had a sedative effect on them as well. This led Dr. James Simpson to invent forceps to help forcibly remove infants when women could not exert enough force to push them out of the birth canal. Another big step in the use of medication during labor and delivery came in 1857 when Queen Victoria of England delivered Prince Leopold. Rather than using ether, her doctor held handkerchiefs soaked with cholorform over her nose every 15 minutes or so and reported that the Queen had a smooth delivery and the prince was born healthy. This led to increased experimentation of different drug combinations including morphine and scorpaline that eliminated pain and actually induced amnesia so that women would forget the trauma of childbirth (Cassidy 2006).

In 1900, over 95 percent of births in America took place at home. By the 1950s this number had completely reversed and over 95 percent of births took place in the hospital. This gives rise to the question, what led to this drastic change? In the late 1800s and early 1900s, it was actually the poor who were most likely to give birth in a hospital as they could not afford to pay a midwife and went to the public clinics for assistance. This practice began to shift though and after the 1920s the middle and upper class began to go to the hospital for delivery. The largest contributing factor to this change was the increase of hospitals and trained physicians in the United States. Women now had a place to go to give birth and with the development of improved diagnostic tools and tests led society to place more and more control of their physical health into the medical field. This movement of birth into the hospitals continued to reinforce the idea that birth was not a natural process but instead was a medical condition. One would think that an increase in hospital deliveries would have immediately led to a decrease in the infant and maternal fatality rates, but the risk of infection from being at the hospital was high, and women and infants that survived the birth died later of an untreatable infection. In 1935 the infant mortality rate was 56 deaths for every 1000 live births (Singh and Dyck 2010). There was a lack of knowledge about how infection and disease spread which contributed to less than hygienic practices such as not washing hands or instruments between patients. Prior to the invention of antibiotics, nothing could be done once infection spread so even the most minor infection could be deadly.

During the 1930s and 1940s hospital births were characterized by being highly controlled by the medical staff. One of the largest fears at the time was infection, and it had taken such a toll in the previous decade, so hospitals took extensive measures to keep out germs. Even though antibiotics had been invented during this time, there was a strong focus on keeping hospitals as sterile as possible which meant that women had to check into the maternity ward alone and were not allowed any visitors during labor including their husbands. Once checked in women were administered enemas, had their pubic regions shaved, and were instructed to lay in a bed while they labored sometimes for as long as three days. Women had little say in the medications that were administered to control the pain and often the doses were so high and the women were so sedated that they had few memories of giving birth. This heavily medicated state became known as Twilight Sleep, and the fact that women could labor and deliver in an almost unconscious state was considered by many to be a positive medical breakthrough. Many women's liberation activists pushed for the availability of Twilight Sleep arguing that the practice liberated women from the physical pain of birth. Some records of childbirth during this era report women being unaware of their reactions while under sedation causing them to lose control of their mental facilities. Reports also exist of laboring women being cuffed to their beds to prevent them from hurting themselves or the nurses and at times even being forced to wear helmets to protect themselves if they fell. Another practice was to strap women's legs into the stirrups for extended times periods, sometimes 12 hours. This led to women having numbness and pain long after their deliveries. Because women had no memory of the events they were not able to complain.

Immediately following the delivery, which often required forceps due to highly sedated women being unable to push, the baby was taken to the infant nursery and the mother was taken to recovery. Contact between mother and child was extremely limited as nurses tended to the newborns while mothers were sent to a postpartum delivery ward. Formula feeding was considered superior to breast-feeding at the time so women's chests were often tightly bound to minimize engorgement and this also meant that women did not need to be with their infants every two to three hours in order for them to eat. Little concern was given to letting the mother and baby bond and instead, the focus remained on preventing infection and getting the mother back to optimal health before discharging her from the hospital. This meant that visitation to the hospital was severely restricted and women spent their time postpartum lying in a bed on a maternity ward recovering alone rather than welcoming friends and family to meet the new baby. Hospital stays were much longer then, sometimes up to two weeks, so mother and baby had limited contact for the first week or two of life.

By the end of the 1950s, there began to be a backlash against the heavily drugged and controlled births that placed pregnant and laboring women in a passive role often unable to even remember giving birth. In 1957, *Ladies' Home Journal* published a letter written by a labor and delivery nurse calling for an investigation into the standard practices in hospital maternity wards. In her letter she described women being strapped onto delivery tables for hours, attempts to delay births to accommodate doctors' schedules, and women in general being treated by nurses and doctors in a cold and impersonal manner. Soon after the publication of the letter, women and nurses across the country began to write additional letters calling for a more humane delivery system

(Cassidy 2006). These complaints and a growing sense of discontent among American women with the birthing process were some of the driving forces behind the shift toward the natural birth movement which was a movement that viewed birth as a natural occurrence that had been occurring since the beginning of time and did not need the intense medical interventions that had become so common.

One of the key players in this movement was Fernand Lamaze, a French doctor who worked to discover a way for women to have painless childbirth without the heavy use of medications that were so common in Twilight Sleep. Adapting techniques he had observed in Russia, Lamaze created a system of muscle relaxing and breathing techniques to help distract women from the pain. What is interesting is that these techniques were developed because during wartime in Russia there was a shortage of anesthetics and women had no medicinal option for pain relief. The techniques Lamaze observed and later adapted had been borne out of necessity. In addition to breathing and relaxation, his method also heavily relied on constant emotional support from the father and trained nurses. His Lamaze method came to the United States in the early 1950s and began to be known as natural childbirth.

The Lamaze method really caught on after Marjorie Karmel, an American woman who was very unhappy with how little she participated in the birth of her first child, was assisted by Dr. Lamaze and used his method during the labor and delivery of her second child. Karmel documented her birth experiences in the book *Thank You Dr. Lamaze* which was published in 1959 and helped to legitimize the method. She also teamed up with Elisabeth Bing, cofounder of Lamaze International, to teach childbirth classes using the Lamaze method. Both of these pioneers in the natural childbirth movement were quick to emphasize that the true contribution of the Lamaze method was not the very specific breathing patterns and sounds to make while breathing, such as the distinctive hee-hee-hee that is so often portrayed on TV and in the movies, but the recognition and affirmation that birth is a natural process and women should be able to work with their bodies while in labor and move and breath in the ways that bring them comfort (Zwelling 2000).

Through the 1960s and 1970s, the natural childbirth movement gained steam and more and more women refused pain medication and worked to have a completely natural birth. Similar to the way that women's rights advocates had argued for Twilight Sleep because it liberated women from pain, many women's rights advocates now pushed for natural childbirth methods by arguing that this allowed women to embrace their natural power and it was a way to celebrate the female body and all it can do. Natural birth methods also gave more control of the birthing process back to women. Even if women did not learn or use the actual Lamaze method, labor and delivery was highly influenced by Lamaze's ideas and things such as having a birth support person—usually the father, taking child birth preparation classes, and the building of birthing centers all arose out of the Lamaze movement. Birthing centers are free-standing clinics generally staffed by trained midwives and offer patient-centered holistic care for mothers and provide them with a variety of birthing options. The number of birthing centers peaked in 1998 and has been on a steady decline since, primarily due to insurance issues and more alternative birthing options available at hospitals. The number of homebirths also began to rise since 2000 and more women chose to deliver at home while attended by a midwife although the number of home births since the 1950s has never been greater than one percent of all births (MacDorman, Mathews, and Declercq 2012).

Completely drug-free births became less common in the late 1980s as the use of an epidural became more refined. Although the technique of inserting medication directly into the spinal cord for pain control had existed for some time, the method had a large list of serious side effects and the insertion of the needle and medication often caused a small amount of spinal fluid to leak causing massive headaches and the need for women to lay completely flat for up to 24 hours after the delivery. Once physicians figured out how to better manage the insertion of the medication and manage the amount of medication being administered, epidurals became increasingly popular to the point that they are now almost routine during labor and deliveries.

Even as there was shift to more natural methods of childbirth and women being more in control of their labors and deliveries, the hospitals were still very much in control of the time that women and infants spent together postpartum. One positive change was that women were able to hold their babies immediately after vaginal delivery and babies were brought to mothers as soon as possible following a C-section. One of the major advocates for giving women and infants time together immediately following the delivery was Dr. Benjamin Spock who published *The Common Book of Baby and Childcare* in 1946. He argued that the first hour after birth was a critical time for bonding and women and children needed to spend that first hour together to start the bonding process (Spock 1946). Other child development specialists also began to weigh in on the issue of mother/child bonding and while there was a general consensus that bonding is an important process in which mothers became more and more attached to their infants, there were mixed ideas as far as the existence of a critical time period for bonding and the importance of the first hours after birth for effective bonding to take place. Spock also encouraged women and infants to spend as much time together as possible during the first months to facilitate the attachment and bonding processes, but hospitals still treated infants and mothers as separate patients and entities. Generally, mothers were taken to their postpartum rooms and infants were taken to the nursery where they spent the majority of their hospital stay except for feeding times. One of the primary goals of this set up was to give new mothers time to rest and recover before going home. Visitation was very strict with established visiting hours and often young children were not allowed to be in the room with the infants as the thought was that the risk of infection was too great. I can vividly remember going to the hospital with my dad and brothers after my youngest brother was born in 1986. My mom came out to meet us in the general visitors' lounge wearing her nightgown and robe because we were not allowed back into her room. We walked over to the nursery and looked through the window where my mom pointed out our new brother to us and a nurse came over and kindly held him up so we could have a closer look. It was not until he came home from the hospital three days later that I was actually allowed to touch and hold him.

This experience was a far cry from what is now the common practice of rooming in postpartum where infants and mothers are encouraged to spend their entire hospital stay together. The impetus for the practice came in 1991 when the World Health Organization (WHO) launched the Baby Friendly Hospital Initiative which was a global initiative designed to increase breastfeeding rates. One of the major components of the initiative was the practice of rooming in so that babies could be breastfed on demand and mothers would gain confidence in their abilities to care for their infants. Even for women who did not breastfeed, the practice of being together in the room was encouraged to promote bonding and to give mothers the opportunity to care for their new babies. Hospitals also began to loosen their strict visitation policies and friends and family were able to visit throughout the day and siblings were able to come to the hospital and interact with their new siblings. Fathers were encouraged to stay at the hospital and many hospital rooms are now designed with couches that can be converted into beds or a cushioned recliner so that fathers have a place to sleep.

Today, deliveries primarily take place in the hospital with just 1.4 percent of births in 2012 taking place outside of the hospital either at home or at free-standing birthing centers. There has been an upsurge in the number of certified nurse midwives (CNM), many of whom work and deliver at the local hospital with CNMs attending 7.6 percent of hospital births in 2012. Hospitals work hard to give women options as far as the birthing process and many obstetricians and hospitals encourage women to fill out a birthing plan that indicates their preferences for a wide range of things from the types of pain medications they would like, if they want an epidural, who will be in the room during the labor and delivery, to even what may seem like minor details such as whether or not they want a certain type of music playing in the delivery room. Additionally, the rate of C-sections has been steadily rising over the past three decades and almost one-third of deliveries in United States are by cesarean (Osterman and Martin 2014). There has been growing concern over this rate as it is generally considered to be better and safer for both the women and infants to have a vaginal delivery. In 2012, and the American Medical Association has instituted guidelines disallowing elective C-sections prior to 39 weeks. Women are also likely to opt for pain medication and 61 percent of women have an epidural during delivery (Osterman and Martin 2011).

Not only were the physical circumstances of how women delivered in the past different, but perhaps even more importantly, the way that pregnancy was viewed was also quite different. In today's society, we think nothing of seeing pregnant women not just out in public but proudly posting pictures of their bare bellies on Facebook or sitting for a maternity photo shoot to commemorate their pregnancy. In the past, women were much more modest and sought to hide their growing bellies rather than flaunt them to the world. While there is some indication that during the Victorian Era upper class women went into confinement during their pregnancies to avoid being seen in a pregnant state out in public, the majority of women continued to live life as normal, especially women in the lower classes who needed to continue to work and take care of the household duties. Modesty was highly valued at the time though and women did not go out of their way to emphasize their pregnant bellies and in many cases wore tight-fitting dresses and corsets to minimize their size—a practice that was hardly beneficial to the mother's health. Pregnancy is directly linked to a woman's sexuality, so great care was taken in dressing in a way that did not emphasize the female body or the results of a woman's sexual activity (Mannering 2009). Those without the money to make or buy specific dresses for pregnancy made do with a large apron or shift with an adjustable tie that could cover the belly throughout the pregnancy.

With time there was a general shift in fashion and corsets went out of style but in terms of maternity dress, the aim was still to hide or disguise the pregnant body as much as possible. An ad for maternity clothes that appeared in *Good Housekeeping* in 1923 extolled the virtues of a dress that allowed women to be "entirely free from embarrassment of a noticeable appearance during a trying period." Additionally, more and more clothing was mass produced rather than hand sewn by a seamstress or at home, and in the early 1900s there began to be a mass market for maternity clothes and companies such as Sears and Roebuck began to specifically advertise their maternity line and several pattern companies promoted their maternity patterns. Maternity clothes at the beginning of the 1900s were loose-fitting dresses or smocks and once pants came into style, fitted pants were often paired with a loose top. Maternity clothes were meant to be functional and while there was an attempt to be stylish, maternity looks were often characterized by feminine and more infantile accents such as bows or flowers, almost as if the clothes were designed to emphasize that they were being worn because a new baby was coming ("What to Expect," 2004).

A real shift in the style and design of maternity clothes came in the 1990s. In their research on the commodification of motherhood, Ogle, Tyner, and Schofield-Tomschin (2013) explained how purchasing and wearing maternity clothes are one of the ways women begin to shift their identities to being a pregnant woman and a mother. In the 1990s, pregnant celebrities began to show off their growing bellies and pregnant bodies, rather than trying to hide from the cameras or wear baggy concealing clothes. In 1991, Demi Moore shocked the world when she posed nude for the cover of *Vanity Fair* magazine when she was seven months pregnant. Her move was applauded by many for choosing to celebrate her pregnant body and showcase its beauty rather than be ashamed of her extra size. Maternity clothes began to be more form fitting and kept up more with the prevailing trends in fashion. Several upscale maternity stores such as Motherhood Maternity and Pea in a Pod opened and pregnant women began to embrace buying and wearing maternity clothes as one of the rituals of pregnancy and motherhood. Today maternity clothing is a growing industry and in 2015, its sales in the United States are expected to hit 4.8 billion dollars ("US Maternity Apparel Market Size $4.8 Bn by 2015" 2010). Many companies such as Old Navy, Gap, and H&M have expanded to offer a maternity line giving pregnant women an abundance of stylish choices (Ali 2003; Bener 2005).

Another major change is in how pregnancy was talked about, if it was talked about at all. In the past, pregnancy was more of a private affair and even though women would speak about their pregnancy and symptoms with other women, it was not a topic they would be comfortable discussing in mixed sex groups. The word pregnant itself was considered vulgar and was taboo until the 1950s, so many euphemisms were used instead including expecting, being with child, being in a delicate condition, and being in the family way. I looked for an explanation of why the word pregnant was taboo and did not find any conclusive answers so all I can speculate is that the term was either too clinical, referred too directly to the female body, or the word made one think too much of the activities a woman engaged in to get in the pregnant condition. Not only could the term pregnant not be spoken in public, but being pregnant itself could get women fired. Prior to 1978 and the passage of the Pregnancy Discrimination Act, employers could fire a woman solely on the basis of her pregnant status. Of course some of this firing was done because employers knew the woman would be taking time off to have the baby or even leaving the work force, but employers could also fire women if they thought it was inappropriate for a pregnant woman to hold a position.

Today, most women have no problem not only saying that they are pregnant, but discussing various aspects of pregnancy symptoms and deliveries with both other women, and in front of men as well. Not only do women routinely take photos to document their growing bellies, but they also share these photos and updates on how their pregnancies and deliveries are progressing with friends and family. Social media outlets such as Facebook and Twitter have made this kind of sharing even easier (Stevens 2011). It is so easy in fact, that many parents and women have been accused of oversharing online. A 2011 *Washington Post* article described the growing trends of women posting ultrasound photos, photos of positive pregnancy tests, swollen body parts, and graphic pictures of the delivery and birth (Anderson 2011). Some women even upload videos of the delivery and will post status updates during labor that let their friends and family know how much they are dilated. The oversharing trend as *Good Morning America* dubbed the increased amount of information being shared on social media has even sparked websites such as STFU parents which poke fun at what parents choose to publish online.

Another ritual that has changed drastically over time is the baby shower. Today the baby shower has become one of the iconic rituals of pregnancy and motherhood and in many ways is seen as a rite of passage for first time mothers as an initiation into motherhood. Fisher and Gainer (1993) explain that the importance of the baby shower lies not in acquiring the paraphernalia needed to raise a child, but in the public acknowledgment of the pregnancy and the baby to be. In the United States, there are no formal rituals that exist to mark the birth of a child or of the transformation of a woman into a mother after the baby is born. Some religions have specific ceremonies to welcome a baby into the faith community such as baptism, infant dedication, or a bris, but there is no universal ritual. The concept of baby showers traces its roots back to the Victorian Era when given the more private nature of pregnancy and the high risk of both maternal and infant death, many women did not publically announce their pregnancy until after the baby was born. After the first few months, women would host tea parties where other women would come to meet the new baby and often these women would bring small handmade gifts such as hand-sewn baby blankets and baby clothes. The term shower developed from this early practice of "showering" the new baby with gifts. Women would sometimes play silly games to predict who else at the party was pregnant or would soon be expecting, a practice that may have led to the tradition of playing games at modern showers.

What we would now recognize as the modern version of a baby shower began shortly after World War II during the baby boom when America was prosperous and consumerism was taking hold. Baby showers were almost always held for a woman who was having her first child as this was when she was in the most need of equipment and supplies. They were held prior to the birth so that women could acquire all of the necessary supplies and equipment they would need to raise a baby such as high chairs, clothing, and blankets.

Showers were almost always had an exclusively female guest list and themes and decorations tended to be baby related such as Noah's Ark, baby animals, blocks, or rubber ducks. Women gathered together to play games, give gifts, and often share stories and impart wisdom to the mother-to-be about delivery and child rearing. During this era the baby shower became a highly anticipated event and one of the important rituals that marked the transition of a woman into a mother.

Baby showers have continued to be one of the important rituals of pregnancy although they have evolved and in some ways become even larger events. Stores began to provide registry service and expectant mothers could carefully select which diaper bag, swing, and burp cloths she wanted. Themes of showers also began to change as more and more women eschewed the traditional infantile themes and instead opted for more trendy or sophisticated themes such as Modern Mommy or a Baby Rave. Couples showers have also become more popular where both men and women are invited to celebrate the coming baby. Baby showers are now just as likely to have barbeque and beer as they are to have rubber ducks and punch. Some couples, especially those who are older and more established may have a simple diaper shower where guests bring just essentials such as diapers and wipes as couples take it upon themselves to purchase their baby equipment and nursery decorations or a favorite books shower where guests bring books to help start the new baby's library (Paul 2007).

Perhaps the biggest reason for the change in the way that pregnancy and childbirth has changed through the years is due to the fact that people have far less children than in the past so the event of being pregnant or giving birth is not as common, and it is something that women will only experience on average two times in her life. Given the decreased number of pregnancies and children, women will often make more of a conscious effort to record and enjoy the pregnancy experience.

Competing Models

While the dominant model of childbirth in the United States from the early 1900s has been the medical model, there are other models and ways of thinking about pregnancy and childbirth. The midwifery model of childbirth has stood as a counternarrative to the medicalized view of birth (Kline 2007; Maher 2003). In this view, pregnancy and childbirth are considered as normal human conditions and experiences as women have been bearing children forever. Pregnancy and childbirth are viewed as natural processes rather than things that need to be controlled by medical professionals and medical interventions. Proponents of the midwifery model argue that taking childbirth out of the medical realm returns power to women and allows them to connect with themselves and their infants, because a woman works with her body and frequently avoids extra medical interventions such as Pitocin or epidurals. Some of the basic tenants of the midwifery model include the idea that pregnancy and birth are natural processes, the role of the midwife is to provide for the physical, emotional, and social needs of the mother and child, viewing the mother as an active participant in her care, the importance of providing continuous care and support throughout labor, and limiting the use of medical interventions. It is important to note that while many midwifes attend homebirths, this is not a requirement and many midwifes practice at hospital in conjunction with other medical staff including physicians. The midwifery model also emphasizes that midwifery is an excellent option for women experiencing normal pregnancies and recognize that when there are complications and a pregnancy is high risk that women need to seek out appropriate medical care (Thachuk 2007; Rooks 1999; Worman-Ross and Mix 2013; Embler 2006).

UNDERSTANDING PREEMIES AND HIGH-RISK PREGNANCIES

As the previous section illustrated, both the physical and social process of being pregnant and giving birth have changed drastically through time. The concept and experience of having a high-risk pregnancy and a preemie have also drastically changed. Medical technology has allowed for greater diagnosis of pregnancy complications so women now know that they have certain conditions that make their pregnancy high-risk that in the past they would not have known about until early delivery. Prior to the use of ultrasound, many women did not know they were carrying twins or triplets until they delivered, and conditions such as in uterine growth restriction (IUGR) were impossible to diagnose. Medical advancements have enabled smaller and smaller premature infants to survive whereas in the past there was little that could be done. This means that more women have the experience of having an incredibly premature baby in the NICU than ever before.

When I learned that I was carrying triplets and later when they were in the NICU, I felt so alone and isolated. I had known in the abstract that women delivered their babies prematurely, but I knew no one close to me had delivered early, and I certainly had no idea as to the extent of the problem and just how many women had a similar experience to mine. The March of Dimes reported that in 2011 that one in eight infants in the United States was born prematurely which is over 450,000 infants a year. Prematurity is defined as any gestation less than 37 weeks ("March of Dimes Peristats" 2014). The percentage of infants born early seemed so high when I first read the statistics, and as it turns out, the number is high when compared to other countries. The

US rate of preterm births is actually the sixth highest in the world behind only India, China, Nigeria, Pakistan, and Indonesia. Despite having one of the most advanced medical systems in the world, the preterm birth rate in the United States is worse than developing countries such as Kenya, Ethiopia, and Sudan. A 2013 article in *Newsweek* decried what it called the full-term crisis. Even though the rate of premature births in the United States has slowly been declining, the rate and numbers of premature births are comparable to countries like Bangladesh and the Democratic Republic of Congo (Harris 2013). This leads to the important question of why the preterm birth rate in the United States, despite some modest declines in recent years, still remains so high, and why it is so high as compared to other developed countries.

Unfortunately, for the most part these questions remain unanswered and researchers continue to search for ways to solve the problem. Although any woman can deliver early, there are several known risk factors that put a woman at greater risk for preterm labor and delivery. One of the greatest risk factors is being pregnant with twins or higher-order multiples (Chism 1997). The average gestation for twins is 35 weeks and for triplets is 32 weeks (Luke 1994). Although many may consider a twin pregnancy somewhat routine, most obstetricians and reproductive endocrinologists consider a twin pregnancy high risk. Although many twins are born full term, many are not, and a twin pregnancy presents serious risks for both mothers and infants (Saul 2009). The rate of multiple births in the United States has increased exponentially in the last thirty years due to both the increased use of fertility medications and treatments as well as a great number of women getting pregnant in their late 30s and early 40s. As women age they are more likely to release multiple eggs during ovulation leading to an increased incidence of multiple births. The number of twin births has risen 67 percent since 1980 and triplet births have experienced an even more drastic increase with a 400 percent increase from 1980 to 1998 (Ventura et al. 2001). Since 1998, the triplet birth rate has actually been on a slight decline as fertility specialists have refined their procedures and are more cautious in performing fertility treatments such as taking precautions when performing inseminations and in limiting the number of embryos they implant during in vitro fertilization in order to prevent pregnancies with higher older multiples (Martin, Hamilton, and Ventura 2013). Even if fertility treatments do not result in multiples, there is evidence that women who have difficulty conceiving are at a greater risk for premature birth (Gupta and Gajilan 2003).

Age is also a key risk factor for preterm delivery. Both older, women over age thirty-five, and younger, females under age seventeen, women have a greater risk for premature labor and birth. Older women are more likely to develop conditions such as preeclampsia and gestational diabetes which can lead to premature delivery. Teenagers, bodies are not fully developed and pregnant teens often do not receive adequate prenatal care. Other factors that place women at greater risk for preterm labor are having certain medical conditions including diabetes, high blood pressure, kidney problems or certain clotting disorders. Certain physical conditions such as an incompetent cervix can lead to premature labor as a woman's cervix starts to thin and dilate too early. Placenta previa is a condition where the placenta lays completely or over the cervix which can lead to severe bleeding and early delivery. Another common condition is preeclampsia (i.e., a condition marked by high blood pressure and protein in the urine) which may lead to an early delivery as delivery is the only way to cure the condition (Luke 1994). There are times when the infant's health leads to an early delivery such as the case of IUGR where the baby stops growing due to poor cord blood flow or for other reasons.

Finally, environmental factors also can contribute to preterm labor and delivery including stress, physically demanding working conditions, and lack of prenatal care (Shapiro et al. 2013; Misra, Strobino, and Trabert 2010). Smoking, drinking, and drug abuse can all contribute to preterm labor and premature birth. There is also a connection between socioeconomic status and the risk of preterm labor of women who are on Medicaid or have a family income of less than 30,000 dollars a year have a 50 percent greater likelihood of experiencing preterm labor than the general population (Whitehead 2012). Experts are unsure of why this is as even those who seek regular prenatal care still have higher chance of premature delivery but hypothesize that it could be due to greater levels of stress or poorer nutrition. Sometimes though there is no known reason and a woman's water just breaks or her body goes into labor and it cannot be stopped.

Even though there are still a lot of unknowns as to why the premature birth rate remains high despite advances in medical treatments and prenatal care, there is much known about the complications preemies can face. Premature birth carries with it significant risks, and infants born at less than 37 weeks gestation face several potential complications such as anemia, jaundice which is a condition where the liver does not function properly, apnea which is when an infant does not breath for twenty seconds or more, and an increased risk for infection due to an immature immune system. They also have a greater risk for long-term health problems including mental retardation, learning disabilities, cerebral palsy, and vision and hearing problems. Infants born at less than 32 weeks are at an increased risk for more severe problems including respiratory distress syndrome caused by a lack of surfactant, the protein which helps the air sacs in the lung to stay inflated, brain bleeds or strokes which can lead to brain damage, heart conditions, necrotizing enterocolitis (i.e., a life threatening intestinal problem), retinopathy of prematurity (ROP), which untreated can lead to vision loss, a Patent Ductus Arteriosus (PDA), a heart condition where the ducts in the heart do not close properly.

Micropreemies are at the most risk for immediate and long-term complications. While different organizations define micropreemie slightly differently in terms of gestation and weight, a general definition is infants who are born prior to 27 weeks or weigh less than two pounds. Micropreemies have not fully developed any of their body systems from their immune systems to their digestive systems and require machines and other medical functions to perform most bodily functions. They are often covered with a fine layer of downy hair and their skin is so thin it is almost translucent and often has a waxy or sticky appearance. Sometime they are covered in plastic wrap shortly after birth to keep their skin moist. The youngest preemies are sometimes born with their eyes still fused shut. They spend most of their day sleeping and have difficulty dealing with most stimulation as their nervous systems are grossly underdeveloped. The risk of a serious level 3 or level 4 brain bleed is even higher which can lead to permanent brain damage, disability, cererbral palsy, and even death.

The majority of premature infants require a stay in the NICU where they can be closely monitored as they grow and receive any assistance they need including breathing, feeding, and temperature regulation. Born with underdeveloped lungs, many premature infants struggle to breathe on their own and required a variety of respiratory interventions ranging from being on a ventilator to using a nasal cannula. The digestive tracks of these babies are poorly developed and many struggle to digest food and often suffer with severe reflux. Even for infants who can digest their food, the suck reflex is not fully developed and infants struggle to learn how to drink as well as how to breathe while drinking. Given their small size and lack of fat, premature infants are unable to regulate their own body temperature which necessitates a temperature-controlled incubator to keep their body temperatures up.

Even after infants are discharged from the hospital and are labeled healthy, there is still the potential for long-term side effects. Many preterm infants suffer from developmental delays and require early intervention including speech, physical, and occupational therapy in order to catch up with their peers. As younger and younger infants are being saved due to advances in medical technology, the number of premature infants with long-term learning issues is growing (Leigh 2005). A study reported in the New England Journal of Medicine found that in infants born prior to 25 weeks, 80 percent had some degree of disability. The average IQ score for these infants was 82 as compared to a 106 for full term infants (Marlow et al. 2005). Many preemies continue to have long-term delays such as speech delays, lower school achievement, feeding issues, difficulty gaining weight, and sensory issues (Odd, Evans, and Emond 2013). It is important to note though that some preemies grow up to have no long-term issues and there is no way to predict which preemies will have problems and which ones will not.

The Costs of Premature Birth

In looking at premature birth, one cannot ignore the costs. The medical demands of a premature infant can place a large financial and emotional burden on families. In terms of financial costs, the average medical costs for a premature infant's first year of life are $32,325 as compared to a full-term infant whose average costs are $3325 (Ante 2008). This means on average, the costs for a premature infant are ten times greater than those of a full-term infant. This is only an average though and the costs of caring for micropreemies can be astronomical with some families racking up hospital bills close to $1,000,000 and the mean cost of an infant born at 25 weeks is $326,953 (Huynh et al. 2013). These costs get passed on to employers, parents, and state and federal governments in the form of higher insurance rates, lost work hours of parents, as well as an increased need for government support for uninsured and underinsured infants (Argus et al. 2009). Average NICU costs continue to rise as hospitals are able to save younger and smaller infants from death who routinely require very long NICU stays and often undergo a variety of treatments and tests (Doyle 2004; Friedman et al. 2002). These costs also do not take into account the costs of treating women with a high-risk pregnancy and preterm labor. During my pregnancy the terbulatline pump and home monitoring had cost me over $1000 a day and then there were the three weeks I was hospitalized prior to delivery, the multiple ultrasounds, and the different medications I was on. After accounting for all of my costs and the girls' NICU stay, our medical bills added up to over $500,000. Thankfully we had good insurance and the majority of these costs were covered, but we still had to pay over $10,000 out of pocket and I cannot even imagine how those without insurance or with minimal coverage deal with the enormous costs. These costs do not even account for the lost work and income of families and mothers. The March of Dimes reported that the societal economic costs of preterm births in 2005 was $26.2 billion ("March of Dimes Peristats" 2014).

Families also must cope with the emotional stress of having an infant that most likely will remain in the hospital and may require intense medical interventions. For many families, the premature birth of their infants is unexpected and parents are forced to quickly face a new reality that is potentially far different than they had imagined. The NICU itself can be a very stressful environment (von Gontard et al. 1999). Many NICUs have open floor plans or pods with multiple infants in the ward or in a pod meaning that there is little privacy and families are exposed to not only the situations of their own child, but also to the difficult situations of the other families in the NICU. Numerous monitors and alarms are constantly beeping and medical staff move from bed to bed dealing with the causes of these constant beeps (Reid et al. 2007). Most mothers are discharged from the hospital prior to their infants which can result in a separation for many families as parents return home without their infants creating both emotional and many times logistical stress (Dimes 2007). This stress is often multiplied when parents have older children at home, have to return to work, or live far from the hospital.

Parents may also be concerned with the potential of their infants having long-term health issues. A mother's bonding with a very sick infant may be compromised because of the fear of losing those infants (McDermott-Perez 2007). Premature infants often look different than a full-term infant as they have thin skin, longer heads, and may be covered with a thin layer of hair making them less attractive to parents than full-term infants (Johnson 2008). The infants often are hooked up to a variety of machines and have multiple wires and tubes going in and out of their isolettes which can be alarming to parents. Most have to stay in a specialized enclosed bed that helps their undersized bodies that lack the proper amount of body fat maintain their body temperature, so there is literally a wall between the parents and the baby (Padden and Glen 1997). When parents can interact premature infants are less responsive and are generally more sensitive to extra stimuli making it difficult for parents to engage with them. Most often, the infants in the NICU do not resemble the infants parents were picturing.

Another common issue is that mothers may feel helpless as they watch medical staff being the primary caretakers for their newborns and may struggle to bond with their infants as many of the normal bonding routines such as holding and feeding cannot take place (McDermott-Perez 2007). The altered parental role can be a source of great stress and confusion for parents. Parents may feel as if the medical staff knows their infants better than they do and some may worry their infants will not be able to distinguish between medical staff and their parents (Padden and Glen 1997). Additionally, many mothers feel guilt over not being able to carry their infants full term and spend a lot of time trying to figure out what they did wrong to cause their early labor (Barshun 1996; Leichtentritt et al. 2005; McDermott-Perez 2007). In her writings about her premature daughter's birth, Barshun (1996) writes, "Needles, plastic tubing, strangers in scrubs. Her first sight of the world is of the NICU, and I am to blame" (37). In her writing she chronicles the overwhelming sense of guilt she felt when she would see her daughter struggling to survive and the long process it took for her to forgive herself and let go of some of the guilt that was weighing her down.

History of Neonatal Care

In looking at the serious problem of preterm labor and preterm births, it is interesting to consider how relatively new the field of neonatal medicine even is. One hundred years ago, there was little that could be done for premature infants other than trying to feed them, keep them warm, and wait and see if they would survive. Being born prior to the 1900s was a dangerous prospect even for full-term infants and the infant mortality rate was as high as 20 percent at some periods in the late 1800s (Philip 2005, 799). The danger continued into the twentieth century and in 1915, 10 percent or 100 out of every 1000 infants died before reaching their first birthday. The development of antibiotics and better prenatal care helped to drastically decrease the infant mortality rate, and by 1997 the rate was down to 0.07 percent or 6.8 deaths per every 1000 live births. When a baby was born too early his or her chances of survival were even lower, and an infant who could not breathe on his or her own had no chance at all.

As the prior discussion of prenatal and obstetrical care described, prior to the 1930s the medical community was not very involved in the pregnancy and birth processes and similarly they were not highly involved in the medical care of infants. One of the first major breakthroughs for the care of premature infants actually came in 1835 when the first incubator was used. This was hardly a sophisticated piece of medical equipment—it was actually a modified egg incubator from a chicken farm, but it was the first time a closed box was used for the purpose of keeping a premature infant warm. Scientists continued to refine the use of the incubator and argue for its utility throughout the remainder of the nineteenth century. One of the ways they did this was actually to have live infants in the incubators on display at a permanent exhibit on Coney Island in New York from 1903 to 1943 as well as a special display at the Chicago World's Fair in 1933. Mothers stood backstage waiting to feed their babies while visitors paid a quarter to enter the Baby Incubator exhibit and peer through the glass sides of the incubators at the tiny babies being kept warm and alive by this new medical technology (Baker 2000; Brick 2005). This seems incredibly barbaric now and in extremely poor taste, but those displays were one of the ways that the world learned about the advantages of keeping preterm babies warm.

The next big development in prenatal care came in 1934 when Julius Hess, an American physician, invented the Hess oxygen box which was the first incubator that was able to administer oxygen while also providing a stable thermal environment. It was during this same time period that the majority of births now took place in the hospital, and rather than leaving infants with their mothers, nurseries were created where nurses could tend to the newborns. Eventually special care nurseries were established to take more advanced care of preterm infants although the techniques used to assist preemies were limited to keeping them warm and providing a steady flow of supplemental oxygen. One of the downfalls to the use of oxygen in this era was the way it was administered which was to blow oxygen into the incubator without controlling the flow or saturation. Physicians later discovered that prolonged exposure to 100 percent oxygen leads to hardening of the retinas and many preterm infants went blind from too much oxygen exposure. Both Ray Charles and Stevie Wonder were born prematurely with sight, but went blind after excessive oxygen exposure caused their retinas to separate from their eyes.

As medical technology was rapidly improving there was also a growing awareness of the many problems that could accompany birth. In 1938, President Franklin D. Roosevelt established the National Foundation for Infantile Paralysis which later became the March of Dimes. The original purpose of the foundation was to raise money and support research to fight polio, the disease that left Roosevelt paralyzed and struck millions of other US infants and children in the early 1900s. It was Eddie Cantor, a popular entertainer at the time who came up with the catch phrase, March of Dimes, which encouraged everyone in the United States to send a least a dime to the White House to help fight polio. The efforts of the foundation were incredibly successful and in 1955, Jonas Saulk developed the polio vaccine and polio was successfully eradicated in the United States. After this success, the mission of the foundation changed to birth-defect prevention.

As the foundation worked to discover ways to prevent birth defects there was also a growing awareness of the problem of preterm birth, low birth weights, and the high infant mortality rate in the United States, and the March of Dimes incorporated the prevention of preterm birth and low-birth-weight babies into its mission. The March of Dimes recognized the need for improved treatments for premature infants, but even more importantly it recognized the need for healthier pregnancies in order to decrease the number of sick and premature infants. One of their initial slogans, "Be Good to Your Baby Before its Born" reflected their focus on the importance of proper prenatal care, good prenatal nutrition, and the importance of avoiding tobacco, drugs, and alcohol during pregnancy. To this day, the March of Dimes continues to lead the fight against prematurity by both funding research and in raising awareness about the problem of preterm labor and birth, risk factors, and ways to prevent it. Its annual March for Babies, a series of walks held across the country, raises millions of dollars each year and continues to raise awareness about preterm birth and the importance of giving every baby at least 39 weeks in the womb.

One of the most notable developments in the 1950s that was funded by the March of Dimes was the creation of the APGAR score by Virginia Apgar. The APGAR score was a simple evaluation tool which allowed physicians to quickly assess newborns' appearance, pulse, grimace, activity, and respiration after birth and provide insight into what the immediate medical needs of newborns are. Another huge development was the adaptation of the ventilator so that there was now mechanical ventilation of infants which allowed infants who could not breathe on their own to survive for the first time (Stern and Markel 2004). The early use of the ventilator was not without its problems though as prolonged ventilation can lead to disease and physicians tended to set ventilators at 100 percent oxygen and exposure of these levels also increased the risk of developing ROP and blindness. Interventions were still limited and up until 1960, babies born prior to 28 weeks were considered previable.

The 1960s was when neonatal medicine really took off and became an official specialty. This was the decade when the term neonatology was first introduced in textbooks and physicians and nurses began to seek special training on treating the smallest patients. It was in this decade that the name of special care nurseries was changed to the Neonatal Intensive Care Unit or NICU and the first official NICU was established at Vanderbilt University in 1961. Greater national attention was brought to the issues of preterm birth and the risk of early delivery in 1963 when Jackie Kennedy delivered her third child, Patrick Kennedy, nearly six weeks early. The nation who had not seen a first lady pregnant in the White House since the 1800s had watched the pregnancy with great interest and excitement. Patrick was over four pounds, but quickly developed respiratory distress syndrome due to the lack of surfactant in his premature lungs. Patrick died within two days and his tragic death sparked increased funding and research into ways to help preterm babies survive.

At the beginning of the 1960s, a baby weighing less than 2.2 pounds had only a 5 percent chance of surviving whereas by 2000, the same sized baby had a 95 percent chance of survival (Jorgensen 2010). Some of the major reasons for the increased survival rate was the improvement of respiratory interventions. Rather than exposing infants to 100 percent free-flowing oxygen, ventilators and C-PAP machines were modified so they were able to be used on preterm babies and the saturation of oxygen could be controlled. The improvements in respiratory therapy improved the survival rate and decreased the incidence of chronic lung disease, a common side effect of extended ventilation support, and decreased the chance of vision impairment. More precise and accurate monitors also let physicians and nurses know when infants were suffering from apnea episodes, desaturations, and allowed for constant monitoring of the heart rate. Any parent who has spent any time in an NICU is all too familiar with the constant beeping and dinging of monitors and although these bells and alarms can be a source of stress, they are an invaluable tool in caring and treating for preterm infants.

The 1980s brought about massive changes in the treatment of preterm babies. A major development in treating respiratory disorders came in the early 1980s when physicians began medical trials of steroid injections in pregnant women to develop the infant's lungs in utero. The trials were highly successful and by the end of the 1980s, steroid injections were routinely used in women experiencing the threat of preterm delivery between 24 and 32 weeks. Respiratory therapies continued to be refined and preemies were treated with a variety of breathing machines including ventilators, oscillators,

Si-PAP and C-PAP machines. Other major advancements included advanced feeding techniques, routine eye exams and surgery to fix ROP, improved neonatal surgical techniques, and the use of ultrasounds to detect brain bleeds.

Following the major breakthroughs of the 1980s the 1990s became known as the decade of the micropreemie as medical techniques were discovered and existing techniques were refined even further, which meant that smaller and smaller, and younger and younger infants were able to survive. The age of viability or the minimum gestation at which infants could survive outside of their mother's body continued to be pushed backed and physicians were now able to save infants born at 24 and 25 weeks and sometimes even babies born prior to 24 weeks. In 2004, Rumasia Rahman was born at 25 weeks at Loyola Hospital in Illinois, weighing just 9.2 oz and set a Guiness World Record for being the smallest infant to ever survive (Carollo 2001). A large contribution to this was the discovery of surfactant and its role in lung function. In the 1980s researchers discovered this key enzyme in the lungs that keeps the air sacs moist and keeps them from sticking when they are inflating and deflating. Researchers worked for a decade to develop an artificial lung surfactant to help premature lungs develop and in 1994 scientists got FDA approval for an artificial surfactant that is administered through the breathing tube. This combined with in utero steroid shots gave these extremely small preemies a chance at survival that they previously did not have.

The improvements in neonatal care did not come without controversy and debate as people began to wonder how small was too small and how far interventions should go to keep the smallest infants alive. Some argued that too many financial and medical resources were being used to save infants who would most likely grow up to have severe medical conditions. Others questioned how ethical it was to subject preemies to so many invasive and sometimes painful medical procedures that might only serve to prolong their lives, but not ultimately save them ("Ethics of Intensive Neonatal Care" 2000). These debates continue today as medical technology continues to make it possible for younger and younger infants to survive. Policy varies from hospital to hospital, but in general, between 23 and 26 weeks is considered a gray zone in terms of viability and it is often left to the parents to decide if they want to use extreme interventions to try to keep their infants alive, a terrible decision for any parent to have to make.

In addition to advanced treatment for preterm infants, there were also advances in the treatment and prevention of preterm labor. Prior to 1960 there was nothing women or doctors could do when contractions started too early other than to place the woman on bed rest and hope for the best. Physicians hoping to find a way to halt labor once contractions had started began experimenting with tocolytic drugs (i.e. drugs that stop uterine contractions). This led to the discovery of using various IV, injectable, and oral medications such as magnesium sulfate and terbutaline that relax smooth muscles and slow contractions. Another common problem that leads to premature birth is a weak or thinning cervix which physicians began treating by sewing the cervix shut using a procedure called a cerclage. A preventative cerclage is placed between 12 and 14 weeks if a woman has a history of incompetent cervix, but emergency cerclages can be placed up until 20 weeks if a problem develops, but are not as effective as cercalges placed earlier. Another discovery was the use of progesterone, a hormone that early in pregnancy prevents the uterus from contracting and later helps with the production of breast milk, to treat a thinning cervix and to prevent labor. Progesterone gel is inserted in the vagina and has been shown to reduce cervical thinning in women pregnant with one baby. Progesterone shots are used in women who have previously delivered prematurely and have been shown to reduce the risk of delivering prematurely again. Although the development of medical treatments has not significantly lowered the overall rate of preterm birth in the United States it has decreased the rate of extremely premature births as women receiving interventions are sometimes able to delay birth by a week or two. Even if labor is delayed for at least 24–48 hours there are tremendous benefits as this allows time for the steroid injections to mature the infants' lungs to take effect.

One of the interesting things to consider in looking at the history of neonatal medicine is the changing role of parents through time. When nurseries and intensive care units were first established, the fear of infection was paramount and the desire to protect premature infants with immature immune systems led many NICUs to limit the interaction between infants and parents. As late as the mid-1970s many hospital policies did not allow parents into the NICU until one or two days prior to discharge (Davis, Mohay and Edwards 2003). Even when parents were allowed into the unit, the prevailing belief was that touching and handling the infants was too stimulating and stressful, and physical contact was discouraged. In the 1960s there was also a push to regionalize neonatal care and locate high level NICUs with specialized staff at regional rather than local hospitals. This led to many mothers and infants being separated after birth when infants were transferred to the regional centers when they required more intensive care.

In the 1970s, some physicians began to question the practice of isolating infants from their parents and ran studies that indicated that there was no greater rate of infection when parents were allowed into the NICU than when they were kept out. Researchers also noted that mothers who were allowed contact with their infants showed more connection to their children and increased confidence in their mothering abilities. This was also around the time that general hospital procedures were also changing as far as mother-infant interaction postdelivery. Increased interest in infant development and the ways children and parents bonded led to an increase in parental involvement in the NICU as parents were encouraged not just to come and spend time with their children, but to take part in their care whenever possible doing tasks such as changing diapers, taking temperatures, and helping with baths. Mothers were strongly encouraged to breastfeed and if actual breastfeeding was not possible due to the infant's size or health, women were encouraged to pump to provide breast milk for their infants. Breastfeeding was strongly encouraged for all women, but it was especially important for women with premature infants whose underdeveloped digestive and immune systems had trouble with formula and needed the extra immunities breast milk provides.

Another big change in the ways parents were encouraged and able to interact with their babies was the practice of kangaroo care which involves holding infants skin to skin and cradling them, much like a kangaroo mother holds her joey in its pouch. This practice was first developed by Dr. Edgar Sanbria in Columbia who was looking for ways to improve the outcome of low–birth-weight infants in his country. This practice was slow to catch on, but it began being practiced in NICUs in the United States during the 1990s. Benefits of kangaroo care for infants include better respiratory status, more consistent heart rate, better temperature regulation, faster weight gain, and shorter NICU stays (Hall and Kirsten 2008). The benefits for parents include increased bonding, improved success with breastfeeding, and lower stress levels. It is important to note that the different NICUs and different medical staff have varying rules, regulations, and beliefs concerning how often kangaroo care should be practiced and how stable an infant needs to be for the procedure to be allowed. For example, some hospitals will not allow babies on a ventilator to be held while others have beliefs that the benefits of parent and child contact outweigh the risks.

Hospitals have continued to work to create as family friendly policies as possible and have looked for ways to help parents bond and connect with their infants. Practices such as rooming in where NICU parents are allowed to stay in empty rooms at the hospital after the mother is discharged allowing parents to stay close to their infants and be able to visit throughout the day and night. Some large hospitals are connected with a Ronald McDonald House so parents who live far from the hospital can stay close to the hospital free of charge allowing them to more frequently visit the NICU. Some newer NICUs are built with private rooms for each infant giving the parents the ability to stay overnight with their children if they want, something they are unable to do in traditional NICUs consisting of an open room or pods where multiple babies are in the same unit. The private rooms also can make parents more comfortable as they interact and care for their babies without feeling like all of the eyes in the NICU are on them. Private rooms also allow for parents to focus on their own babies and are not constantly hearing the alarms and complications of the other babies in the unit, which can compound the stress parents are feeling.

Another innovation that has the potential to really change how NICU parents observe and stay in contact with their children when they are unable to be in the NICU is Baby CareLink, an internet-based program that uses webcams so that when parents are not in the NICU, they can log into the system and observe their child or children at any time. Parents can also check on their child's stats such as weight and number of ounce eaten. The system also gives parents and providers an additional avenue for communication as parents can send messages directly through the session and with the web capabilities, physicians and nurses can conference and educate parents who cannot be at the hospital. The program was first piloted in 1997 and controlled studies of the system found that parents who had access to Baby CareLink were overall more satisfied with the care of their infants; there was a reduction in the stress and anxiety levels of the parents, and infants were actually able to be discharged earlier due to the additional educational and emotional support of parents which could also result in cost savings for insurance companies (Gray et al. 2000; *Wall Street Journal* 2000). In 2002, the University of Iowa hospital system implemented the Baby CareLink system and found that not only were parents happier and more informed during the NICU stay, but readmissions to the hospital following an infant's release were decreased as parents were able to ask better questions and stay more informed about various health issues and conditions by using the system. One of the mothers I spoke with was from Iowa and found this system invaluable. Not only did she and her husband have to return to work, but they also lived over an hour away from the hospital and the system allowed her to stay connected to her son and feel like she and her husband were still involved in his care and were an important part of the team, even when they could not be there.

More attention is also being focused on the emotional needs of parents and things like NICU support groups and parent mentor programs are in place at some hospitals to help guide parents through this difficult time. Hospital social workers and volunteers from the local March of Dimes chapter are some of the people who can provide much needed emotional support to parents during this incredibly stressful time. Many women I have spoken with talked about things like weekly dinners for NICU parents or weekly breastfeeding support group meetings that gave parents and mothers a chance to connect with each other and share their concerns. This is an area that continues to develop though the amount of formal emotional support varies widely from NICU to NICU. Since 2010 more and more research has been done indicating that NICU parents and women who deliver early are at a high risk for developing post-traumatic stress disorder which has prompted increased interest in intervention programs (Shaw et al. 2009; Feeley et al. 2011).

Understanding the history and context on prenatal care helps to put the situations that women experience when they have preterm labor, preterm birth, or spend time in the NICU into perspective. Women experiencing pregnancy, preterm labor, and preterm birth have a much different experience than women fifty years ago. In many ways the labor and delivery experience has improved as far as keeping women active participants in the process and allowing for parents to spend time and bond with their newborns. The outcome for premature infants has also improved exponentially and babies who would have never survived fifty years ago now have an excellent chance at survival. Some of the changes have led to different expectations of what pregnancy, birth, and early motherhood will be like, and those changing expectations have made experiencing a high-risk pregnancy in some ways exceedingly difficult as certain expectations cannot be met. For those who work with and are attempting to support women whose pregnancy, birth, and early motherhood experiences look nothing like what they had expected, there is a question of how to best help women. What can someone say or do that will help lessen some of the emotional pain women feel or even if the pain is there, how can someone help a woman work through her disappointment? The following chapters will further explore the impact of unmet expectations on women and offer suggestions for dealing with them.

Chapter 4

This Wasn't Supposed to Happen to Me

When Shelley found out she was pregnant with twins after three miscarriages she was excited, but also anxious as she went in each week for monitoring, constantly worried that she would miscarry again. Around 11 weeks she started to have severe cramping and fearing that she was losing the twins she went straight to the hospital. An ultrasound quickly revealed that one of the twins had implanted in her fallopian tube while the other had implanted in her uterus. She was rushed to surgery and although both she and her doctors thought she would lose both of the babies that day, the doctors were able to extract the ectopic twin, a boy named Colin, from the tube and pushed the other twin, a girl named Riley, back into the uterus and closed the incision. Doctors considered it a miracle that Riley had survived the surgery at all, and warned Shelly that the likelihood that she would stay pregnant long enough for the pregnancy to be viable was extremely slim as there were not many cases of a woman delivering a surviving twin after having an ectopic pregnancy. Despite the enormous odds against her, she recovered from surgery, was discharged from the hospital, and continued on with the pregnancy. Each day she feared it would be the last, but she and her daughter both kept fighting and after 17 weeks of bed rest, frequent appointments, and ultrasounds, she delivered Riley at 28 weeks and 1 day. Throughout the pregnancy Shelly had a very hard time accepting what was happening to her and constantly questioned why it was happening. She could not understand why she had lost so many babies to miscarriage, had lost her daughter's twin, and now there was a very high chance that she would deliver Riley before she had a chance to survive. Often the things the doctors were telling her about her daughter's chance of survival seemed surreal and more like fiction than reality. As she put it, "our story would make a perfect Lifetime movie." The events happening to her were so rare and so crazy at times that it felt like she was living in a bad dream that would not end. Luckily she eventually was able to wake up from her nightmare. Even though her daughter was born very early, she survived and after over 100 days in the NICU she came home. Today, Riley is a happy little girl who is meeting her milestones and is otherwise healthy and not a day goes by that Shelly is not cognizant of just how lucky she, her husband, and her daughter are.

Cassidy (2006) writes in her introduction to her book *Birth* that after learning she was pregnant with her first child, "the women of my family gave me three things: new born outfits, advice, and accounts of their own birth experiences" (p. 1). This sentence pretty much sums up so many women's experiences. There is something about pregnancy, childbirth, and motherhood that makes women want to share their stories and through those stories women come together. Being a part of a large family full of aunts and cousins—my mom has twelve siblings and my dad has eleven—I grew up hearing women talk about their pregnancies and deliveries and each time someone announced they were expecting the stories started all over again. As an adult I have had extensive conversations about pregnancy complications and symptoms with random strangers in line at Target or while watching my daughters swim in the pool. It is amazing how women are willing to share some incredibly intimate and personal details about themselves when it comes to pregnancy.

Mercer (1995) argues that the telling and sharing of stories is a critical way that women learn about pregnancy and childbirth. In the past, as we saw in chapter 3, women and girls were present at their friends' and family members' birth and this is where they got a firsthand education about the labor and delivery process. Once labor and delivery moved into the hospital, girls and women had to rely on others' accounts to learn what would most likely happen. These stories helped women to develop expectations for what pregnancy, delivery, and the first moments of motherhood would be like. So many women grew up hearing these stories about pregnancy and birth and many spent a lot of time imagining what it would be like to have a child based on what they observed and heard. From the stories women learned to expect a certain level of pain discomfort. They had heard countless stories about fatigue, body aches, and morning sickness, but those discomforts in the stories were always outweighed by the joys and excitement of pregnancy. Over and over women heard that you forget all of the pain and the not so great parts of pregnancy and delivery once you hold that little baby in your arms.

Expectations are formed not just about the physical aspects of pregnancy and birth, but about the social experience of being a pregnant woman, being a mother, and having an infant. When talking about their pregnancies, especially if it was their first, many of the women I spoke to talked about their initial excitement about getting to do all of the things you get to do when you are expecting like decorating the nursery, registering for shower gifts, patting their rounded bellies, and wearing stylish maternity clothes. Women anticipated the attention and friendly questions that pregnancies often solicit such as "when are you due?" or "is this your first child?" Women wanted to be that cute woman in line at the grocery store that elicited smiles from the other people in line. So what happens then when something occurs in a pregnancy and everything a woman had thought about, imagined, and dreamed about does not happen? This is the experience of so many women who are diagnosed with a high-risk pregnancy and give birth to preemies. Often, the small milestones and moments that were so greatly anticipated never occur or are far different than women had presumed they would be like. How do women deal with the shattering of expectations as they are thrust into a world and situation they had never seen themselves facing? How do women reconcile reality with their dreams? This chapter explores how women come to understand and cope with the unexpected events of their high-risk pregnancies in light of the expectations they had developed from the stories they had heard.

In looking at high-risk pregnancies and preterm deliveries there are two general categories of women. There are those who are diagnosed with a high-risk pregnancy early on and are aware of the risk of delivering prematurely and there are those who suddenly go into labor or experience other complications and have to deliver early with no warning. In either situation the news that one's pregnancy is not going to go as planned is usually shocking and women struggle to comprehend and come to terms with their new realities. Over and over as I have met and talked to women who have shared their stories with me and the most commonly repeated phrases were "this was not supposed to happen" and "this was not the way it was supposed to be." Not only do women have to deal with their fears and concerns over their baby or babies' health, but they also have to deal with the difference in how their pregnancies and births will be from what they have previously envisioned. Sometimes those differences can cause a lot of pain and can be as hard to get over as the fear and trauma of early delivery and the ongoing worries about the health of their children can have lasting impacts.

For the first group of women, their first indication that their expectations will most likely not be met comes the day they receive a diagnosis of a high-risk pregnancy with the risk of a premature birth. So many described the moment when they learned their pregnancy was high risk either because they were carrying multiples, or something was wrong either with themselves or the baby. It was often too much at that moment for women to process that they most likely would not deliver a healthy full-term baby. For example, Julie described what it was like when she learned at her first ultrasound that she was carrying triplets. She had been feeling very sick from the start of her pregnancy, so she had a feeling that she might be carrying twins. When she looked at the screen as the ultrasound started she immediately saw three circles and all she could think was, oh no. She knew that she was at an increased chance for having twins because she had used Clomid, but never thought she would get pregnant with triplets. She started crying hysterically and all she could think was that there was no way she and her husband would be able to handle this. During the appointment her doctor came and spoke to the couple about selective reduction which she and her husband quickly said no to and then they were informed that she needed to be transferred to a high-risk doctor. Julie had gone from being ecstatic that she was pregnant to being absolutely terrified in just a matter of minutes. That first ultrasound was supposed to be a happy milestone, but instead, her doctor was sitting there discussing everything that could go wrong and the possibility of terminating one or more of the babies. This was hardly the scene she had imagined. She then spent the rest of her pregnancy which lasted until she was 26 weeks and 3 days being constantly anxious about the future for her children and her family. Again, this was nothing like how she had imagined what it would be like to finally be pregnant and preparing for her baby's birth, but she did at least have some time to think about and prepare for what it might be like to have preemies.

Other women had almost no time to mentally prepare for the fact that their babies were being born far too early as they simply went into labor and their babies were born or their blood pressure suddenly spiked which necessitated an emergency delivery. They went from experiencing what they thought was a perfectly normal pregnancy to going to the hospital and being told they were having their baby. Sometimes women deliver three to four months early and have to go from just starting to feel like they are past the halfway points and really can start getting ready for the baby to having the baby be born in a matter of hours. One of the most shocking stories I have ever heard was from Jennifer who was pregnant with her first child Whitney. Given that it was her first pregnancy, she had no idea what to expect and what was normal as far as pregnancy symptoms were concerned. Everything was going along great until around 28 weeks when she started to have severe pain in her abdomen that wrapped around to her back. She called her OB's office and the nurse told her to come in to get checked. Her regular doctor was not there, so she saw the physician on call who checked for the baby's heartbeat with the Doppler monitor which was strong. After listening to her symptoms and seeing where the pain was he diagnosed her with a likely kidney stone. Because she was so far along in her pregnancy there was little that could be done to get rid of the stone if there was one, and they did not want to do any kind of scan to confirm, so they sent her home with a prescription for some pain medication and told her to wait for the stone to pass.

Jennifer went home and started the medication which at first helped to lessen the pain. After about 24 hours though, the pain came back and continued to get worse so she figured she was getting ready to pass the stone. She had heard from others that kidney stone pain was worse than labor so even though her pain was intense and terrible, she did not question it and tried to cope with the discomfort as best she could. At one point she got up to go to the bathroom and when she was about to wipe when she was done, she felt something dangling down that then retracted back into her. Panicked, she yelled for her husband who rushed her to the hospital. As it turns out, what she had thought for the past two days was kidney stone pain was actually contractions. No one at her OB's office had checked her for signs of labor and because she had never been pregnant before she had no idea. She had been in labor for two days and her water had broken without her knowing. What she felt when she went to wipe was actually her daughter's foot that was hanging in the birth canal. Without her knowing it, she had gone into full blown labor and her daughter was making her way out. As soon as the ER doctors checked her she was rushed to emergency surgery. With not even enough time to start a spinal block, she was put under and when she woke up she learned that her daughter had been born at 28 weeks weighing exactly three pounds.

As she was being rushed to the hospital and being told that she was headed to delivery she could not believe that this was happening to her and all she could think was that this was way too early, and her daughter could not be born yet. Having never even thought of the possibility of delivering early, she had no idea what to expect and was completely overwhelmed when she was first able to visit the NICU and see her tiny daughter. She was just so small and looked nothing like Jennifer had imagined. She had never in a million years thought that her daughter would be anything but a healthy newborn and she struggled to not only come to terms with what had happened, but even to comprehend it. She was so confused by the fact that her daughter came early that for the first few days after the birth she continued to worry about her kidney stone and if it would pass until her doctor finally explained to her that she had never had a kidney stone and her pain had been misdiagnosed. Even though Jennifer's delivery was incredibly traumatic and her daughter spent several weeks in the NICU, she is now a toddler and doing very well. Although there were many things that went wrong and the first months of her life were incredibility difficult, Jennifer and her husband are just thankful that their daughter is alive. If much more time had passed, her daughter would have likely died while trying to be born.

Sometimes women had trouble accepting that they were experiencing complications or that their child was born early because they had already been through so much in their lives such as having a preemie before, previously dealing with infertility, having miscarriages, or even losing a child and could not understand why another terrible things was happening to them. An example of this is BethAnn. On a personal note, I met BethAnn when her son was in my husband's fourth grade class and we attended the same mom's group. She was the first triplet mom I had met in our town and we instantly connected over the shared trials and joys of raising triplets and I was secretly thrilled to see that people survived the toddler years. As I got to know her better she shared all of her incredible story with me and I was amazed at all she had been through and her strength to just keep going every day. BethAnn and her husband started trying to have a baby shortly after they were married and struggled to conceive for a while before they went to a doctor and started the process of undergoing fertility treatments. The treatments worked fairly quickly, and they were both overjoyed when they learned she was pregnant with twins, as they were eager to start their family.

Everything was going fairly well until 19 weeks when she started to feel like she was having painful contractions. She went into the hospital where she learned that her water had broken and because she was so early, there was nothing that could be done to stop the delivery. Her sons who they named Austin and Brandon were born later that day and shortly passed away, being too young and small to survive. They were able to hold the boys and take photos, and it was an absolutely heartbreaking loss for the couple. While they mourned the loss of their sons, they knew they wanted children so they tried fertility treatments again and were shocked when they found out after the next round of IVF that she was pregnant with triplets. Rather than elation and excitement this time though, BethAnn felt fear. She described feeling almost detached from the pregnancy and her babies as a way of coping with all of the anxiety and stress. She thought that if her body had not worked well enough for her twin sons to survive, there was no way that she would be able to carry triplets long enough to bring them home. When she started experiencing contractions and a shortening cervix around 17 weeks she could not believe it was happening again. She had already been through so much in terms of infertility and the loss of her twins and yet again things were not working out. She was convinced that she was going to lose even more of her children.

Because of her shortening cervix and prior history, BethAnn was admitted to the hospital at 18 weeks and remained there for the next 10 weeks on strict bed rest as well as a variety of medications to stop or at least slow down her contractions. Throughout this time she did everything she could to keep her pregnancy going, but she admits that she continued to feel a separation from her triplets. It was too hard to become attached to them when the fear of losing them was so large. At 28 weeks her water broke and her triplets Emily, Alison, and Jacob were born. Even after they were born at 28 weeks, very small, but well past the point of viability, it was still hard to believe she would be taking all three of her babies home with her and it was not until one of the nurses mentioned something about being prepared for their discharge that it sunk in that her triplets would survive and she needed to start buying things and getting things ready at home. Even now she says she still can't believe it sometimes that she lost her twins and that she has triplets even though they are now in middle school. It might be that the shock of going through such an extraordinarily difficult pregnancy may never completely go away. Even though BethAnn still does not understand why her children were all born so early, she told me that she believes that there is a reasons and even if she does not know that reason now, she will one day.

The first few years of her triplets' life were both busy and difficult as they navigated doctors appointments and early intervention, but BethAnn never forgot how grateful she was to have three healthy children. Unfortunately for BethAnn and her husband, their trials and challenges were not over. When the triplets were about three years old, BethAnn's husband John was diagnosed with cancer. After aggressive treatment he went into remission and they were hopeful that the cancer was behind them. Feeling thankful to have his health again, John and his brother-in-law trained to run the Cincinnati marathon and raised several thousand dollars for the Lymphoma Leukemia Society. The day after the marathon John woke up with a fever and tests revealed that his cancer had returned throughout his body, and just two weeks later, John passed away from cancer-related complications when his triplets were just four-years-old. BethAnn later remarried and had another daughter. One might think that given everything she has endured she might be a sad, angry, or bitter woman, but instead she has a deep appreciation for what she does have, because she knows how easily the people and things one loves can be lost.

UNMET EXPECTATIONS

For so many women, their sadness and grief over their high-risk pregnancies and early deliveries was not just because of their health or the health of their children, but because of all of the experiences, moments, and emotions they did not have. As chapter 3 described, there are several customs and rituals that frequently accompany a pregnancy and many women look forward to taking part in these activities as they are unique to pregnancy and motherhood. Additionally, many women had an idea of what their labor and delivery might entail and even if they were not focused on the birth, they had ideas about how their first moments with their child would be like. These expectations came from prior deliveries of older children, from talking with other women, reading, and watching TV and movies. Often women did not even realize they had some of these expectations until they were not met. When you think about it, it is not at all surprising that women have so many expectations of pregnancy, delivery, and motherhood. Think of how many little girls like to play house and play with baby dolls acting out their earliest ideas of what having a baby and being a mother will be like. There are constantly scenes of birth and motherhood on TV and in the movies, and as the first chapters documented, stories about pregnancy and childbirth are frequently shared among women.

The first set of expectations women have surround the pregnancy itself. So far this chapter has focused a lot on unmet expectations which makes one think of positive expectations that do not come to be, but of course not all women's expectations are positive, especially when it comes to the physical aspects of pregnancy. Women are exposed to countless stories about the physical discomforts of pregnancy and many anticipated with a lot of dread bouts of morning sickness, fatigue, body aches, and having to go to the bathroom constantly. Christine, whose daughter was born at 33 weeks after her water suddenly broke, heard a lot of stories about morning sickness prior to her pregnancy and although she expected to feel nauseous she found herself feeling great during the early stages of her pregnancy. "People would tell me how bad their nausea was and it was like I felt bad because I felt great, but that was the main one, that was the main story I would hear and you know they would just wake up with the most terrible nausea known to man." Her experience did not meet the expectations and she felt almost guilty early in her pregnancy that she did not have the physical symptoms that made so many others miserable. Morning sickness, although incredibly unpleasant, is one of the things that is unique to pregnancy and is for many women a part of the pregnancy experience. Not having morning sickness is in no way a bad thing, but it is often expected and anticipated. When some women did not have a common symptom like this, she felt that her pregnancy was in some way different or not the norm as it did not conform to what she thought pregnancy would and should be like.

Other than concerns over physical discomfort, women pregnant with only one infant and no other medical complications generally had only positive expectations for their pregnancies and deliveries as they heard and read countless stories of uncomplicated pregnancies and most expected to carry their infants without complications to around 40 weeks. Even if they were aware of potential complications, many women either ignored information about what could go wrong or even if they did hear or read something they did not get too concerned because they figured that the chances of something going wrong were so small or that early delivery was something that happened to other people. The idea that bad things like premature birth and complicated pregnancies happen to others is an excellent example of the natural human tendency to believe that bad things are more likely to others than oneself, a tendency psychologists have termed the optimism bias (Sharot 2011). Numerous studies have shown that often people will grossly underestimate their likelihood of being involved in a serious health situation or being exposed to a serious threat including skin cancer (Borschmann, Lines, and Cottrell 2012; Bränström, Kristjansson, and Ullén 2006), adverse side effects from prescription drugs (Anh, Park, and Haley 2014), car accidents (M. J. White, Cunningham, and Titchener 2011), and workplace injuries (Caponecchia 2010). These women had no reason to be overly concerned that something would go wrong. Having this expectation made their experiences of having major complications or giving birth prematurely shocking because no stories had personally prepared them for the possibility of their water breaking at 33 weeks or for suddenly developing a life-threatening condition such as preeclampsia.

For so many preemie moms who suddenly developed complications or went into labor early the possibility of preterm birth was not even on their radar. For example, Heather gave birth to her son at 34 weeks after contractions began and couldn't be stopped. She had no complications prior to this, so there were no indications that her son might come early. Her first son had been full term and her own story as well as the majority of others she had heard or read gave her the expectation of having a similar outcome with her second pregnancy. She never considered that her son might be born early or require an NICU stay. Another woman who was completely shocked by her early delivery was Jamie who developed a rapidly progressing case of preeclampsia when she was 27 weeks pregnant with her daughter Aubrey. Her pregnancy had been fairly typical until this point. After a few days of a terrible headache that would not go away she called her OB's office who recommended that she go to the hospital to have some labs drawn which revealed that she had extremely high levels of protein in her urine. The hospital staff then prepared to transfer her to a different hospital that had an NICU and told her that because of the risks to her health from the preeclampsia she would be delivering her daughter that day. "I kept telling them I was only 27 weeks so this couldn't be happening," she told me. "This was my first baby, I had read the books, but prematurity does not happen to you. No one told me I was going to have my baby early. I had not considered that as a possibility." Even though she had read about different complications, she never thought she would be the one experiencing them.

Even women who knew there was a risk of premature delivery sometimes chose to ignore or avoid information about potential complications because it was easier mentally and emotionally to not consider what could go wrong. At times, stories women heard or read set up negative expectations for what the pregnancy or birthing experience would be like, but instead of preparing themselves for a negative possibility they chose to ignore or disregard the story. Danielle turned to several pregnancy books after learning that she was pregnant with twins as she at first wanted to have as much information as possible. One book was particularly upsetting to her as it had stories with outcomes that scared her. She explained, ". . .and I got that really early on and I started reading it, and it was just very, it was written by a doctor and a mother of twins. She's both. And the book was very, very medical and very you know, 'you are going to go to a specialist and you are going to go to a perinatologist and this one, and this one,' and it just didn't feel right. I stopped reading it." This book set the expectation that a twin pregnancy would involve a high level of medical intervention, an idea that scared her so she put the book aside and hoped she would be one of the twin moms who carried her twins to full term with no complications.

In talking to women who delivered prematurely one of the things that I noticed was the degree to which women mourned the loss of their last trimester or weeks of their pregnancy. Some women who deliver prematurely never even make it to their third trimester or if they do, it is very truncated. The third trimester is an important period of the pregnancy as this is when women really start to grow and their bodies are completely transformed. As the end of the pregnancy comes closer there is more and more anticipation of the birth of the new baby. Given that many women are anxious for the third trimester to end because of physical side effects and their desire for the baby to be here, it may seem strange that some of the women I spoke with felt cheated out of the discomforts of the end of pregnancy. Angie whose first son Noah was born full term was very upset by all that she missed out on when her daughter was born at 27 weeks. "I didn't get to be huge and fat and uncomfortable, I was robbed of that, we had lost all of that because Izzy came so early."

Now some may questions why a woman would bemoan that she did not gain a lot of weight and feel physically uncomfortable, but it is important to consider these physical changes and discomforts for what they represent; a typical, healthy, normal pregnancy. Gaining weight, being sore, and having your belly so large that it is hard to do things are all a part of the experience of being pregnant and although many women do not enjoy these side effects of pregnancy while they are occurring, when they do not women often feel like something is missing from the experience. One mother I spoke with Astrid, was on bed rest from 18 to 34 weeks and left her home only to attend weekly doctor's visits. She admitted it seemed like a strange thing to be upset about, but she felt like she missed out on a big part of pregnancy because she never had people comment on her size or never needed to ward off strangers at the store who tried to rub her belly. Had she had a typical pregnancy she might have found some of the things annoying, but she never even got the chance to see what it would be like to be a pregnant woman in public.

Another thing that many women had looked forward to during their pregnancies was getting to shop for and wear maternity clothes. This desire was not so much about wearing a-line tops and pants with elastic waistbands, but about being pregnant in public and dressing in a way that showed the world that she was expecting. As was described in chapter 3, the act of buying and wearing maternity clothes is an important rite of passage in the United States and is one of the ways that women publically declare their pregnancies. Women who delivered prematurely or who were placed on bed rest early in their pregnancies felt as if they missed out a large part of the pregnancy experience because they never got to wear the maternity clothes they had because they never got big enough or they never left their bed, so there was no reason to get dressed. For women who have not delivered early this particular complaint can be hard to understand and relate to. When I was working on my dissertation one of the professors on my committee told me this complaint about maternity clothes was one of the most surprising things I had found. "Maternity clothes were awful," she exclaimed to me, "Why would anyone want to wear them and get all big and fat?" I completely understood her reaction, but I knew that what she had not recognized was that even if maternity clothes are not the most fashionable option and the extra weight may not be flattering, maternity clothes are a sign that a woman's body is doing one of the incredible things it is made to do, growing a child. The only time women can wear maternity clothing is during her pregnancy and they are a part of the overall experience of having a child.

One mother I met spoke for a long time about the experiences she missed out on in her pregnancy, especially getting to wear maternity clothes. Jen is the mother of twins who were born at 29 weeks. Early in her pregnancy her cervix started to thin and she was placed on strict bed rest at 15 weeks meaning that she only left her home for doctor's appointments. While we were talking, she described still being sad over many of the pregnancy traditions and rituals she missed out on. One of the things that saddened her the most was that no one saw her pregnant other than her husband and her physician. She described her sadness,

> It's something I deal with a lot, I feel very sad about. You know, I remember going out shopping for maternity clothes really early. I was still working and I got big fast. Like I couldn't fit into any of my work clothes after eight weeks. And I was working on Wall Street so I had to wear a suit. So I went out and had to go to Anthony and Lock which were the only reasonable maternity clothes for working women. You know, I spent hundreds of dollars on those maternity clothes and I was on bed rest shortly after I did that. . . . It is one of the things that causes me sadness. Like sometimes more than their NICU time. . . . But I rarely got to you know, go to the grocery store and have people be like, and you know, being able to walk around in cute little outfits and to be pregnant in the world.

She so badly wanted to have people see her that she would beg her husband to at least wheel her around the grocery store after her weekly doctor's visits, but her husband would never take her insisting that she needed to get back home and lie down. She of course is thankful that her time on bed rest allowed her to carry her twins to 28 weeks, but there is a deep sense of regret that she did not have the pregnancy she had hoped for.

Catt, mother of surviving triplets, also mourned that she did not get to be pregnant out in the world. Surviving triplets is the term used to describe the triplets who are alive after one or two of their siblings pass away. Catt was placed on bed rest at 17 weeks when two of her triplets were diagnosed with twin-to-twin transfusion syndrome. So much of her pregnancy had been incredibly difficult including the loss of one of her triplets, premature delivery, and weeks in the NICU, but that did not minimize the sadness she felt about not getting to do normal pregnancy things like wearing maternity clothes. She explained, "And the other thing. I had like two pairs of maternity pants and pair of maternity shorts. But you know, after seventeen weeks of being on bed rest, no one's going to see you. So you know, what's the point?. . .So I feel like I missed out on a lot."

One of the driving forces behind wanting to wear maternity clothes and look pregnant was that others would recognize she was pregnant and ask a woman about her pregnancy. Pregnant women can attract a lot of attention and questions. Although some women find these types of questions intrusive, many women enjoy the extra attention and don't mind talking about their pregnancy and the new baby. Some women never got approached by strangers though because they were never out in public due to bed rest or they delivered so early that they were not showing very much. It felt like they missed out on something because they never got the public attention or the chance to field those types of questions. One woman I met told me she would have loved to tell strangers to stop touching my belly, but she never got the chance because she was never out walking around with a large round belly in front of her.

Another ritual or milestone women looked forward to was having a baby shower or in many cases two or more baby showers. In the United States, the custom is to throw baby showers a month or two before one's due date. Because many preemies are born between one and three months early, a lot of preemies are born before the date of a scheduled shower, and when a baby is born around 24 weeks, it is often before a shower date has even been set. Women who are placed on strict bed rest often miss out on the traditional shower experience because they are unable to get up to attend. In some cases, women who have experienced loss before or are extremely worried about the outcome of the pregnancy refuse to have a shower because they do not want to have a pile of presents and supplies that they might have to return if their baby or babies do not survive. Others worried that having a shower and amassing baby items was almost like a jinx and preferred to wait until their baby was here and healthy before they celebrated. BethAnn the mother of twins who passed and triplets mentioned earlier, was one of the women who refused to have a shower or to buy anything during her second pregnancy. She had bought some things in preparation for her twin boys and returning unused baby items was one of the most difficult things she ever had to do and she was not willing to put herself through that again. When her triplets were born she had nothing and it was not until weeks later when she finally started to believe that they would actually come home from the hospital that she began to frantically gather all she would need.

Sometimes showers are held after the baby is born while he or she is still in the NICU and mothers in these situations described how difficult these experiences were. Monica delivered her son at 28 weeks exactly after she developed severe preeclampsia. Her shower had been scheduled for March 4 when her son was still in the NICU. She had contemplated having her friends and family cancel the shower as she was not sure if it was a good idea to leave her son, but the nurses encouraged her to go and enjoy it and take a little time for herself. She did go and was thankful to her friends and family for throwing the shower and bringing gifts, but it was so different than what she had imagined. She had pictured herself big and pregnant, excited about her upcoming delivery, eagerly anticipating the days when here baby would be able to use all of the new gifts. Instead, she was no longer pregnant and her son was in the NICU almost two hours away from home. She remembered opening a lot of clothes and wondering if her son would ever even get to wear them, because she was still afraid that he might not survive. Other women have their shower after their babies are born and home from the NICU and while they all expressed a great deal of appreciation for the party and the gifts, they all commented on how strange it was to have the baby at the shower. Again, this violates the traditional story of what a baby shower is, which in American culture is a celebration that takes place before the birth to help celebrate the pregnancy and help the mother to get ready.

Samantha attended her baby shower while her twin daughters who were born at 25 weeks were still in the NICU. She was incredibly thankful to the friends and family who came to celebrate her daughters, but the entire time she felt like something was off. Her daughters were stable in the NICU by this time, but it was still a stressful situation and there were still a lot of worries and unknowns. A few of the guests had recently had babies themselves and brought their infants to the shower. Samantha remembers being almost irrationally angry that those babies were there while her daughters could not because they were still in the hospital hooked up to machines. For Nicole, the disappointment over everything that went wrong during her pregnancy has led her to stop going to other's baby showers. The experience of seeing the celebration she never got is just too much for her. She explained, "I can't go to baby showers. It is just so much of a reminder of what I did not get. That is because I was in the hospital and I felt like we can't do anything because what would happen if they die? At a shower everyone talking is so excited and the pregnant person says something about how they can't wait to deliver, and it is just too much." She tried to attend a few after her twins were born and always came home feeling the pain of her traumatic pregnancy and premature delivery as if it had just happened. She always sends a gift and a card, but for now baby showers are something she just avoids.

A major reason that some of the expectations women had of being pregnant had were not met was because they were placed on bed rest and had a highly restricted activity level. One of the things that consistently came up when I spoke with women who were on bed rest at some point during their pregnancy was their belief that bed rest is very misunderstood by the general public. More than once women recounted stories of friends or family making comments to them about how nice it would be to have some time to rest before the baby or babies came or told women how much they wished they could be on bed rest so they could get a break from their job and household responsibilities. These comments were often infuriating, as bed rest was rarely something women described as pleasant or even relaxing. Astrid, mother of triplets born at 34 weeks explained that for the first day or two it was nice to just lie in bed and watch TV, but after that the days were long, tedious, and hard. Her husband worked all day, so she was alone except for an occasional visitor. She could read and go on the computer, but after a while even those activities grew wearisome. On top of that she was physically uncomfortable and could not change positions in a way that relieved much of the pressure her triplets were placing on her body.

Beth, delivered her daughter Emily full term, but spent over 20 weeks on bed rest at home said bed rest was the most grueling thing she has ever done. Around 18 weeks she went to her doctor as she was experiencing mild contractions. She was diagnosed with premature labor. She was given medication to slow the contractions, but nothing would completely stop them so her doctor placed her on strict bed rest. Her daughter Emily is now eighteen years old and when Beth was pregnant with her she did not have a laptop or wireless internet, so she could not use the internet to distract her self as many women in the recent times did during pregnancy. She did not even have cable, so she was at the mercy of whatever was on basic TV which meant a lot of her time was spent watching soap operas and talk shows. Her days were very long as her husband was working 12-hour shifts, so she was mostly alone. Here insurance would not cover a terbutaline pump that would provide continuous medication so she instead set her alarm for every eight hours and made sure that she took her medication round the clock. When her mother-in-law would take her to her weekly doctor's appointments she would beg her to drive around for just a little bit longer so she could enjoy being outside of her house, but her mother-in-law always gently reminded her that she needed to get home and lie flat again. When she was 36 weeks pregnant, her doctor lifted her activity restrictions and although she was eager to be up and about, her muscles were so atrophied from her many weeks of activity, that she found it tiring and difficult to get around. She does not regret one second of bed rest as it resulted in a healthy, full-term baby, but she also finds that few people understand just how long and trying those 20 weeks were.

One of the saddest things women described was barely getting to feel their baby or babies kick inside because shortly after they started to feel movement and kicking they delivered. Yvette, was 40 when she got pregnant with her twins Madison and Joshua. She was hospitalized at 24 weeks after she started bleeding heavily. Doctors started her on an IV of magnesium sulfate to slow her contractions and complete bed rest for the next 22 days. At 27 weeks she was rushed to an emergency C-section after Madison's heart rate dropped and did not return to normal. In terms of her pregnancy and delivery, there were so many things that did not go the way Yvette had thought they would. Being an older mom, she had always thought her difficulties would be in getting pregnant, but after easily conceiving, her difficulties were in carrying her twins. Due to her complications, there were several things she felt like she missed. "I don't think I can ever get over the NICU. You can't put into words that kind of loss and even though I have two beautiful children. It's a loss that I never felt them kick. I had an emergency C-section, no one was there." She did not get to enjoy her pregnancy, share the delivery with her husband, or hold her newborns against her chest.

Nicole was another mom who never really got to feel what it was like to feel her twins moving and kicking inside her. She delivered her sons who were monochorionic-diamniotic (mono-di) twins at almost 25 weeks. Mono-di twins are when identical twins each have their own amniotic sac but share a placenta putting them at risk for twin-to-twin transfusion syndrome. She feels like when she is comparing stories with other women she can't relate to a lot of what they talk about because her pregnancy never got to the third trimester. One time a woman told her she was lucky that she delivered so early because she hardly gained any weight and did not have a baby belly to lose after the pregnancy. Nicole was so taken aback that she had to just walk away hardly believing that someone could say something so insensitive. She told me, "I never got to feel the babies kick. We have one picture of me with a slight belly. You feel like you walk around with an asterisk." She was pregnant, but her pregnancy was so different than a typical one, that she feels like her story does not fit in with the norm and her pregnancy is more of a cautionary tale.

Another set of expectations women had involved the labor and delivery process. Again, women had both positive and negative expectations based on the stories they had heard and the births they had seen on TV as well as any prior births they had experienced. A lot of women had fears about the pain of labor and delivery as they had listened to other women's stories about terrible and excruciating pain, watched countless scenes of women screaming in agony as they attempted to push, and had heard about things like tearing and episiotomies. Others looked forward to the birth with excitement, curious about how the process would work or excited to embrace a natural delivery without using any medication or other medical interventions, believing that it was best for them and the baby.

One thing that many women commented on when I spoke to them was that they had heard, read, and seen multiple stories of vaginal deliveries and had imagined this when they thought about the labor and delivery process. Even though nearly one-third of women in the United States give birth via C-section (Osterman and Martin 2014), most women, especially first-time mothers anticipate a vaginal delivery. Due to the nature of their high-risk pregnancies though, many women gave birth via C-section which surprised them as they had expectations of long labors and pushing their infants out. Jana explained how she had heard so many detailed stories of vaginal deliveries so she had an idea of what to expect, but had never heard any stories of the details of a C-section. She knew that she was going to have a C-section for her twins, but she had never heard or seen really detailed accounts of what a C-section was like and this lack of stories left her unprepared for the procedure. She commented that she had never thought about being awake for the surgery, and this freaked her out at first. Jana has Crones disease and has had multiple surgeries in the past, but she had never been awake or aware during a surgery so when they started prepping her, she was a little alarmed that she would know and be aware when they were cutting into her. She also had no idea what it would be like in post-op in terms of her recovery time and her ability to be with her sons and what the physical recovery of a C-section would be like.

Several women were unprepared for the emergent nature of their deliveries. They had anticipated enduring hours of labor or even checking into the hospital for a C-section, but few had imagined themselves having less than 30 minutes between the time they were told the baby or babies were coming and the birth. Often once the decision was made that the baby or babies were being born, women were rushed to the OR for an emergency C-section either because the baby or babies were still breech, the infants were in distress and needed to be delivered immediately, the mother's health was at risk, or the babies were so small that their bodies could not handle the stress of a vaginal delivery. Sometimes the delivery was so unexpected that women went into the delivery room alone because they could not wait for their husband or support person to get there. If things were especially serious or the anesthesiologist had any trouble inserting the spinal block, women were put under for the procedure so they not only went into the surgery alone, but they also woke up with no memory of giving birth. When women were put under it was often hospital policy to not allow anyone into the OR who was not a medical personnel including the father, so women did not even have their partner's firsthand account of the birth to go by. Other women were alone, because no one had time to get to the hospital for the delivery. Heather was hospitalized at 27 weeks after she started to bleed heavily. When her doctor made the decision to deliver her daughter at 28 weeks there was no one at the hospital and her husband who worked almost an hour away did not have enough time to get there. Before going in to the OR, the nurses warned her that her daughter would most likely come out not breathing and she found it difficult to stay calm. She is incredibly thankful for the kind anesthesiologist who talked her through her incredibly frightening and stressful delivery. She remembers him gently rubbing her arms as she shivered from both fear and cold.

In general, when women delivered early, it almost never matched their expectations. For example, Sarah was admitted to the hospital while pregnant with her son Conner when she was almost 25 weeks pregnant after it was discovered that she had almost no amniotic fluid and an ultrasound showed no fetal breathing. She assumed she would be in the hospital for a while but in the middle of the night at 25 weeks and 2 days she was awoken by nurses who told her that Conner's heart rate had dropped for the past five minutes and she was going to be taken in for a C-section now. Prior to this moment she says she was in so much denial that she really never considered that he might be born so early, and when they came to tell her they were taking her in for a delivery she just kept asking why because she knew it was way too early for him to be born. The delivery itself was so crazy that she does not remember a lot of it, but she does remember that as soon as they told her they were taking her to deliver she started shaking all over consumed with fear. When she got to the OR there were what seemed like a million people in the OR and after Conner was born a nurse quickly brought him over for her to see and several people in the delivery room commented on how big he was at 1 pound 8 ounces, which was still incredibly small. The one thing Sarah vividly remembers is telling anyone who was close by that his name was Conner. "I really needed them to know his name," she explained through her tears, "because you can't ask baby X not to die." Despite his early arrival, Connor did not pass away and after 142 long days in the NICU he was able to come home.

Cora also had an incredibly traumatic delivery with her first child Lily. She was having a completely normal pregnancy until she reached 29 weeks and she noticed that the baby was not moving. After trying a bunch of the things they found on the internet to make her move such as drinking juice and doing jumping jacks, Cora and her husband decided to head to the hospital knowing that if something were to happen they would never forgive themselves. Once at the hospital, Cora was quickly hooked up to the monitors and Lily's heart rate kept plummeting so they got an ultrasound machine and started looking for specific movements. The nurse and doctors left the room and she knew something was wrong, but she had no idea how wrong until five minutes later when an entire delivery team came into her room. At this point Cora describes herself as being a complete mess. She knew they had seen no movement and a million thoughts were running through her head. "I knew she was going to be so tiny, I just kept telling them I don't want to see her, I don't want to see her." Cora is a pediatric hospice social worker, so her previous exposure to premature children had been with children with serious disabilities that ended up being fatal so she was terrified by what her daughter would look like and what kinds of medical issues she might have.

She was wheeled into the OR and the anesthesiologist had trouble getting the epidural in and he told her that he had to move fast because was the baby was dying and if they did not get her out soon, she would die and be stillborn. Cora told them to just get the baby out and to knock her out if needed, but they were able to get the epidural in and Cora was awake and heard a tiny yelp when they pulled Lily out. "I could see the look on the nurse's face," she told me, "and it was terrible." Her husband followed the baby to the NICU and she later learned that they made him touch the baby because they were concerned that she was not going to survive. It took a long time to get Cora stitched up and out of recovery and it was not until early the next morning that she heard anything else about her daughter's condition. This delivery was so far from what she expected that she still wakes up and has nightmares about it.

The differences between what women expected and what actually happened often led to feelings of anger, bitterness, and envy. Marie described how she viewed other women's noncomplicated pregnancies and births, "The way I view them is like, wow they have it so easy, they have a few contractions, they go in, they push a baby out, and they're holding their baby immediately, they're breastfeeding their baby, everything is fantastic, everybody is healthy and everybody goes home. They have people bring them cooked meals and everything is great." For Marie this was the ideal and she had expectations that this is how the process should be and had trouble reconciling her own experiences with those expectations. She explained what it was like for women with a high-risk pregnancy, "For us it's like, you just have all of these different scares and all of these different worries, and you want all of your concerns to be addressed, but then you don't even want to think about it. You are just trying to stay positive. Then you have all of these rush of hormones. Good grief! How do you deal with all of that? I don't know. I think it's a little different. You just have a lot more to think about than a normal pregnancy." Obviously Marie knew that even noncomplicated deliveries can be long, hard, painful, and even traumatic, but compared to what she had been through it all seemed so easy. Prior to her triplet pregnancy these stories were integrated into the stories she told of what might be. After her triplet pregnancy and the birth of her girls, these expectations introduced a note of bitterness and longing into her story as her own experience was so different than the norm. Many women describe listening to hear their baby's first cry as they know this means that their child has come out breathing on his or her own. Sometimes mothers are rewarded with a small cry that many describe as sounding like the tiniest kitten crying, but unfortunately, sometimes the baby's delivery is followed by nothing but silence—one of the scariest and worst sounds or lack of sounds for a mother to experience. What so many women had envisioned as being the happiest moment of their lives turned out to be one of the hardest and most frightening.

Women often heard stories of what giving birth would be like in terms of the process and this created expectations of how they would spend the first moments of their infants' lives. Most women expected to hold and begin bonding with their infants immediately following birth. Due to the early arrival of their infants, many preemie moms were able to do nothing more than catch a quick glimpse of their small infants before they were whisked away to the NICU. The birth of their infants and the time immediately after did not meet their expectations and many of the women felt sadness and grief over the loss of the initial bonding moments with their infants. Psychologists have termed experiences like this as ambiguous loss, which is a loss that is unclear, confusing, and traumatic (Boss 2009). Ambiguous loss is difficult to cope with as those experiencing it are often unable to articulate to themselves or others what it is they are mourning and they are therefore unable to get the emotional and psychological support they need (Betz 2006). The loss felt after a premature birth is not a loss in the traditional sense of a death or a separation, but women and their partners go through a grieving process even though their child has not passed away. It is a hard grief for women to deal with because they often have trouble identifying what specifically they are mourning the loss of, but is most often the loss of the pregnancy, birth, and infanthood they had imagined. Because there is not a concrete loss, it can also be a difficult grief for others to understand. Ambiguous loss can be difficult to overcome as there are no formal ceremonies or rituals to mark the loss such as funeral or memorial service.

Researchers Golish and Powell (2003) were interested in further studying the experience of ambiguous loss among parents of premature infants in order to better understand their grieving process and to identify strategies for providing emotional support and assistance. Their study found that parents mourned a loss of a healthy pregnancy and a healthy infant, and their grief was often compounded by fears surrounding their baby's health and future. Additionally, many parents felt caught between the tension of joy and grief as they felt guilty for mourning something when their child was still alive. Parents were often unsure of what exactly they were mourning and this lead to additional confusion and stress as they did not know what their feelings were about and therefore were unable to adequately deal with their grief. One of the promising things that Golish and Powell found was that there were factors that helped both mothers and fathers better cope with their loss and move more healthily through the grieving process. Some of these factors included having strong support from one's partner, feeling a sense of teamwork with one's partner, learning more about the technical issue of prematurity, and choosing to focus on the present rather than thinking too much about the past or future.

Jana who had two high-risk pregnancies explained how stories she had heard and read had shaped her expectations, "You know that you've seen the *Baby Story* or heard from your friends, and you've seen the pictures on their blog in the hospital of them delivering the baby and holding the baby right away and being able to bond with the kid for that two day period." Women had high expectations of the moment when their infants were born and they would be able to hold and bond with them. They had seen enough depictions on TV, heard enough stories, and seen plenty of their friends, pictures posted on social media to formulate an idea of what birth would be like. The stories they saw and heard set up the expectations of the baby being placed immediately on the mother's chest, the mother exhausted but elated as she holds her new child, counting his or her fingers and toes, welcoming this new little life into the world. Frequently these expectations include shedding some happy tears, sharing smiles with their significant other, showing off the new baby to excited friends and family, and feeling an overall euphoria. As was discussed in chapter 3, after births were moved to the hospital in the early 1900s, the relationship between the mother and newborn was not a high priority. It has only been since the 1950s when Dr. Spock wrote his groundbreaking book that there began to be a real push for giving women and their infants time to bond immediately after birth as Spock argued that the first few hours after birth were a critical window in which bonding occurred. Women who delivered early not only felt robbed of their first moments as a new mother, but also worried about the long-term impact the lack of initial bonding might have on their babies.

One mother I spoke with, Merillat, was extremely upset that she and her son had to be separated immediately after he was born at 32 weeks and felt that it was in many ways a traumatic experience. Merillat started to have contractions right before she hit the 32 week mark and after receiving a dose of indocin to slow contractions, she was sent home to be on bed rest. Unfortunately the medicine did not work and the next day her water broke and she went into active labor and six hours later her son was born and was taken immediately to the NICU. After he was discharged from the NICU, she started a support group for women who were separated from their children at birth either because of prematurity or other medical conditions. When I spoke with her, even though her son is now three years old and healthy, the memories of his birth were still so fresh that she cried as she spoke of the experiences she and her son did not have. She explained it in this way,

> I think that from the time I started wanting to have children it was the one experience in life I could identify as being a spiritual experience, the carrying and bearing and raising of a child. I had read a lot about what happens in a woman's body. You give birth to your baby and at the moment of the birth this is the biggest rush of hormones you will ever have, and they put the baby on top of your and your eyes meet and it is the indelible spiritual moment. I did not get that at all and he had to be taken away and I will never get over that.

Not only did Merillat not get her first moments with her son that she had so eagerly anticipated, but for his first week in the NICU she was only able to hold him once a day for a few minutes because he was jaundiced and needed to be under the lights for at least 23 hours a day. Even though she was there with her son each day in the NICU, it was difficult to bond with him in the way she had imagined given that he was under the care of NICU staff and she was unable to stay at the NICU 24 hours a day. When she was finally able to bring him home she spent the next few months mostly lying in bed with him by her side allowing him to nurse throughout the day, and through this close contact and special time she felt she was able to bond, but she still is sad and angry that his birth did not go as she had expected.

Unfortunately, when premature babies are born they almost always need immediate assistance so for many women their first moments with their premature babies are nothing more than a quick glance as the baby is held up for the mother to see or the incubator is quickly rolled by her bedside. Sometimes when the preemies are more stable, women are able to quickly touch a hand or foot, but almost always, the preemies are quickly transported to the NICU and women are sent to recovery and sometimes will have to wait almost 24 hours before they themselves are stable and healthy enough to go and visit the NICU. For Jolee whose son Noah was born at 24 weeks, just being able to get into the NICU to see him was a challenge. Three different times her nurse wheeled her down to the NICU, and each time they were sent away because the medical team was busy working to save him. When she finally was able to come in she said that he was covered with so many tubes and wires that she could barely see him.

Leslie's twins were born at 25 weeks. During her emergency C-section, the surgical team delivered her daughter first. After her daughter was out, her uterus started contracting and collapsed around her son, making it difficult to get him out. It took the team a few minutes to get her son out, and when he was removed he was not breathing and required immediate intervention. It was several hours then before Leslie was able to go and visit her twins in the NICU. Her husband had taken some pictures for her and she had looked at pictures of babies at different gestational ages while she was pregnant, but she was still not prepared for what she saw when she first looked at her children and especially her son. She told me that she would never tell her twins, but when she looked at her son she thought of the scene from the Harry Potter movie where Lord Voldemort is at his weakest and is nothing more than a pile of flesh. Her son was completely black and blue all over his body from the birth trauma and he was curled up in a tiny ball hooked up to what seemed like a million machines, wires, and tubes. It was the most frightening and heartbreaking things she had ever seen.

Many women who deliver early are so bothered by the pregnancy and birth that they described wanting to have another child so that they would be able to have the same experiences as others or replicate prior experiences they had with full-term delivery. Women felt cheated or robbed of the joy and excitement of normal pregnancy and birth and were envious of those who had those experiences. Denise, mother of triplets, explained how her envy of her friends' experiences made her at one point consider trying to have another child. When I met Denise her triplets were thirteen years old, but she still vividly remembered how she felt after they were born. At the time, my own triplets were only eighteen months old and we shared pictures of our children as we chatted while sitting in a mall food court. While we talked she told me what it was like after her children were born,

> Afterwards, when my kids were about the age of yours, I went through this phase where I really wanted to get pregnant again because I felt like I got gypped out of a pregnancy. You know, because I didn't get to wear maternity clothes. I wore like a t-shirt, my husband's 3X t-shirt. And you know, I didn't get to go out shopping and I didn't get to do all those things. So I went through a lot, because my friends who had been through pregnancy I got to see them, you know, experience that. They got to take pregnancy exercise classes and all that and I didn't get to experience that. So I went through a phase where I really wanted to be pregnant and wear cute little bib overalls and all that.

Her desire for another child arose more out of a desire to have the experiences she saw around her than a desire to add a child to their family. Eventually, Denise came to terms with her experience and decided against having another child, but still feels a twinge when she thinks about the things she missed.

Many mothers also expressed envy of mothers who were able to keep their infants with them following their deliveries rather than having to visit their infants in the NICU. Women recalled sitting in their hospital rooms and being able to hear other infants crying on the floor and wanting so badly to have a crying infant to hold. My sister-in-law Jessica has type I diabetes and my nephew Michael was born at 37 weeks exactly weighing in at an enormous 11 pounds 13 ounces. He was taken to the NICU right away for monitoring and the staff had a difficult time getting his sugar regulated and he spent his first three days in the NICU. He was my sister-in-law's second child and she told me how terrible it was to know that she had a baby, but he was not in the room with her. Her first daughter Abby had also been taken to the NICU for monitoring because of Jessica's diabetes, but her sugar was quickly regulated and within a day she was brought into Jessica's room. With Michael, she was alone in her room and she could hear all of the other babies on the floor and she wanted so badly to have Michael with her, especially when friends and family came to visit and they had to make the trek down to the NICU where only a few people could go in at a time.

Nancy, mother of twins born at 34 weeks, described having similar feelings when she was alone in her hospital room without her infants,

> Yeah, I think that was a weird thing too, like at night when you are trying to recover from the last weeks at the hospital and my room happened to be right across from the newborns' so everybody was coming up and I could hear them going on about their own babies and getting to take them back to the room and I'm like stuck here and like no baby you don't get the pomp and every time the nurse opened the door I'd snap at everybody.

Nancy was upset that her twins were born early and were in the NICU and hearing the other infants and mothers around her made her situation more upsetting. Because she was a patient in the hospital and had no control of where her room was, she was unable to avoid the happy mothers around her. Her response was to become angry with those around her, even though they had done nothing wrong.

Another moment that many women talked about as traumatic and not living up to expectations was the first time they saw their baby or babies after delivery. When describing the first time they saw their children after they were born many women described feeling completely overwhelmed with fear and sadness. While they had imagined exclaiming over tiny fingers and toes, they had never imagined seeing a baby so small that a wedding ring would fit around its upper arm or a baby attached to so many tubes and wires that it was difficult if not almost impossible to see the baby's face. Even if women had toured the NICU before or had done research about what a premature baby at a certain gestation would look like, over and over women told me that there was no way that someone could be prepared for what it would be like the first time they walked or were wheeled into the NICU and saw their child hooked up to the machines and monitors with wires running out of their heads and feet and tubes going into their mouths and noses.

Jennifer talked about how devastating it was when she was finally able to see her daughter. Jennifer is the mother who gave birth early after what she thought was kidney stone pain turned out to be labor. She was not awake for her delivery so she did not even get to see a brief glance of her daughter before she was taken to the NICU. After she had left recovery and the physician gave her the go ahead, she went to the NICU for the first time, and she was completely overwhelmed by the experience. She had been told about her daughter and her husband had shown her a picture, but she could not believe how small her daughter actually was. She told me "I just wanted to hold her. I just felt awful like I failed her and I couldn't hold her. I felt so awful and I wanted to say to her, this is not what I was supposed to do and I was supposed to keep you in and you were supposed to come out healthy and happy." Jennifer like many mothers had imagined holding their babies when they were born, It was three days before Jennifer was able to hold her because she was under the lights for jaundice and had an IV going through her belly that the medical staff did not want to be moved. A nurse finally let Jennifer hold her and the entire time Jennifer just sat and cried and thought to herself, "This was not what it was supposed to be."

Another woman, Brooke, told a similar story of being devastated by her daughter Olivia's birth at 30 weeks after Brooke developed preeclampsia. Brooke had been admitted to the hospital where she planned to deliver and was put on magnesium sulfate to try and reduce her blood pressure, but as time went on her pressure began to rise and she developed a severe headache as her brain began to swell. The doctor started her on Pitocin to induce her labor and finally after 12 long hours, Olivia was born. Unfortunately the hospital where she delivered did not have an NICU, only a special care nursery, so Olivia had to be immediately transferred by ambulance to another hospital about 30 minutes away. Brooke was ready to get up and ride with her in the ambulance, but her blood pressure was still dangerously high and she was in no condition to be released from the hospital. The hospital where Olivia was being transferred was full, so it was not an option for Brooke to be transferred as well and her doctor convinced her to stay and not sign herself out against medical orders. Her husband and in-laws left to be with the baby and Brooke worked on staying calm so that her blood pressure would be low enough that her doctor would let her go. After about 24 hours with her blood pressure still high but not high enough to cause a stroke, Brooke's doctor agreed to discharge her from the hospital so that she could go and visit her daughter.

It was after midnight when she got there and Brooke explains that she is not normally a crier, but as she sat next to the isolette she started sobbing and could not stop. Her daughter was so small and was on C-PAP and under the lights to help with her severe jaundice. All Brooke wanted to do was pick her up and hold her, but she was not allowed to due to Olivia's unstable condition. It was a horrible moment for Brooke as she felt like there was nothing she could do and she felt so guilty that her baby had been born early. Her first time spending time with daughter was nothing like she had ever imagined.

Along these same lines, the day they were discharged from the hospital was a very difficult day for some women. This was another one of the iconic scenes that women had imagined. They saw themselves sitting proudly in a wheelchair holding their new baby and being rolled to the front door of the hospital where their husband or partner would be waiting with the car and together they would carefully load the baby into the car seat and drive away, ready to start their lives together at home. So many women expressed how wrong it felt to be leaving the hospital without a baby because that was not how it was supposed to be. You went to the hospital, had your baby, and a few days later you all went home together. Many women stayed at the hospital as long as their insurance would allow and then the day they were discharged, they stayed as late as possible to avoid leaving their babies behind. Leaving for the first time was often always the hardest time as this was often a moment when women realized just how wrong things had gone and how different their birthing story was from what they had envisioned.

For example, Heather delivered her daughter at 28 weeks after her doctor found that the baby had stopped growing. She had two older children at home, a nine year old and a four year old, and her husband worked 12-hour shifts. They had recently moved to the Las Vegas area and had no family nearby and knew very few people. The day she was discharged from the hospital her husband told her that she would not be able to come back to the hospital and visit every day because their house was 45 minutes away and they could not afford the gas money. They also had no one to watch their other children and her husband had to go back to work because they needed the money. Not only did Heather have to leave the hospital without her daughter, but she also had to leave thinking she would not be able to get back very often to see her and she was devastated. What happened next seems like something you might see on TV, but Heather had always entered a lot of contests and sweepstakes online. The day after she got home she got an email informing her that she had won a contest she entered to win diapers for a year. Rather than sending actual diapers though, the company mailed her a $1000 check and she was able to use this money to visit her daughter every night after her husband got home from work. It was still a very stressful and difficult time for her as she was home with her kids all day and then would drive herself to the hospital through busy Las Vegas traffic each evening so that she could spend a few hours with her daughter. Her husband was working overtime so he was not able to go to the hospital often and Heather was split between her world at home and her world in the NICU.

Another mother, Jennifer, whose daughter Whitney was born at 30 weeks, described the day she was discharged from the hospital as being almost as difficult as the day when she first held her daughter. The volunteer who came to her room with the wheelchair did not speak very much English and kept telling Jennifer that she needed to go get her baby so she could take her home. She tried to explain that she was not taking her baby home because she was an NICU mom and the baby had to stay here, but the volunteer became more and more adamant that Jennifer's baby needed to be found. It was the first time Jennifer had ever referred to herself as an NICU mom out loud and she says it struck her as she said it that this is what she now was. Finally a nurse came and clarified the situation so that the volunteer would let her leave. As she was being wheeled out to car though, there was a woman next to her being wheeled out who was holding her baby and Jennifer had to look away. She was again struck by the thought that this was all wrong and not what was supposed to happen. The woman next to her was getting to do what you were supposed to do, and Jennifer's story was all wrong. There was nothing happy or exciting about this moment and Jennifer could hardly believe she was driving away and leaving her four-day-olddaughter behind.

Women also had an idea about what it would be like to parent a newborn either from stories they had heard if this was their first child or from prior personal experience with older children. When a baby is early and goes to the NICU, parenting takes on a very different shape, and this shape is usually not one that women had thought about or considered. Because their stories did not match with the other stories they heard or read about typical pregnancies and childbirth, many women had a hard time figuring out how to be a mom to a baby in the NICU. Because they had no other stories to pull from, many women felt their reactions and behaviors were unique, as if they were the only mother who had ever acted or felt a certain way, which lead to feeling like they were alone in their experiences and feelings. Marie, the mother of triplets tried to explain how it felt to be a mom in the NICU, "I just felt like I was visiting some babies and I wanted to hold them and I wanted to love them and I wanted to be with them, but I was just like, I don't know because I don't have anything or experiences to compare it to, but it was definitely, like I didn't spend my whole day there. . . ." Her prior knowledge of early motherhood made her feel as if she should constantly be by her daughter's side and not be able to leave the hospital, where in reality she went to visit often, but also went home to recover and rest. Although she had trouble articulating her exact emotions, as she talked it became apparent that her connection to her triplets while they were in the NICU was not what she thought it would be and did not meet her expectations of what it would feel like to be a mother.

Another mother of triplets, Angie, described how she was also surprised by how strange she felt being a mother while her children were under the hospital's care, "We felt like the babies were ours the moment we first saw them. The frustrating part for us was not being able to scoop them up and snuggle them, or smell them, or soothe them. Even diaper changes and bathing are part of what makes you feel like a parent, and we weren't allowed to do that for some time. The bond was certainly there, but being limited in their care was very tough." Some of the basic parts of being a parent such as holding a baby when it cries or rocking them to sleep cannot happen when babies are medically fragile and many parents struggle to figure out what it means to be a parent to a baby that they are unable to physically care for.

Catt, mother of surviving twins, talked about her frustration in not being the primary caretaker for her son and daughter. She is a pediatric nurse, but as a parent of NICU babies her role in caring for them was very limited. She explained, "You know, there is so little you can control in that environment. And you know we were there at night and I wanted to do the bath and they would be like, we're not doing the bath today. And it would crush me not to be able to give him his little bath, and when he was finally ready for one of those. It felt like, I was finally the mom and I found that it was almost like getting the most common experience. . . . But yeah, yeah, it was very surreal." Another mother of triplets, Jessica, described how difficult it was to see her infants in pain and not being able to do anything to comfort or soothe them. She explained the difficult time she had standing by during various medical procedures. "Another thing that really got me was not being able to comfort them when they were being poked or getting an IV in her head or crying so hard because they were in so much pain and you could do nothing. It was so hard I had to leave on more than one occasion." Mothers struggled to take on the role of mom as they were unable to perform many of the basic caretaking tasks associated with motherhood such as feeding, holding, bathing, and comforting.

While many of the expectations women had involved their personal experiences, they also had expectations as far as how those around them would behave and react, and sometimes those expectations were not met by a woman's family and support system. Cynthia's story is slightly different. She delivered her twins at 39 weeks via a vaginal delivery after a difficult pregnancy. For many twin mothers, her pregnancy and its outcome were ideal, she carried her babies to full term and was able to bring them home from the hospital with her. Cynthia's struggles came from the role her husband played in her pregnancy, delivery, and in caring for their twins. Cynthia and her husband used fertility medications to conceive, and her pregnancy actually began as quadruplets. She made the difficult decision to reduce the pregnancy to twins and had to travel to New York City to have the procedure done as no local physicians would perform a selective reduction. Her husband wanted nothing to do with the reduction procedure even though he wanted her to have the reduction but he refused to travel with her and to this day will not speak about it. She understands why the topic was and still is difficult for him, but she carries some resentment over how she had to handle such a difficult situation without his support.

She also was disappointed with his support during her twins' birth and during the aftermath. She described going to the hospital for her delivery, "He came into the delivery room and promptly said he felt faint. He was laying down on the floor with two nurses helping him. I'm like, are you okay, while I am having a C-section." Her husband chose not to stay overnight with her at the hospital after their twins were born because he was feeling fatigued. He went home to sleep and left her alone with their twins. She described it, "I was just alone in a room with these two kids and was just so sad." For her, watching programs such as *A Baby Story* or *Bringing Home Baby* were difficult because she was envious of the way the husbands on the programs acted toward their wives and their infants. One of her high school friends was featured on the program and she described her reaction to watching her friend,

> So it was really interesting to see you know, her. And at the time I was really jealous because in watching her, her husband was so supportive, or at least appeared to be on the TV, and that's not what I was getting at all. So that was actually one of the hard things actually. Seeing, oh honey, I'm so glad, and you know, thank you. Give a hug and kiss. You know some type of appreciation, something positive, and I didn't get any of that.

Cynthia was envious of other women whose spouses were more supportive of their stressful and complicated situations.

One of the reasons it is important to understand the impact these unmet expectations have on women is that in addition to being difficult emotionally, the unmet expectations play a large role in shaping the stories women tell about their pregnancies and deliveries. When talking about their experiences of having a high-risk pregnancy or having a premature infant, women often talked about what they had missed out on and what was lacking from their experiences. Jana, who had two high-risk pregnancies, described what she felt she had missed. She told me,

> I have talked to other people who have had kind of difficult pregnancies and they all say kind of the same thing. You do feel kind of robbed of the story of your pregnancy, especially with your first pregnancy. Everything is supposed to

> be new and wonderful and exciting and you get to plan all of this and the baby shower is supposed to be wonderful and it is supposed to be this kind of fun-filled exciting time, and that is sort of clouded over by your concern for your children and your children's health and your own. And you kind of just feel a little bit robbed of that experience. You know that you have seen *Baby Story* or you have heard from your friends, you've seen the pictures on their blog in the hospital, of them delivering the baby and holding the baby right away.

Women who experience high-risk pregnancies as well as others who interact with these women need to be aware of the expectations that exist and how not meeting those expectations may influence women's experiences and their stories. For example, women who had the expectation of immediately bonding with their newborns frequently told stories of disconnect and trauma if their infant was taken to the NICU immediately following delivery. Now the solution is not to give all women time to hold their newborns, as the obvious priority is the health of the babies, and babies in respiratory distress require immediate intervention. Instead, in these situations, women and those supporting them need to find ways to create new expectations for what will occur or alternative ways to meet those expectations. One way to accomplish this is for women to be exposed to the stories of others in similar situations. This could provide women with a better idea of the events and feelings they will experience. Women who have been told beforehand that they will not be able to hold their premature infants will be prepared for the situation. This is not to say that she will not experience disappointment, but she will least have more accurate expectations going into the delivery. Additionally, if possible, allowing women to see their infants or reaching out to touch their heads would be a way to assist women in starting to connect with their infants. Many hospitals do this as part of the standard procedure and every woman who was able to do this commented on how much even just the quickest glance meant to them.

Because their ideas of what pregnancy and childbirth would be like are often so ingrained, women may need assistance to either change their expectations or find alternative ways to fulfill their expectations. One important expectation many women had was being pregnant out in the world and they wanted to be seen by others when they were pregnant and to have the opportunity to participate in the many rituals that surround pregnancy including showers, shopping for the new baby, and planning the nursery. Friends and family members could help women fulfill these expectations by visiting women on bed rest and assisting in shopping for and decorating the nursery. Many of the women commented on how nice it was when friends and family hosted a shower even if it was in the pregnant woman's home and she never got up from bed. The shower was about much more than getting supplies and equipment for their infants. It was about the acknowledgment and celebration of a new life and sharing their happiness and excitement with family and friends.

Another thing women looked forward to was shopping for and wearing maternity clothes. When women were advised bed rest, they were unable to go shopping and because they rarely left their homes, many did not see the need to purchase maternity clothes and instead lived in stretchy yoga pants and oversized t-shirts. Instead of going to the local store though, women could use the internet to purchase clothes and could wear their clothes for medical appointments or when they have visitors. Some would argue that spending money on clothes that were rarely seen was frivolous, but even just a few cute items could go a long way in allowing women to experience this pregnancy ritual. Women also could be encouraged to create new rituals and ways of marking and documenting their pregnancies. Activities such as journaling, blogging, or taking weekly pictures could be ways to remember and record the pregnancy experience as well as provide them with a way to share their pregnancies with others. Even though a weekly photo shared through social media is not the same as walking through the store, it is a way for others to see and comment on a woman's pregnancy.

In addition to new expectations, it would be helpful if women could hear stories of how different experiences of pregnancy, birth, and becoming a mother can lead to similar outcomes such as a loving bond between mother and child. Women may need help to appreciate that even though the initial moments of their infants' lives may not be as they imagined, they can still form an important and lasting bond with their infants. In her book on helping parents cope with premature infants, McDermott-Perez (2007) offered the stories of many adoptive parents as a counternarrative to women's beliefs that the first moments of life are essential to the bonding process as has been presented by some physicians and child-rearing experts (Spock and Needlman 2004). Many adoptive parents are not present for their children's births and might not even meet their children for several days, months, or years. These parents still feel connected and bonded with their children despite not holding them immediately after birth. Stories such as these could expose women to other possibilities. Instead of telling stories that focused on the moments that were lost, women could focus on the special moments they had with their infants when they were able to bond such as the first time they held their infants in the NICU or the first time they were able to feed them.

Women need access to alternative stories about motherhood and the journey to becoming a mother. With such a narrow set of expectations, women whose pregnancies and births do not conform to the norms are bound to be disappointed. No mother wants to have a difficult pregnancy or birth, but the knowledge that this is how many women become mothers may be of comfort to women as they recognize themselves in these stories. These alternative depictions should include mothers who struggled with the early months of motherhood for a variety of reasons including postpartum depression, poor maternal health, and poor infant health. Again, knowing that other women have walked a similar path can be comforting and make mothers feel less alone.

When women's babies were born early and their expectations were not met, they felt a myriad of emotions including extreme guilt, constant fear, or lack of connection to their infants which are not emotions typically associated with motherhood. Many of the women commented they were unable to enjoy or be excited about their pregnancies once they learned they were high risk. Instead of being excited and filled with joy, they lived with constant fear and anxiety about their unborn infants' survival and health. After enduring a stressful and emotional pregnancy, many mothers had to face the challenges of having infants who required time in the NICU. This also was a time of stress as women tried to physically heal and worried about their infants' health and progress. These overwhelming emotions combined with surges of hormones made the initial weeks after delivery emotionally challenging for many women. Some felt withdrawn, depressed, irritable, or angry and in turn did not feel the joy, love, and bonding they had expected. Because these emotions did not match women's expectations of pregnancy and motherhood, many women felt isolated and ashamed to talk about their emotions. The feelings that they needed to keep quiet about their negative emotions for fear of external judgment were similar to those that women who suffer from postpartum depression have reported. Feeling sad or depressed about the events surrounding a child's birth does not fit with the societal ideal of a "good mother." Often women choose to hide or keep quiet about their feelings for fear that they will be judged for having less than motherly instincts or feelings, (Knudson-Martin and Silverstein 2009) which means both that they may not get the social support they need because their support networks are unaware of the problem and because of the lack of social support, the symptoms and negative feelings may increase.

This silence also creates a vicious cycle as women believe they are one of the only mothers who has felt sad, anxious, or depressed about their situations because they had not previously heard or read stories in which women experienced similar feelings. This led to many women feeling ashamed of their feelings. Over and over women told me that having a baby was supposed to be a happy thing, and there was no room for sadness and anger in these events. So instead of talking about their feelings, many chose to keep quiet, which meant that other mothers were not able to learn about their struggles. Their silence also limits their ability to connect with others who would be able to relate to their stories and provide emotional support. The issue of connection to their infants actually came up often in the interviews and women seemed eager to share their experiences. Unfortunately, many of the women explained that their eagerness to share their stories in the interview situation was unique, and they rarely felt comfortable discussing their negative emotions in other settings. The feelings of isolation and guilt were perpetuated as women had nowhere to go to find stories that showed them that their feelings were not rare, but were quite natural.

Due to the stories women see, read, and hear, they develop expectations about what their pregnancy and birth experiences will be like. When preterm labor and premature birth occur, women's worlds are often turned upside down as the things they anticipated doing and feeling and saying, do not happen. While disappointment and grief are natural and human reactions to situations like this as no one wants to see their baby born sick, struggling to do basic things such as breathe and eat, women's sadness and grief is often compounded by the loss of the experiences they had imagined. Women have to let go of their wishes for a perfect baby shower, holding their newborn, and bringing home their baby from the hospital with them. Additionally, when a baby is born early, most women find themselves in uncharted territory as they have no idea what it is like to parent a preemie, have a child in the NICU, and live with the constant anxiety that something will be seriously wrong with their child. Women need ways to both cope with unmet expectations and to develop new expectations for what their experience will be like.

Chapter 5

The Comparison Game

Ambrosia and I met one morning at a funky little coffee shop just south of Indianapolis. As mothers of young triplets we were both excited to meet each other and exchange stories and we were nearly giddy about the thought of enjoying a few child-free hours. When Ambrosia who has triplet sons learned she was pregnant with triplets she was not only overwhelmed at the thought of having three babies at once, but she was terrified of what might happen when they were born too early. She was not very optimistic about what the possible outcomes would be and admits she was convinced that her boys would have serious medical issues as she could not conceive of her story ending with three healthy babies. As nervous as she was, she did get some comfort from finding stories about other triplets and multiples pregnancies with positive outcomes. In particular, one story stuck in her mind throughout her pregnancy. "I actually had a student whose mom had triplets and they were 19 at the time when I heard about them, and they were spontaneous, but they were all normal. You know and I think that was one of my other fears. I think I had read too much about how preterm babies are more likely to have cerebral palsy, so I was always worried." Knowing there were triplets who had been born and suffered from no long-term complications and that a woman had successfully carried triplets to a point where they not only survived but were completely healthy allowed Ambrosia to see the possibility of her sons growing up and leading normal lives. She realized that it was not definite that her sons would be disabled and she was able to consider a positive life and future for her sons. Whenever the negative thoughts began to take over, she thought about that mom and her triplets and reminded herself that her story could have a good ending.

It is human nature to compare ourselves to others, and pregnant women and preemie moms are not immune to this tendency. Comparing ourselves to others gives us a sense of how we are doing and where we fit into this world. It is through comparison that people determine if their actions, circumstances, and thoughts are within the realm of normal. A woman who is pregnant for the first time may have no idea what to expect and can listen to and read about others' experiences to try and determine if a symptom she is having is typical or something she should be concerned about, if she is gaining too much or too little weight, or if her fears and concerns are just what every other expectant mothers has or if they are an indication that her anxiety level is too high. The results of these comparisons can be reassuring if it seems like everything is at par for the course, but when one comes up short in the comparison process it can be cause for alarm, concern, and even disappointment. Sitting next to a woman who describes gaining only 22 pounds during her pregnancy can be a little disheartening for a woman who is currently seven months pregnant and has already gained 30 pounds. On the other hand, a woman who is worried that she hasn't felt her baby kicking yet at 20 weeks might feel some relief after polling her friends and learning that several women did not feel movement until the 24th week.

The impact of comparisons on one's sense of self can be explained by Festinger's (1954) Social Comparison Theory. According to Social Comparison Theory, individuals make assessments about their own opinions and desires by comparing themselves to others. It is through comparison to others that individuals learn about themselves by discovering how they are similar and different from those around them. Social comparisons are frequently prompted by uncertainty when individuals are in situations where they lack objective standards to assess themselves. A new mother might be unsure of what she should be feeling and doing, and therefore will look to other new mothers as a way to gauge herself and see how well she is handling her new role. Pregnancy itself is full of a lot of unknowns, but when a woman is experiencing a high-risk pregnancy the degree of uncertainty is even higher. Women often have no idea what is happening or might happen as they have no frame of reference or knowledge about their conditions, so comparisons to other women with similar complications become a critical way that they learn what to expect and how to evaluate their situations. When Festinger first developed his theory, he asserted that individuals will typically make upward comparisons to those who are superior as these types of comparisons show a person areas where he or she can improve. Subsequent work however, has shown that individuals will compare themselves to both superiors in the process of upward comparison, but also to inferiors in the process of downward comparison (Wills 1981).

In upward comparisons, individuals compare themselves to a superior who is doing better than they are doing, that they perceive as having better qualities, or who has achieved more. As a classic example, consider how women will pour through fashion magazines looking at the images of beautiful models. This upward comparison can be a positive experience as the superior individual can serve as a role model or provide inspiration as women might aspire to look like one of the models and be motivated to take actions such as exercising or using different makeup to achieve that goal. Comparing oneself to someone who is superior can also have the complete opposite effect and lead to negative emotions when an individual feels they are inferior or will not be able to match the progress of the superior individual. Going back to the model example, it is easy for a woman to get down on herself if she feels that she will never be able to obtain the perfect body and flawless skin of the women featured in magazines. Given the tremendous amount of airbrushing and photoshopping that takes place and the incredibly high standards that models are held to, it is very likely that the majority of women comparing themselves to women featured in magazines ads will have some negative impacts from the comparison. In terms of pregnancy, upward comparisons might involve a first-time mother comparing herself to an older woman who has successfully given birth to four healthy babies or a woman who has an incompetent cervix comparing herself to a woman who also had an incompetent cervix but carried her baby to 38 weeks.

The opposite of upward comparisons are downward comparisons which are comparisons that are made to inferior others. Generally these types of comparisons serve a self-enhancing function because when individuals see they are doing better than someone else they often feel better about themselves. This process works in two ways. One is purposely and directly comparing one's progress or situation with another's. For example, if a student is upset after receiving a B in an exam, he or she might compare themselves to friends who got lower grades and feel better about his or her own result. In terms of pregnancy, a woman who is experiencing extreme fatigue might compare herself to a friend whose morning sickness is so bad that she is vomiting throughout the day and determine that her own side effects are not so bad. The second way is more general and this happens when people unintentionally come across the stories of inferior others and through the process of social comparisons both feel better about themselves and their situations. This for example might occur when watching the news and seeing a story about a town that was recently destroyed by a natural disaster. A common response to stories and images like this is a recognition of how fortunate one is to be in a town that was not stuck by tragedy and an appreciation for one's situation and circumstances. This comparison is not related to being better or worse than a person as far as personal traits or accomplishments are, but instead comparing life situations.

Downward comparisons do not automatically lead to happiness though. Research has demonstrated that downward comparisons also can create negative affect in situations where individuals feel empathetic to the inferior person (Michinov 2007). Going back to the example of the natural disaster, seeing people who are in dire situations can lead to feelings of sadness and grief. One might recognize how fortunate he or she is to not be in that situation, but the empathy felt for the families who have lost everything will very much outweigh any positive feelings they have. Others may feel guilty when they think about how much they have as they view images of people who have lost everything. Downward comparisons can also lead to fear and anxiety as one becomes concerned that they too could be in a similar situation. The next time a storm hits it could possibly be in his or her hometown and the awareness of what the tragedy and destruction might look like can be overwhelming.

There are several factors that influence how likely one is to engage in social comparison. During times of illness and medical situations social comparisons are more likely because of the uncertain nature of illness and because medical situations can be completely new experiences and outside of one's existing knowledge. One's self-esteem can also influence the direction of comparison as well as one's reaction to it. Those with higher self-esteem tend to have more positive reactions to social comparison whether upward or downward due to their propensity to view themselves in a positive light. Those with lower self-esteem not only tend to make more social comparisons, but they tend to feel more negative after those comparisons. Another factor that influences social comparison is individuals' sense of control. If individuals feel as if they can control situations, then they are more likely to make upward comparisons as they seek out information that will assist in self-improvement or provide inspiration (Taylor and Lobel, 1989). In contrast, when a situation feels like it is out of one's control, people tend to avoid upward comparisons as they do not want to look at what can feel like an unattainable ideal. A woman's beliefs as far as how much she can control how her pregnancy is progressing will often determine if she engages in social comparison and what type.

Because social comparison is so common in medical situations, there have been some research studies conducted that specifically looked at the comparisons pregnant women make and the impact of those comparisons on their well-being. Dias and Lobel (1997) reported that pregnancy can be highly conducive to social comparisons as it is time of great uncertainty and there is such a wide variation in what is considered normal. Women's pregnancies are all unique and are accompanied by a multitude of physical and emotional changes. When a pregnancy becomes high risk or a woman starts to experience complications her pregnancy seems even more confusing, as high-risk pregnancies can be so different than a woman's other experiences with pregnancy or the experiences of those she knows. Women experiencing complications and the threat of premature delivery may also feel like they have less control over the situation, a factor that has been associated with greater amounts of social comparison. Dias and Lobel (1997) found the social comparison activity of medically high-risk pregnant women was similar to that of groups facing other health threats such as cancer or AIDS. The researchers also discovered that women who were pregnant for the first time made the most social comparisons, which makes sense considering that this is a new experience and they do not know what is normal, and those with higher self-esteem made more upward comparisons. An interesting finding was that women who made the most downward comparisons had the lowest levels of anxiety, a finding that supports the ability of downward comparison to generate positive emotions as women's anxiety was reduced when they found that their pregnancies were not as problematic as other women's pregnancies.

A 2008 study of pregnant women who had been admitted to the hospital with hypertension found that the women in the study actively engaged in both upward and downward comparison to help manage their emotions. Examples of upward comparison included thinking about women they knew who had also been hospitalized during their pregnancies who had delivered full term and brought a healthy baby home from the hospital. Stories like these gave women both hope and comfort as it was evidence that everything could end up perfectly fine. Women also thought about and compared themselves to stories of women who had much worse outcomes such as losing a baby during the pregnancy or having a baby born with serious medical conditions. These comparisons provided a sense of perspective and allowed women to recognize that even though they were in a frightening situation, it could be much worse. Some upward comparisons did result in negative emotions as some of the women felt bad about themselves or more concerned with their circumstances when they saw or heard about other women without complications delivering healthy infants (Helen, Hainsworth, and Thornton 2008).

Social comparison also plays a role in parenting premature infants. Padden and Glen (1997) found that mothers of infants in the NICU frequently used downward comparisons to make assessments about their child's health situation. Women often engaged in downward comparison both intentionally and unintentionally as they saw many infants and families around them in the NICU that were in poorer health and in worse situations. As a result of seeing families and babies with greater struggles, women were able to reappraise their situations and many referred to themselves as lucky to have a healthy infant as compared to other babies in the unit. Women also engaged in upward comparison toward other babies in the unit or babies they knew who had been born full term and these comparisons made them feel worse rather than providing a sense of hope or inspiration. One woman commented on how seeing a set of triplets bigger than her single infant made her feel worse about her situation as her one infant was so small. Rather than giving her hope or something to aspire to, the larger infants made her feel bad because her own infant was not as big or doing as well as in her mind it seemed that a single baby should be better off than a set of three.

So it is known that women will most likely make comparisons to others, but who will they compare themselves to? This question does not concern whether women will engage in upward or downward comparisons, but who are the actual women they will compare themselves to. A common experience of women with high-risk pregnancies and preemies is that they often did not have a lot of people within their direct social circle who had experienced a high-risk pregnancy or given birth to a preemie so they have to go outside of their personal contacts to find stories. Some women met other mothers with high-risk pregnancies by joining something like a parents of multiples group, but more often women turned to the internet to find websites, message boards, and forums to find similar women to learn from their stories. One of the remarkable things about the stories they found on the internet was that women were able to find incredibly detailed accounts. Many women described becoming engrossed in what they found and spending a lot of time reading stories on blogs of women who had high-risk pregnancies or pouring through the messages on forums. Frequently they found themselves amazed at how far some women carried their infants despite extreme circumstances or overwhelmed by how much families had been through before they were able to bring their baby home from the hospital. In addition to reading about pregnancies, they read blogs of families with preemies to see and learn what life with a preemie might be like. A third common way that women encountered stories was by hearing them secondhand from friends and family. These are the stories that often begin with something like "my neighbor's cousin's water broke at 25 weeks. . .,"or "a woman I used to work with had a preemie." Additionally, medical staff such as nurses or obstetricians often shared stories of other women with high-risk pregnancies they had treated who had had positive outcomes or of others infants who had spent time in the NICU and are now doing remarkably well.

COMPARING FOR HOPE

One of the benefits of social comparison is that it can provide a positive role model, the possibility of a positive outcome, and encouragement for individuals as they work to achieve their aspirations. One of the first things many women did after they learned that their pregnancy was high risk or they would deliver early was to try to find stories and examples of people who had been in similar situations. The primary motivation was to see what happened to others and how they managed, but at another level these stories gave other women situations to compare themselves to and they hoped that the stories they found would provide the possibility of a happy ending. Women wanted to know what could happen, but many also wanted to check and see if there were others with the same complications that had good outcomes. As many women reported, physicians often focused on facts and statistics when talking to women about the possibilities which meant that many women were given a somewhat bleak outlook for what was to come. In order to regain a sense of hope and to put a human face to the numbers and facts they heard, many women used positive stories as sources of encouragement and motivation. For example, hearing or reading the story of a mother pregnant with triplets who delivered at 36 weeks and was able to take her babies home from the hospital with her made without spending any time in the NICU made some women pregnant with triplets feel better as they saw a successful outcome as a possibility.

In talking with mothers, it became apparent that many of the upward comparisons that resulted in positive emotions such as hope took place early in their pregnancy when women had just been diagnosed with a problem or learned they could possibly deliver early, but prior to the women experiencing major complications. When women were in the early stages of their pregnancies they were able to look to those who had already experienced positive outcomes and aspire to be like them. Because they had yet to experience numerous complications that lowered their chances of a successful outcome, they still had hope and believed in the possibility that they could also be a success story. Shortly after being diagnosed with a high-risk pregnancy, many women described turning to books and the internet to learn more about what the best possible outcome for their condition could be. For example, women pregnant with triplets wanted to know the average gestational age at which triplets are born as well as how long a woman could possibly carry triplets before birth. Women then used those stories as evidence that a good outcome was possible. This was especially important for women who had been told by physicians of the likelihood of a negative outcome. Hearing or reading success stories allowed them to envision success stories for themselves. These stories let them know their pregnancies were not doomed to certain failure, but instead, there was hope for positive outcomes.

These upward comparison did not just inspire hope, but they gave women practical information about coping with a high-risk pregnancy or taking care of a premature infant. They also tried to learn what these women had done during their pregnancies to have such successful outcomes so they could emulate those successful women. Astrid, mother of triplets born at almost 34 weeks made it her goal to carry her children as long as possible. She spent a lot of time reading books as well as researching online to determine the best ways to meet her goal. In addition to reading medical sites she read the stories of women on both blogs and message boards who had carried their triplets at least 34 weeks and adopted many of their strategies.

Due to prior exposure to or experience with premature infants, some women had trouble conceiving of any type of positive outcomes. Catt was one of those women. She is an ICU nurse at the local children's hospital and deals with the sickest children every day at her job. Prior to learning she was pregnant with triplets, her interaction with multiples had only been with very sick children who were on her unit. At the beginning of her pregnancy her fears regarding her unborn infants' health consumed her. She explained, "It terrified me. Like my initial feeling was, 'am I going to have three severely damaged babies?' and then I was like, 'what if they are all handicapped? How does that work? Am I going to have to take on most of that. Not take it on, but emotionally. . . . And then it wasn't fair to bring them into the world that way." When she imagined her children's future it always involved them having long-term health issues and pervasive developmental delays. Early in her pregnancy Catt was able to attend a few meetings of a support group for mothers with higher-order multiples. At one of the dinners several mothers had brought pictures of their children to share with the newer members of the group and as Catt poured over the photos she was shocked but in a good way. She explained, "and we looked at them and there wasn't a single, you know special needs child or handicapped or anything there. And I mean, I was like, "How can this exist?" I mean, when your perspective is what happens in the hospital. . . ." After spending time with these other women and listening to their stories she began to believe that it was possible for her triplets to be healthy.

Unfortunately, Catt, who was carrying a set of identical twin girls and one fraternal triplet who was a boy, learned that her twin girls had twin-to-twin transfusion syndrome. As her pregnancy progressed it became apparent that her case was extremely severe and twin A was taking almost all of the nutrition and blood from the placenta, so twin B who was unable to grow. Catt and her husband were told that if the pregnancy continued twin B would die which would cause twin A to die as well because the girls had so many shared blood vessels. Catt looked for hopeful and positive stories for inspiration, but was unable to find any success stories for twins with such a severe case of twin-to-twin. The only option they had was to perform a selective reduction which is a procedure where potassium chloride is injected into an infant's heart in utero causing it to stop beating and the infant to die. In their case the potassium chloride would be injected into twin B's heart as this was the weaker twin and the hope was that by terminating twin B, twin A would have a more normal blood flow and survive. It was a horrible option, but Catt and her husband opted to try to save at least one baby rather than definitely lose both.

Because she was so far along, 21 weeks, there were very few doctors in the country who would perform the high-risk procedure so Catt and her husband who live in Ohio had to travel to North Carolina to have the reduction procedure done. The procedure itself was short and as she lay on the examination table Catt could only hope that by saying good-bye to one of their daughters she was giving her other daughter the gift of a chance at survival. The ultrasound was on as the doctor located twin B and Catt and her husband listened with tears in their eyes as they heard the tiny heartbeat and then after the injection, it slowly stop. After returning home from the procedure Catt spent the remainder of her pregnancy on bed rest and despite the chances of her losing twin A and even the entire pregnancy she carried her children to 34 weeks. Even though she lost one of her daughters and still grieves for her, she is incredibly thankful every day for her surviving triplets who are healthy and have no long-term complications or delays due to their prematurity. Some may argue that her earlier upward comparisons to women with healthy triplets and quadruplets had given her false hope since she lost one of her daughters, but given that her surviving children were typically developing children, Catt was still thankful for the early hope and inspiration.

Sometimes women were so convinced they would be able to emulate the outcomes of the positive stories they heard that they were blindsided when things did not go as they had planned. Some women developed positive expectations for how their high-risk pregnancies would progress after hearing or reading the stories of other women who had been in similar situations. Donna described how her sister's stories about her pregnancy with twins set her expectations for how her own twin pregnancy would progress,

> My sister had twins 20 years before and she worked in a dental clinic up until she delivered and the day she had her babies, and she went in for an appointment and they said, oh, you are contracting. Yeah, you are having these babies today and she had them at 38 weeks instead of the 39 weeks scheduled C-section. And so I was like, you know that's what I am going to do. And I had no idea that we would have a NICU stay or anything like that. Not to mention having surgery when the baby is ten hours old.

Donna incorporated her sister's story of carrying twins successfully into her own in her assumptions that her experience would be the same. In the beginning stages of her pregnancy she was not concerned or worried about twins and her story was one of excitement. When she went into labor at 30 weeks and delivered the next day, she had trouble reconciling her story with the expectations she had created from her sister's tale.

Similarly, Kari, whose triplets passed away after being born at 23 weeks, talked about hearing the stories of a distant cousin with triplets and how those stories shaped her understanding of her triplet pregnancy. When talking with her I asked if she had known anyone else who had triplets prior to conceiving her own and she responded, "I did. Actually, I think that was part of my being naïve. But my, it's like my distant cousin on my mom's side had triplets, had spontaneous triplets actually. She carried them and delivered them with a C-section. They didn't even stay in a neonatal unit or anything. They were just born in this small hospital in Terre Haute." This cousin's story, a great triplet pregnancy, had set an expectation for Kari that her pregnancy would be similar as this is what she knew. When her pregnancy ended so early due to an infection she was blindsided as she had only really compared herself to this cousin as she had not spent a lot of time seeking out other stories so she did not fully grasp everything that could wrong with such a high-risk pregnancy.

Another common time when women actively sought out stories and particularly positive stories to compare their situations too was when their infants were born early and they looked for stories of other infants who were born at the same gestation. Particularly, women wanted to find success stories of infants who were born the same number of weeks early and those who were born with similar health issues. These stories helped women learn how others managed and often helped to reassure them that their infants would be okay or at least gave them the belief that their children possibly could be okay. Frequently women saw posts on internet forums posted by women asking for stories of infants born at different gestations or with different health issues. These types of posts did not ask for any specific information, but simply asked for women to share their story when their infants were born at a certain gestation or with a specific medical issue. Some of the participants even posted these types of questions themselves as a means of gathering similar stories. Getting connected to these other stories gave women the information they were craving, hope when the stories had good outcomes, and a sense of being connected to others.

Kiera was a woman who craved a connection with other mothers who had similar experiences or could at least relate to her situation. Kiera's triplets were born at 25 weeks and one of her daughters, Zoe, suffered from extensive complications including hearing loss and needing continued oxygen support leading to a ten-month NICU stay and her coming home on oxygen and a feeding tube. Kiera often worried about her daughter's health and how she would relate to her two sisters with fewer medical issues. Because her situation was both rare and extreme, she did not have anyone in her personal circle she could turn to. Through friends though, Kiera was connected to another woman in her town with eight-year-old triplets who had been born at

25 weeks as well. One of this woman's triplets had cerebral palsy, yet continued to make strides and overcome her limitations. Hearing that this triplet was able to play golf and keep up with her siblings brought peace and hope to Kiera as she was able to imagine a future for Zoe where she would thrive alongside her sisters.

Women did not only look to compare their children to other children, but they also looked to other mothers to try and find examples of women who were able to successfully cope with difficult and stressful situations such as having multiple infants or a preemie as well as older children. These stories gave them hope that they could survive their experiences without losing their sanity. Often the women in these stories served as role models and inspiration. Helene, mother of triplets, described meeting and becoming friends with a local mother of quintuplets and how encouraging this was to her. She talked about meeting her friend through their local multiples group.

> I met Candice and she has quintuplets and hers are two years older than mine. Hers were born at the exact same time, they were 28-weekers. We go to their birthday party every year. And so I figured to myself, and this sounds terrible the way I am going to phrase this, but I thought, if she can do it and she has five of them, I can certainly do this. And it wasn't belittling her intelligence or her ability to be a parent, it was just, she has two more than me and no helpers or anything.

This upward comparison helped Helene to realize the possibility of being a successful mother to premature triplets and helped her story become one of ability rather than inability.

When Jenny learned she was pregnant with triplets she found that a lot of people shared stories of others triplets they had known and one of her co-workers even put her in touch with a woman in the neighboring town who had triplets and Jenny was able to call her and ask about her experiences. Her friendship with this mother and the stories she heard became very important to Jenny when she was admitted to the hospital for preterm labor and was started on an IV of magnesium sulfate. She was miserable as the side effects of the magnesium sulfate reared their ugly head. She was hot, nauseated, weak, and seeing double, but she kept thinking back to her friend who had been on magnesium for six weeks when she was pregnant. Not only had this mom suffered through being on the drug for six weeks, she was much older than Jenny during her pregnancy, so Jenny kept telling herself that if this other mother could do it, then so could she. This fellow triplet mom's story was a source of motivation for Jenny as she strove to stay pregnant and endure the terrible pain and discomfort brought on by the medications she was on.

Recognizing the transformative power of positive stories also encouraged some women to share their stories with others. Marie, who had a positive outcome with her triplet daughters, described how she tries to provide encouragement to other triplet mothers whenever she can. "Now I take my girls back about every six months and we visit our NICU nurses and everybody and they'll bring, if there are any triplet moms in there, they'll bring them out and I'll talk to them and just try to encourage them and tell them you're going to get through this." She also spoke about trying to be encouraging on the message boards by letting women know that it was possible to have a healthy pregnancy and have healthy infants.

COMPARING FOR PERSPECTIVE

During a high-risk pregnancy, preterm labor, and time spent in the NICU women invariably came across a number of stories which prompted downward comparison as the women or children in these stories were doing worse or had worse outcomes. This type of comparison could also improve women's emotional states and feelings as they were able to reconsider their own situations in light of others' experiences. One of the most common reactions women had to hearing a negative story was a sense of gratitude or relief about their own situations. In hearing or reading what could have been, women felt thankful for the positive aspects in their situations. For example, after finding out she was pregnant with triplets, Angie began reading about the potential outcomes and was determined to make it to at least 35 weeks and possibly avoid any NICU time for her sons. When the boys were born at 33 weeks she was devastated that she had not met her goal and very distraught about her sons' health and NICU experience. For the first couple of weeks she was so angry at herself that she had not met her goal and was upset that by delivering her sons this early she had not given them a good start and a good chance for healthy development. As she spent more time in the NICU and saw other struggling infants who were born far earlier and were far sicker, her story began to transform from one of her sons' early birth being the worst possible thing that could have happened to a story of gratitude that her sons were okay and only experienced the normal complications of prematurity. In describing how her sons' time in the NICU actually helped her to feel better about her situation, she explained, "They were not as bad as some of the other babies, the singleton babies that were in there. There were people, I mean there were people and this was their first child and it had been born at 24 weeks. So I guess I felt relieved that they, and as I said, I was so scared about them being on a ventilator." Even though her sons were in the NICU, they were breathing on their own and doing better than many of the other infants in the NICU. Recognizing this helped eliminate some of the distress from her own story and added an element of gratitude.

Carla, mother of twin boys born at 34 weeks, talked about how the stories of her friends who had premature infants at much earlier gestations influenced her outlook on her situation,

> My two friends in Chicago, they each had singletons, but one was like two pounds. And when I saw her, I think she was actually lower than her birth weight. And I remember going, when I went to see that baby, the mother, my friend told me, I hope you never see another baby this small in your entire life. And I remember walking in and she was in the totally enclosed bed. . .and I just remember thinking, oh my God. So with my kids, I felt they were big, and things were so much better compared to that experience. And then my other friend, her daughter had a very rare blood disease and had to have bone marrow transplants. . . . So I was like, my kid doesn't have cancer. My kid is not two pounds.

Even though her twins were born early and only weighed five pounds at birth, in comparison to her friends' infants, her sons were doing very well which made her see her situation in a positive light.

Hearing or reading stories with outcomes that were worse than their own provided women with stories of what could have been or what could be. Knowing how bad it could get and did get for others, made women's own situations seem more bearable. Marie, mother of triplets, was a mother who purposely avoided stories with poor outcomes during her pregnancy because she did not want to make herself even more worried about the possibilities. After she gave birth to her girls at almost 35 weeks she began to open herself up to more stories and found herself reading and listening to stories of infants born at very early gestations who have very serious health problems. She explained, "My husband and I talk about this now, I don't think I realized how many risks there were when I was pregnant as I do now. I have now learned about or know about what could have happened or now I hear about some of these 23 to 24weekers and I am like, oh my gosh, I didn't realize that at 24 weeks, what that meant if they came out then." This realization helped her to be more positive during her daughters' time in the NICU as her daughters were in such better shape physically than so many of the other babies.

Another mother of twins, Maggie, echoed these sentiments as she described how observing other infants and families in the NICU made her see the positives in her situation. During her son's time in the NICU, she struggled with the lack of control she felt over what was happening every day and she also had concerns over one of her sons' heart condition. She was completely overwhelmed emotionally and was having a difficult time dealing with her sadness, anxiety, and fear. As she spent more time in the NICU and started being more aware of other babies and families she saw that some of the infants were very sick and many of the families were struggling in multiple ways. Seeing and hearing these families' stories gave her some perspective. One thing she observed while sitting with her twins in the NICU was many women who visited their babies alone and appeared to have no one to help them out as they navigated the turbulent world of the NICU. Watching these other situations every day gave Maggie a sense of gratitude for her outcome as well as for the support of her husband and family. She described her experience by saying,

> There were people and it did help me realize that there were people that had it a lot worse. I mean they are really clearly struggled you know. I remember there was this one set of twins. And the father would just not leave the daughter's side and the poor mother was very needy and wasn't getting any attention from him, and he just sat by his daughter's isolette the whole time. It was very strange. And I didn't feel like she got a lot of support. There were people that made me realize, wow, we are pretty fortunate.

Although her NICU experience was still upsetting, seeing these other families and a hurting mother whose husband was unable to give her the emotional support she needed to help her to evaluate the severity of her complaints and concerns. Although her situation was not what she had wanted or hoped for, she saw that it could have been far worse and this helped her to let go of some of her frustrations.

The idea of perspective taking is one of the major benefits of downward social comparison. In most situations, women were always able to identify at least one if not many women or families who had a worse experience or worse outcome. For many of the women, the experience of having a high-risk pregnancy or experiencing preterm labor was unexpected, unsettling and traumatic. Women spoke about how easy it was to get wrapped up in their own bad situations and becoming focused on everything that was hard and wrong. Seeing and hearing about women and babies who had even larger problems shifted women's focus from their own struggles and discomforts to others' hardships, which in turn altered their understanding of their situations. For many women, their situations were not ideal, no one wants a baby in the NICU, but they were better than someone else's situation and this knowledge helped them to find at least a few positives to be grateful for.

For example, Astrid, mother of triplets, was placed on complete bed rest at 19 weeks when her cervix started shortening and she remained on bed rest for 15 weeks until her delivery. She was allowed up to shower every third day and could use the bathroom, but otherwise she laid on her right side all day and night. Her days were filled with watching TV and surfing the internet and she tried to keep her mind occupied, but as any woman who has been on bed rest can tell you, lying in bed day after day is extremely difficult, and before long you start to feel like the walls are closing in on you. One way she coped whenever she started to feel really down was reading stories on the internet of women who had been admitted to the hospital for bed rest. Because she was doing well enough that she could remain at home and did not need constant monitoring or IV medication, she saw she was doing better than many women in similar situations, and this made her situation seem not as bad. Even though she did not leave her room for days at a time, she took comfort in the fact that she was in her home in the comfort of her own bed and not dealing with life in the hospital where she would be checked on throughout the day and night by nurses.

Another woman who benefited from comparing her situation to others was Heather who gave birth unexpectedly at 34 weeks to her second son. She had no complications prior to the delivery, so she was completely shocked by the early arrival of her son Tanner, and completely unprepared for his time in the NICU. She had a typical birth experience with her first son, and had a difficult time dealing with how different this second birth was. It was hard for her not being able to take him home from the hospital when she was discharged and each day she was anxious for him to be discharged. She was frustrated because it seemed like he was doing better as far as breathing and eating were concerned, and then he would have a setback which would keep him in the unit longer. As her son's time in the NICU passed she noticed other infants who had been there just a few days being discharged and this was hard as she was so upset that her son was in the hospital and not at home with her. After a while though, she also began to notice infants that had been in the NICU much longer than her son and were still in poor medical condition. In particular there was a baby boy who had been born at 25 weeks and was so sensitive to stimulation that his isolette had to be covered with a blanket and three weeks after his birth he still could not be held. Recognizing the struggles of these infants and families helped her to be more accepting of her situation. She explained that she was still sad that her son was in the NICU and was disappointed when his discharge date kept getting pushed back, but she also actively tried to appreciate how fortunate her family was for their son's relatively good health. She also watched the other parents who came day after day to visit their infants and seemed to have upbeat attitudes and tried to mimic their positive demeanors and strength. The birth of Heather's second son was very different than the birth of her first child and this upset her as she found the experiences to be so different. As she spent time with other mothers in the NICU and learned their stories, she slowly began to change the way she thought about her son's birth and his subsequent stay in the NICU. She still wanted Tanner home and was sad that he was born early, but she also began to find the things that were going well for Tanner in terms of his health and began to focus more on those positives. By learning more about what other mothers and babies had gone and were going through she gained a different understanding and acceptance of her situation. Although the birth of her son and his stay in the NICU was not ideal, it was the not the worst-case scenario either, and for that Heather chose to be thankful.

COMPARISON MAKES IT WORSE

The previous sections illustrated how one's natural inclination toward comparison can be a great tool for feeling better about a given situation as well as a way to foster hope and gain inspiration. Both upward and downward comparison can also have detrimental effects on one's well-being and emotional state though. Theodore Roosevelt once said that "comparison is the thief of joy" and for many women this is certainly the case. For example, a woman pregnant with twins who is placed on hospital bed rest at 28 weeks might hear the story of a mother also pregnant with twins who never had any activity restrictions and walked into her scheduled C-section at 39 weeks. In comparing herself to this woman with a very successful pregnancy outcome, the woman in the hospital may experience negative emotions if she perceives herself as falling short in comparison. Even though she is still pregnant, the knowledge that other women had better outcomes can lead to feelings of inadequacy, despair, and guilt. Another women whose baby is struggling to drink from a bottle may observe another baby in the NICU drinking away and feel more concern about her child's eating than she had previously.

Women experiencing a high-risk pregnancy will often compare themselves and their situations to women who experience a typical pregnancy, but more frequently they compare themselves to other women with high-risk pregnancies or who had preemies. This makes sense, as individuals tend to compare themselves to those who are similar to themselves (White et al. 2006; Festinger 1954). That being said, it is important to note that similarity is a fluid concept and an individual's conception of what is similar can change from situation to situation and can also change in order to suit one's needs. For example, a pregnant woman could find herself similar to any pregnant woman due to their pregnant status. However, if she is pregnant with her first child she might find herself dissimilar to a woman pregnant with her third child. Women can use their assessments of similarity and difference to their advantage. For example, a woman with an incompetent cervix may find several similarities with another woman with an incompetent cervix such as age or height who carried her pregnancy to 38 weeks, but find several differences between herself and another woman with an incompetent cervix who delivered at 26 weeks.

When some women began to have complications or delivered very early, they felt like they were suddenly surrounded by stories of other women with similar complications. Women inevitably made a comparison to see how they measured up and there were times when they felt that they fell short because they were not as successful in keeping their pregnancies going. Often women felt envious when they heard or read the stories of women who had experienced positive outcomes and these stories led them to question why some women had better outcomes than others. This is consistent with research that shows that people who engage in more frequent social comparisons, especially upward comparisons tend to be less happy and satisfied with themselves and more likely to have persistent feelings of envy and guilt (White et al. 2006). Catt, the mother of surviving twins who were born at 34 weeks, described meeting a woman pregnant with twins at one of her mothers of multiples club meetings. This woman came to a meeting when she was 38 weeks pregnant. Catt was happy for the woman, but at the same time she could not help but compare her own outcome with this woman's and the comparison left her feeling upset. She explained, "And I just sat there and was like, 'how did you?' And you know, that's horrible. It's like two and a half years later and I am like, 'that is so not fair." Meeting this woman led Catt to question why her own outcome, which included the loss of one of her triplets, was so different and seemingly so unfair. Catt's experience illustrates that often the comparisons do not stop after the pregnancy is over or even when one's babies get out of the NICU. Many preemie moms continue to think about their pregnancy and what went wrong long after the pregnancy and delivery, and whenever they hear about another mother with similar complications they almost automatically start to compare themselves to see how they compared in terms of weeks carried and the health issues of their children.

Another common emotional response to upward comparisons was guilt for not having a good outcome for the pregnancy and questioning one's abilities as a woman and a mother. Laurie, mother of identical twin boys, described her guilt over her difficulties with breastfeeding her sons. Not only was it hard for her physically, but she did not enjoy it and really had an overall lack of desire for doing it after her boys were born. She tried to breastfeed her sons while in the NICU and they struggled to latch so she pumped milk for them but had a hard time getting enough supply to keep them fed. I met Laurie when her twin boys were four years old and she still felt bad that she had not breastfed her sons. She explained, "there are plenty of people out there who breastfeed their twins with no problems, so I wondered what was wrong with me. I just never really wanted to do that. I was really happy to stop pumping at three months. . . . It never seemed natural for me. So you know, I felt guilty about that." Hearing or reading of other women who were easily able to breastfeed twins and enjoyed the process left Laurie feeling guilty. Even though she did not enjoy breastfeeding and her sons were perfectly healthy thriving boys, when she compared herself to women who breastfed twins until they were one or pumped for over ten months she felt that she had not been a good enough mother to her sons. Her regret stemmed not just from the fact that her sons were formula fed after three months, but primarily from the fact that she did not feel that her maternal instincts and abilities matched up to other women. Her story became one of regret because she felt that she should have been able to do better and that she should have had more of a maternal instinct about breastfeeding.

A common situation that sparked feelings of guilt in women was after their deliveries when they would meet someone or hear a story about another woman who had similar complications but was able to carry her baby or babies to a longer gestation. In comparing themselves and falling short, women began to feel guilt over what they had or had not done during their pregnancy that could have contributed to the early birth of their children. For example, Christine's daughter was born at 33 weeks after Christine's water broke unexpectedly. The more she has talked with other women who have carried infants to term after experiencing preterm labor she has begun to question the events leading up to her water breaking. Although her daughter is doing well now, she did have a four-week stay in the NICU. Specifically, Christine expressed guilt over possibly not recognizing the signs of premature labor. She often thinks back to the time shortly before her water broke and replays the events in her mind, trying to determine when she should have said something to her physician, and wondering if she would have been able to change the outcome.

One of the reasons it is important to look at how women engage in and respond to comparisons is because those comparisons can have such a strong influence on how they think about and make sense of their experiences and how they eventually tell their stories to themselves and others. When upward comparison resulted in negative emotion, women incorporated their guilt and disappointment in themselves into their stories as they described how their pregnancy had failed and the role they played in that failure. Helene, a mother of triplets born at 28 weeks, included in her story, "I totally felt like a failure after my kids were born at 28 weeks. I thought, I have failed them miserably." She knew that it was possible for women to carry triplets much further than 28 weeks and when she was unable to meet her goal of 34 weeks she constantly compared herself to other women who carried their triplets longer than she did and she always came up short leading to continued feelings of guilt and self-hatred.

Sometimes women found themselves comparing their infant's progress to other babies in the unit as they worked to get out of the NICU. Janet, mother of triplets, experienced envy when her triplets, who were born just prior to 32 weeks had a difficult time in the NICU as compared to the other babies she saw. She struggled with hearing stories about other premature infants who were born at the same gestation and were experiencing fewer complications than her triplets.

> Well, they told me they will probably be home around 35, 36 weeks, once they were born. You know they said once, they said plan on the due date, yeah, but you know realistically they come earlier, that is what I had seen all along. You know, I was seeing all these moms online that their babies were born about the same gestation as mine and they were all home, so it was like, what is wrong with my kids? Why can't they get it together?

She was upset that her infants were still struggling with basic issues such as eating and breathing when she knew about other infants born at 32 weeks who were released from the NICU after just three weeks. Her triplets had a lot of struggles and ongoing health issues and her triplets were discharged from the NICU after five, eight, and ten weeks. It was very difficult for her to have them in the NICU for so long and to have some home and some still in the hospital, and it seemed even more difficult when she heard about or observed other infants who were healthier and progressing more quickly.

Nikki was another mother who struggled when she compared her daughters' progress to other babies in the NICU. Nikki's identical twin girls suffered from twin-to-twin transfusion syndrome and were born at 33 weeks. The smaller of her twins was born with half of an arm missing due to amniotic band syndrome, a condition that had nothing to do with her being a twin or being born early, and then contracted necrotizing enterocolitis and had to undergo emergency surgery to have part of her bowel removed. Her daughter then endured a ten-week NICU stay while her larger twin sister suffered fewer complications and was discharged after just three weeks. The entire situation took an emotional toll on Nikki and she often felt as if her daughter was the sickest in the NICU and had been there the longest as she daily saw the other infants in the NICU get discharged. Because of this, Nikki sometimes found herself not wanting to hear about the other infants and families in the NICU whose problems were less severe than her own. "Like we saw everyone come in and go, come in and go, come in and go, and we were like, when is it our turn to go? When's it our turn to leave with our baby?" She commented specifically on a family who she had a hard time being around or hearing about. "There were a set of triplets in there, in the NICU with Clair that were going home with their parents. They were all like six pound kids and I'm like, go away." It seemed logical to Nikki that triplets would have a harder time than twins and that a twin mom should be able to carry her babies longer, but this was not the case, and often is not the case. Premature births rarely are logical or make sense. It was not that she wanted the other babies in the unit to be sick and struggle and she knew that any amount of the time spent in the NICU was difficult, but it was still frustrating to compare and the fact that other babies on the unit were stronger and healthier than her daughter made Nikki feel worse about her situation and jealous that they were not one of the families that had an easier time in the NICU.

One of the reasons that women sought out positive stories or others shared positive stories with them was because those stories provided the possibility of positive outcomes and provided a potential story that was hopeful for women who were living with uncertain and difficult situations. In hearing or reading positive stories, women were given access to the best possible scenarios. When their outcomes matched those stories it was great, but sometimes they did not. When their own scenarios did not match the positive stories they had encountered, many women came to understand their stories as negative and were not happy with their outcomes. Even when infants who were born early had good long-term results, women still compared themselves to others and cast the story of their pregnancies in a negative light as they continued to wish they could change the stories of the births of their children. In these cases, upward comparison resulted in women experiencing negative emotions such as guilt or sadness.

Comparing themselves to superiors and finding that they fell short was not the only way that comparison led to negative emotions. Earlier the chapter showed how downward comparisons could give women a sense of relief and encouragement as they saw that there outcome or circumstances were not the worst. Downward comparisons did not always have a boosting effect on women's emotions though. Several women talked about encountering stories of woman they perceived as having worse outcomes or experiences than themselves, and having a very negative emotional response to that story as they felt things like fear, sadness, and guilt. For example, sometimes women would see a television program that featured a traumatic story about preemies such as twins born at 25 weeks, weighing less than a pound each. Rather than having a boosting effect because her own situation was in some ways better, she would feel a deep sadness for the pain that family was going through, or experience fear as she worried that even if her current situation seemed better, there might be a possibility that her situation would take a turn for the worse. Sometimes a woman would see another family in the NICU whose child was struggling to fight off a life-threatening infection and she would be feel deep empathy and grief as she could all too closely relate to what this family was going through. Even if her own baby was not nearly as sick, she often knew how close she had come to having a very similar story to that family.

Downward comparisons that sparked fear frequently occurred during the beginning stages of women's high-risk pregnancies, close to their infants' births, or after receiving a negative diagnosis or news. For example, a woman in the beginning stages of preeclampsia might hear the story of a woman who was rushed to an early delivery at 26 weeks due to her preeclampsia. The woman who is still pregnant and hoping to continue her pregnancy as long as possible would hear this story and then be frightened about having a similar outcome. Similarly, a woman pregnant with twins might not have too many concerns until hearing a story from a friend about someone this friend knew whose twins were born eight weeks early after her water broke. When women were suddenly faced with stories with less than positive outcomes they were forced to confront the idea that things might not have a good outcome. This brings up the important issue of how much information women want and need when facing difficult medical situations.

For example, when Nikki learned at 18 weeks that her identical twin girls suffered from twin-to-twin transfusion syndrome, a potentially fatal condition in which one twin takes nutrients from the other, she had never heard of the condition. After learning of her diagnosis she quickly went home and jumped on the internet to find more information and quickly found the Twin-to-Twin Foundation website where several people had posted their stories about their twins. She explained the fear some of the stories aroused in her, "Well, the woman who created the foundation, she lost a baby to twin-to-twin. So reading her story was really scary and I tried, I tried to tell myself all of the measurements were coming out good and they were monitoring me very closely." The stories she read gave her several negative possibilities that she tried to negate with the positives of her own situation and her girls seemed to have a more mild case than the woman from the foundation, but the story and the possibilities were always in the back of her mind, and the fear never completely subsided.

Often, stories of those with poor outcomes such as very premature infants or the loss of a child evoked sadness and grief in the women. Many of the women felt deeply connected to other women who had experienced high-risk pregnancies and premature birth and were able to empathize with their pain and grief. Women knew they could have had similar outcomes and although they were grateful for their better situations, they were profoundly sad for the women and families who had not been as fortunate. Maggie, a mother of twins born at 33 weeks, recalled routinely being sad for other infants and families in the NICU, "Yeah, and you just feel really sad. I have great admiration for those nurses. I was there one evening when a baby died and that was obviously so hard for them. Just the whole atmosphere was just kind of somber for a while. I remember being so emotional. I think that was the hormones and everything. I was just a wreck." Hearing the stories with negative outcomes often reminded women of just how dangerous their pregnancies were and gave them a glimpse of what could happen. These stories helped them to understand the gravity of having a premature infant and they knew that it easily could have been them with the very sad story to tell.

Hearing stories about other preemies and high-risk pregnancies with not so great outcomes often results in conflicting emotions as women felt gratitude for the positives in their own stories, but they still experienced emotional distress over the sad stories they heard. Marie, the mother of triplets born at almost 35 weeks who used downward comparison to feel better about her situation, also found that the downward comparison also brought up feelings of sadness and grief. As 35-weekers, her daughters were some of the healthier babies in the unit who just needed to grow and learn how to eat before they could come home. In comparison, there were babies in the NICU who had already been there for months or who were looking at a lifetime of complications. The mixed emotions she felt were sometimes difficult to deal with and she told me, "to be honest, I was just so grateful that ours were so healthy compared to many of the babies that were in there. . . . I think I was just literally looking at wow, some of these babies are near a pound and I worry about them, but I was just so blessed and grateful for where we were and the doctors were telling us they're great, they are healthy." After seeing and learning the stories of these critical infants, Marie could not just put them from her mind and despite all that was going well for her, she could not be completely happy as she felt such a deep sense of sadness for the babies and parents around her that were dealing with so much and were experiencing such a great amount of pain and suffering.

Sometimes, hearing or reading the story of another woman with a poor outcome of her pregnancy made women feel guilty as they struggled to understand why such terrible things happened to some people. Some women described sitting in the NICU and seeing many infants and families that were worse off than their own and being filled with guilt over their good outcomes. Amy, mother of twin girls, described feeling guilty for complaining about her situation when she saw other sick infants in the NICU. A particular situation she remembers was being in the NICU one evening and see a group of people gather around one of the infants' isolettes to pray. Several of the people were crying and Amy knew that something was very wrong with that baby. She was so happy her twins were doing so well, but at the same time she felt terrible that other parents were feeling so much pain and felt guilty for complaining when she knew it was just a matter of time before her girls went home with her. She explained, "I would feel guilt at the same time, we would be like, 'Oh my god, we are so grateful.' You know because these other people are experiencing, you know unhealthy babies, going through whatever," so on one hand the downward comparisons prompted gratitude, but at the same time that gratitude was tinged with a mixture of guilt and sadness for those other families.

Ambrosia, the mother of triplets who clung to the story of healthy triplets to give her hope while she was pregnant, echoed these sentiments and described a sense of guilt that she described as being similar to survivor's guilt. She saw herself with three relatively healthy infants next to families who had one infant who died or with one infant weighing just over a pound who had constant medical emergencies. She recalled hearing Kate Gosselin, mother of sextuplets who had her own reality TV show on TLC, describe her guilt that she had six infants who were born at 30 weeks and were doing well while other families in the NICU went home without a child. After her triplets were born she understood Gosselin's feelings. She and other women felt guilt over their good fortune as compared to others. This guilt also prompted women to lessen their complaining and feelings of self-pity as they tried to appreciate the positives of their situations. Even though these women still had babies in the NICU and had often endured hard pregnancy and labors, they still saw themselves as the fortunate ones as compared to many other people they came across, and they sometimes felt as if they did not have the right to complain because other people had such larger problems to face.

Due to the open format of many NICUs, women were easily able to observe and hear the stories of the other patients in the NICU. When they encountered a particularly sad or troubling story, many of the women found themselves saddened, concerned, and wishing they could do something to help. A situation that frequently troubled women was infants who appeared to have none or very infrequent visits from their parents. Women described being in the NICU day after day and seeing infants who never had a parent by their bedside or who had a mother who only came to visit once a week for about an hour or so. Jessica, mother of triplet boys, described her concern for other infants in the NICU, "there were babies where no one ever came to visit and I would ask, like can I hold this baby? It was heartbreaking." Another mother Nicole described her NICU which was in an inner city hospital. All visitors to the NICU actually had to go through a metal detector before they were able to enter. Several of the babies in the unit were drug addicted babies who either never had visitors from their parents or they had been taken away and become wards of the state. Babies born addicted to meth, crack, and heroine had to be kept in the dark and receive as little stimulation as possible as even a soft voice or a touch was too much for their impaired nervous systems to handle. She described how the drug addicted babies would just cry and cry and her heart would break for the lonely babies who were in pain and could not be comforted. One day she was sitting next to her daughter and overheard nurses talking about a set of twins that were in the same pod. They had been cleared to be discharged from the NICU and the nurses were having a hard time contacting the parents so that they would come and pick their children up.

Nicole, wasn't just sad for these babies, but she was mad for them. She described the NICU where her daughter was, "eight babies were in drug withdrawal. Those were the mothers who I wanted to reach across and kill. They took everything for granted. They could have prevented their child from being in there." It was so hard for Nicole to accept that when she had tried so hard to stay pregnant and would have done anything to give her daughter even one more day in the womb, that there were women who did not take care of themselves and abused their bodies with drugs and caused their children to be born not only early, but also drug addicted and in pain.

Another thing women saw that was hard on them emotionally was incredibly young mothers or mothers who did not appear to have the ability or means to care for their children. One of the things that puts women at a higher risk for premature birth is being under the age eighteen, and this accounted for many of the young teenage mothers with babies in the NICU. Women who were older when they had their preemies or were married often wondered how a teenage girl could possibly cope with having a premature baby when they themselves were struggling so much to cope with the NICU and having a preemie. Anna, whose son Ryan was born at 30 weeks was often taken aback by the things she saw and heard from the young mothers in the NICU. She once overheard a teenager asking a nurse how much marijuana exposure she could have before it would go into her breast milk. The nurse of course told her that she should completely avoid using any type of drug, but Anna worried for the baby and wondered how good of care this mother would really be able to provide. There was another mother who was just 16 and was having a very difficult time with breastfeeding. One day she was working with one of the nurses. The girl's mother was there and told her daughter that she had better figure out how to do it quick, because there was no way she could afford formula once the baby was discharged from the hospital. Again, Anna felt deep sympathy for this young girl who was clearly not ready to be a mother and for the baby who was going to be raised by a young girl without a lot of resources.

The comparison game does not stop for most women once they leave the NICU because now women found themselves frequently comparing the progress of their children to other preemies as well as babies and children born full term. Almost any parent, not just the parent of a preemie, can tell you how easy it is to compare children and their development even though they have been told countless times that you cannot or at least should not compare children. The human instinct though is to compare, especially when a situation is new or uncertain, and raising a preemie was usually a very new and uncertain experience for women. Not knowing what to expect made women more likely to look to other mothers and children to try to gauge how well or poorly they were doing in terms of raising a preemie and coping with the challenges as well as how their child was doing.

A major concern for many preemie parents is that their children are not meeting their developmental milestones as failure to meet this can be indicators of larger problems. Until preemies are two-years-old physicians and therapists use a child's adjusted age to assess their development. Adjusted age calculates a child's age based on his or her due date, so a baby who was born at 32 weeks would have an adjusted age of two months when he was four months old. Even accounting for adjusted age though, many premature infants still struggle to meet milestones for a variety of reasons including being a multiple, having spent a long time in the NICU, having brain bleeds, or having other health issues, and some parents find this to be very stressful. Parents know in their minds that it is normal for their child to be behind, but that does not stop them from comparing their children to other children and being upset when the comparisons fall short.

Yvette was a mother who talked to me a lot about the ongoing challenges of raising her twins. She was hospitalized at 24 weeks during her twin pregnancy and spent the next 22 days in the hospital on an IV magnesium sulfate to slow her labor. When her daughter Madison's heart rate started dropping and not returning to normal she had an emergency C-section at 27 weeks and her twins were born. Her son Joshua weighed 2 pounds 1 ounce and Madison was the complete opposite weighing just 1 pound 2 ounces. After a long stay in the NICU Joshua came home and ten days later he was joined by his sister. The twins are now four and as Yvette explains when you look at them they look like perfectly normal, healthy preschoolers, but what you cannot see until you spend some time with them is their moderate to severe delays in their speech, fine motor skills, and gross motor skills. Her daughter Madison also has severe sensory processing disorder. Yvette spends a lot of her time working with her twins and taking them to therapy and to the special preschool program they qualified for due to their delays. In speaking with Yvette it was obvious how much she loves her children, but also how difficult it sometimes is.

She explained that she does not go to a lot of playgroups or outings with other moms with typically developing children anymore because it is too hard for her emotionally. When she had gone to groups in the past, it felt like the entire time she was there she would see what her children's peers could do and for her it was just a way to point out all of the things her kids were not doing yet such as being potty trained or riding a bike. She also found herself comparing her day-to-day life with the other mothers and found it hard to relate to the things they were complaining about. She did not want to discount their problems and concerns, but often she found their complaints minor compared to the daily struggles her children faced and she spent a lot of time wishing that she could have their problems instead of the problems she deals with on a daily basis.

Another mom talked about how difficult it was when she started comparing her daughter's progress and development with her nieces and nephews who had all been born full term. One particular challenge her daughter had was her eating as she had a very poor suck reflux and therefore took almost 45 minutes to finish a bottle. She tried not to get upset when she watched her sister's baby gulp down a bottle, but it was hard because it emphasized that her daughter still had issues from her prematurity. She also found her family was constantly comparing her daughter's size to her cousin who was born a few months later and she found the comparisons frustrating as she had to constantly remind her family and herself that her daughter was a preemie and was still working to catch up on the growth curve.

Keeping Quiet

Women were very aware of the types of comparing they did and how it made them feel, and because of this, many became more in tune to how the stories they told about their own experiences might influence other women. Women who had stories with poor outcomes such as losing one or more of their infants due to complications of prematurity or giving birth prior to 30 weeks recognized that those who were experiencing a high-risk pregnancy or were having signs of premature labor might be upset by their stories and tried not to frighten another woman unnecessarily. Helene, whose triplets were born at 28 weeks, described how she avoided sharing too many details of her pregnancy with those who were still pregnant with twins or triplets. She felt that her story would be upsetting and instead she chose to encourage women by telling them of other women she knew who had carried their infants for a long time.

No matter what type of comparison women engaged in, downward or upward, they often wanted to find women and situations that most closely matched their own. Women often sought out stories from women that they saw as similar to themselves believing that similar women might have similar outcomes. Astrid, mother of triplets, described very specifically the kinds of stories she looked for, "I want to follow somebody who is in the same situation I'm in. I'm looking to find the same thing, for the medicine that I'm on." When she found stories with similarities she could more easily take information from the stories and apply it to her own situation. Janet, another mother of triplets, who also had an older son, described trying to find other mothers on message boards she visited who had an older child as she wanted to see how these women coped with their high-risk pregnancies while still attending to the needs of their older children. When she read stories of women who were on strict bed rest, but had no other children at home, she tended to discount what they said and its utility to her as these women did not have the same obligations and needs to be as mobile as possible for their other children. Jodi, who was 38 when she was pregnant with her twins, belonged to online fertility groups for women over 35. Sharing stories with other women of advanced maternal age who were struggling with infertility was useful to Jodi as the women in the group had similar concerns and she wished she had belonged to a similar group during her pregnancy. Other mothers described trying to find women with similar features such as height, weight, and number of total pregnancies. In general, the more similar other women were, the better.

All of the stories and research reports in this chapter have demonstrated that women are constantly comparing their own experiences to those they heard and read about and making assessments of how their pregnancies were progressing based on those comparisons. The ways their stories compared to the stories they heard or read influenced the stories they told. Women's roles changed as they saw themselves as heroes, protagonists, victims, and even villains. The overall tone of their stories changed as well from positive to negative and at other times from negative to positive depending on the results of the comparison.

It is important to note that these narrative comparisons had both positive and negative results as is consistent with Social Comparison Theory (Festinger 1954). One practical application of this is to be cautious in the tendency to purposely give women stories to compare themselves to as a common form of social support. For example, many women and their friends and family thought that hearing success stories of other women or stories of very premature infants would be motivating and boost their morale. Interestingly, the results of the comparisons were not always what the storytellers or listeners anticipated. A common event that many women recalled being told stories of one-pound infants who survived or of women who were on bed rest for 18 weeks and gave birth to full-term infants. These upward comparisons, of women and infants who had beaten the odds were intended to be a source of inspiration. However, some women had the opposite reaction. Rather than feeling inspired or more hopeful, women found the stories depressing, frightening, or even as a condemnation of themselves. Some women did not want to think about the possibility of having an infant born so early and hearing a story about an infant born at 25 weeks made that possibility all too real. Other women found themselves discouraged and angry at themselves for having such difficulties carrying their infants to full term when they heard stories about other women who did not have the same struggles. The miracle and success stories at times invoked an opposite reaction than was intended or expected by those who were hearing, reading, or telling the stories.

Many of the comparisons women made to the other stories they heard and read assisted them in characterizing themselves and defining their role in the story. Often it was important for women to see themselves and have others see them as the "good mother" character. When women's bodies struggled to carry their infants to a safe gestation, they felt less like a good mother as they saw it as their responsibility to provide a safe and healthy start for their infants. These feelings often were exacerbated when they heard or read of other women who were able to carry their infants longer. For example, many of the mothers of triplets mentioned hearing stories about women who delivered close to 36 weeks and were able to bring their infants home from the hospital. This caused women to question why their own bodies were struggling and they often judged themselves harshly for what they saw as their personal failure. Women struggled to see themselves as good mothers when their infants were born too early and often cast themselves as villains in the stories finding fault with themselves and blaming themselves for their outcomes. Women felt they were at fault for the premature delivery because they believed they should have been stronger or more in control of their bodies to keep their infants gestating longer.

Women who deliver prematurely need constant reassurance that they did all they could to keep their infants as healthy as possible. This reassurance can come from medical staff, spouses, family, and friends. Physicians or nurses could take time to explain to women why they delivered early and during the explanation reiterate that it was not the women's fault. Additionally, the exemplar stories should be prefaced as that, exemplars. These stories do represent the best-possible outcomes, but they are rare stories. For every story about women pregnant with triplets heard or read about a woman delivering triplets at 36 weeks, there were dozens more about women delivering triplets at much earlier gestations. Women may need help keeping their situations in perspective and assistance in understanding the physical factors that lead to their early deliveries. Many women tended to find fault with themselves, even when forces outside their control were responsible for their early deliveries.

Interestingly, none of the women judged other women whose outcomes were not as positive as their own. Instead they expressed feelings of sorrow and pity for women whose infants were born at very early gestations. Women did not fault these women for their weak cervixes or irritable uteruses, however, women did not have the same nonjudgmental attitude when they considered their own situations. When telling their own stories, some women cast themselves in a villain role as they placed the blame for their situations on themselves and believed that something that they did or did not do was the cause of their premature labor and delivery. Women should be encouraged to consider how they positively judged other women in similar situations and apply the same understanding and sympathy to themselves. This encouragement could come from family, friends, and medical personnel. In addition, books written about high-risk pregnancies and premature births should include a section about the need for self-forgiveness. In terms of downward comparisons, this could improve women's mood, but, having faced similar fears and challenges, women could empathize with other mothers who had poor or tragic outcomes and could easily put themselves into these mothers' place. Women could easily imagine having similar experiences and at times this made it difficult to hear or read others' stories. Many women also knew how close they had been to being involved in a story of a tragedy and this added to their grief. Women also may need help letting go of the survivor's gift as well as may need to find positive ways to channel their empathy for less fortunate families and infants by doing things such as serving as a parent mentor or even writing encouraging notes to women on bed rest or other NICU moms.

The big takeaway from looking at the ways in which women compare themselves, their children, and their stories to others is twofold. First, comparisons resulted in both positive and negative affect. Not only did comparisons affect women's emotional state, but the comparisons also developed women's understandings of their experiences and in turn shaped the stories they told. One of the ways that the negative stories women heard and read became integrated into women's stories was that they added an element of fear and sadness. Many of the women were privy to firsthand accounts of the terrible things that could happen when an infant was born too early or when infants were born with serious medical conditions. These negative stories tempered some of the excitement and joy women expressed over being pregnant as they knew that a positive outcome was not guaranteed. The comparisons they made sometimes inspired fear in woman. Finally, women were saddened as they empathized with women who had been through such difficult time and this sadness crept into their own stories in giving them an extreme sense of gratitude, but also an awareness of just how difficult and hard life can be.

Chapter 6

Tell Me More. . .But Wait, Don't

When Janet learned she was pregnant with triplets she was both shocked and happy. She and her husband had been doing fertility treatments because they had been unable to conceive on their own, so she was overwhelmed by the thought of three babies, but also incredibly happy that she was pregnant. One of the first things she did when she got home after that first ultrasound was to go online and start searching for information about triplets and triplet pregnancies. During her search she quickly found the website Triplet Connection and started reading the posts on the message forums to learn more about what the future might hold. Janet had an older son who been born full term, so this was a completely new world to her. She had no idea how this pregnancy would differ from her first or what having babies in the NICU would be like. In an effort to prepare herself for her triplets arrival, she tended to read anything she could find, even when it was sad or frightening. When she spoke about reading others' stories and gathering information she told me, "I actually felt more empowered when I was reading it because I was learning more about what actually happens to triplet moms versus reading what a general pregnancy with a singleton would go through. I thought that a triplet mom would have a different experience so I liked reading about that." Even when something was upsetting or caused her anxiety she still read it because she wanted to know what different people had gone through and what kinds of complications people experienced. Because she desired so much information, her research included stories and information about micropreemies, children with disablities and women who lost one or more of their children. For her it was about being prepared for anything that could happen. She of course read a lot of positive stories with great outcomes, but she also thought that if she read about the negative things that people experienced she would not be completely caught off guard when something happened. With this mentality she researched every possiblity and did not avoid or censoe any information she came across. She of course hoped for the best and tried to remain positive, but she also felt like she needed to know what she might be facing. When her triplets were born at 32 weeks she felt at least somewhat prepared for the different issues they faced in the NICU as she had read about the different complications and was at least familiar with what the conditions were, the terminology used to describe them, and some of the treatments for Janet, all information whether positive or negative was welcome as the more information she had the more in control she felt.

After meeting and talking with countless women, I have found that when it comes to finding more information about high-risk pregnancies and the risks of prematurity, there tend to be three types of women. The first are information consumers who look up as much information as they can find, wanting to know anything and everything. The second are the information avoiders who actively try not to expose themselves to too much information and essentially operate on a need-to-know basis, figuring that if information is relevant and pertinent they will hear about it or seek facts about it, but otherwise they do not actively seek out information about what could go wrong. The third type are women who are in the middle and seek out certain types of information while actively avoiding others. In talking with all of these types of women it becomes obvious that their information seeking and avoiding behaviors are very much a coping strategy and there are benefits and drawbacks to all of these methods. The costs and benefits of being exposed to information leads to an interesting tension between having enough information to be adequately informed and aware, but also not having so much information that women experience stress anxiety, and information overload.

The information consumers are women who described themselves as being open to all information and stories. In addition to not avoiding information, these women actively sought out information because they believed having as much information as possible helped them to be aware of what was happening and what could happen. Having knowledge made women feel more in control, in what were often out of control situations. Astrid, mother of triplets, was a mother who was open to getting as much information as possible and spent a lot of her time once she learned she was pregnant finding as much information as she could. She explained, ". . .maybe I have a morbid sense of curiosity, but I read it all. Oh yeah, I wanted to know the possibilities of everything that could be. . . . I wanted to know it all. I wanted to see it all." She read stories about triplets who had passed away and premature infants with severe complications because she wanted to mentally prepare herself for any possible outcomes. Although she described herself as someone who was very determined to have a successful outcome and had a very positive attitude about her pregnancy, she was also a realist, in part because she had miscarried an earlier pregnancy at 19 weeks. She had experienced firsthand one of the worst possible outcomes of a pregnancy and wanted to prepare herself for the possible outcomes of her current pregnancy.

Women who actively sought out stories attempted to get as many types of stories from as many sources as possible. One of the primary sources women mentioned when asked where they went for information was medical personnel, usually their phsyicans, neonatologists, or nurses. They referred to literature they were given at their physicians' offices as well as different advice and orders they were given about their pregnancies or the care and treatment of their premature infants. Women tended to focus on the factual information they were given as far as risks, probabilities, and procedures when it came from their doctors but women did report that their physicians would often would share stories of other women and families when giving advice or explaining their reasoning behind their recommendations. For example, many of the physicians shared stories with their patients of other patients with good and poor outcomes and discussed how different treatment options had worked for prior patients. Women who were unsure about having certain procedures such as a cerclage or different treatment options such as progesterone shots were often presented with stories of other patients who had the procedure and how the procedure worked. These stories helped women to make better sense of what was sometimes confusing information full of complex medical terms and percentages and statistics.

In terms of information in general, many women commented that they relied on their physicians more than they generally would due to the high-risk nature of their pregnancies. With so much at stake, they tried to follow medi cal orders and felt they had to put their trust in those taking care of them and their infants. Women generally deferred to medical advice and orders unwilling to take any additional risks or to follow the advice of friends and family as they might have if they were having a typical pregnancy. With the stakes so high, in many cases life and death, women found themselves relying on those with the most medical expertise. This finding is unique because studies report that up to 40 percent of patients do not fully comply with physician orders (DiMatteo 1994; DiMatteo and Lepper 1998; Resnik 2005; Robinson et al. 2008; Smith et al. 2005; Vermeire et al. 2001). It is important to note that the strict adherence to medical orders is quite possibly limited to the women I met and spoke with as there are certainly many women who deliver prematurely who do not follow doctor's advice and suggestions, as is evidenced by the larger number of infants who are born prematurely due to lack of prenatal care or the mother's smoking or other drug abuse.

Women's strict adherence to medical advice is desirable as adherence to medical orders is linked to better health outcomes (Berntrop 2009; Fuertes, Boylan, and Fontanella 2009). Because women rely so heavily on their physicians, it is important for them to have an open and good working relationship with their physicians so they feel comfortable asking questions and raising concerns. Women who do not feel they can talk with and question their physicians should be encouraged to find physicians with whom they feel comfortable and can build a sense of trust. One concern that women had when selecting a physician was whether or not to see or consult with a physician who specialized in high-risk pregnancies. While some obstetricians will automatically refer patients to a high-risk doctor if the scope of complication is beyond his or her expertise, some physicians leave that decision to the patient and some doctors will work with a high-risk specialist who will consult on different issues. Having access to information about the different types of physicians could assist women in choosing medical care. This information could be provided by women's general obstetricians or in some cases by their reproductive endocrinologists if a woman was doing fertility treatments. It is most often these physicians who make the initial diagnosis of a high-risk pregnancy and could provide information to help women make decisions as to how to proceed with their medical care. In addition, information about the types of physicians who specialize in high-risk pregnancies as well as information about specific physicians and practices in an area could be posted on internet sites women might consult after diagnosis.

Women often felt that they had to rely on their physicians because there circumstances were so unique and they had no other resources to turn to for advice. Cynthia, mother of twins, turned to her physicians when she learned she was pregnant with quadruplets and was making a decision about whether or not to reduce the pregnancy to twins or triplets. The stories her physicians told her were especially important for her because she did not feel comfortable discussing the issue of reduction with even her closest friends and family as she feared their judgment. She did not know anyone in her personal life who had been in a situation to make a similar decision, so she had no one to talk to and hear their stories. Having only her physician to rely on for stories and information about reduction and the potential outcomes of a quadruplet pregnancy concerned Cynthia as she felt like she was only hearing one side of the story which was the medical side that focused primarily on the risks and complications of a quadruplet pregnancy. Most of the stories her doctors told her painted a pretty bleak picture of the outcomes of a quadruplet pregnancy. She did make the decision to reduce her pregnancy to twins, and after the procedure she was comfortable with her decision and is happy that her twins were born full term. She does wonder though if she would have had made the same decision to reduce had she been able to read or hear more stories from other mothers of higher order multiples, especially those with healthy children and successful outcomes to balance out the more negative stories her doctor told her.

Women who spent an extended amount of time in the hospital prior to giving birth or whose infants had spent had a lengthy stay in the NICU were the most likely to talk about hearing stories from hospital and medical staff as they had the most interaction with them. Donna is a mom whose twin sons were born prematurely. One of her sons, Daniel, spent five months in the NICU due to a variety of birth defects. During this time she developed a relationship with many of her son's nurses and learned about former and current patients in the NICU. "I was at Children's Hospital for a good five months and because I had seen a lot and had really gotten to know the staff, they would always tell me things about other people's babies." Hearing the stories of other infants in the NICU helped Donna to put her son's challenges into perspective and reminded her that she was not the only mother who had experienced such trauma. She had access to these stories because of her prolonged interaction with the NICU staff and the relationships that she built with them.

Because of the amount of time women spent with the nursing staff both before and after delivery, nurses became an important source of stories about other women and preemies. Several women were surprised to learn that many of their nurses had themselves been through a high-risk or difficult pregnancy and had experience with being on bed rest or having an infant in the NICU. Hearing these stories was reassuring to the women as they felt both an emotional connection to their nurses because they felt that their nurses had an intimate knowledge of what they were going through. Some women told me that learning of what their nurses had been through made them seem even more empathetic and relatable. Many women also thought that nurses' personal experience with preemies and high-risk pregnancies made them better nurses, especially when it came to working with and teaching parents. It was also encouraging to women to hear some of the nurses' stories and then hear about how well their children were now doing and to see firsthand that people survived the NICU experience.

Sometimes women knew medical personnel personally outside of the hospital environment, and although they were not treating the women, the women still listened to their stories and considered them to be a valuable resource given their medical background and training. Women sometimes trusted friends or family with medical backgrounds more than their other friends and family when it came to taking advice. When asked about who she went to for information, Christine, whose daughter Anna was born at 32 weeks, mentioned some women she knew who were nurses, "And then my friends Laura and Cara are both OB nurses so I turned to them right at first and I kind of communicated to them via e-mail. I felt like I had a lot of really good resources." Even though she trusted her other friends and enjoyed hearing their stories, her friends Laura and Cara were seen as the best sources because of their nursing experience. Even though this may seem obvious that someone might trust someone with a medical background more than someone without, it points to the fact that not all stories are equal and neither are all information sources and the teller of a story can influence how a woman will respond to and use that story.

Although physicians and nurses were the most frequently mentioned source of information, for many women, the stories they heard from medical personnel were not enough and they sought out additional information about everything from pregnancy symptoms to how to feed a preemie. When asked where they went for extra information almost every woman laughed as she answered, "Google." The internet was an invaluable resource and tool for women as they could use Google or another search engine to conduct searches, to find webpages, forums, blogs, and articles. It is sometimes hard to believe that less than 20 years ago, in 1998, Google was first introduced to the public and it completely transformed the ways people find and use information. Prior to the explosion of the internet women had to rely on their physicans, books, and family and friends for information. Now women can access everything from articles from medical journals to popular websites to find almost anything they are looking for. The use of interenet for information and support during pregnancy is of course not unique to women who have high-risk pregnancies. The Listening to Mothers III survey, a survey conducted by Childbirth Connection, an organization dedicated to assisting women and physicians in making informed maternity care decisions, reported that 82 percent of pregnant women access the interent for pregnancy-related information at least once a week. Smart phones have allowed women to access information at anytime no matter where they are and two-thirds of pregnant women reported using their phones to access information at least weekly. Women listed the most valuable source or information as pregnancy-related sites such as What to Expect or personal blogs followed closely by forums, sites with online videos, Facebook, and Wikipedia. In addition to actively searching for information, 67 percent of women signed up for weekly email updates from sites like Babycenter.com that were tailored for their pregnancy based on their due dates (Corry 2013).

The reasons and advantages that all women in the survey listed for using the interent were very similar to those mentioned by women with a high-risk pregnancy when I asked them why they used the internet. The number one advantage of the interent was the flexibility it offered. Women could access information when they wanted to and process the information at their own pace. They did not have to wait for a physician's office to return a call or make a trip to the library or bookstore to get a book. The internet provided support and reassurance, especially between medical visits. When a new symptom developed, a quick internet search could let women know if it was normal or something more serious. Another huge advantage women noted is that the internet is free as opposed to books that had to be purchased. Some women questioned purchasing a book when they could get so much information for free online. While it was not mentioned as frequently, some women appreciated that they could be anonymous if they wanted when asking questions or reaching out to others especially if their questions were extremely personal. The information women found most often validated and clarified what their doctors had told them and sometimes relieved some of their anxiety when they found stories that showed them that a symptom was normal or someone with a similar complication had a positive outcome. It also made women feel more empowered when they were making decisions and their increased knowledge of complications and treatment options helped them to ask more informed questions (Lagan, Sinclair, and Kernohan 2011).

In addition to allowing women to ask better questions, the information and stories they found also helped them to feel more informed about their pregnancies and their progress. Jodi, mother of twins, described her use of the internet during her pregnancy, "I spent way too much time on the computer. You just, you are just going through everything online. To see what was going to happen and where they were in their development. Gauging what the ultrasound said with what the internet said and just following along and making sure they were developing like they should." The information and stories she found on the internet gave her comfort and also gave her medical information she did not know. When she found other stories of women pregnant with twins it gave her something to compare her experiences to and with those comparisons she felt she was better able to monitor her own pregnancy. When her own experiences matched those that she read on the internet she felt more secure that her pregnancy was progressing well.

Stacy, mother of twins, explained that she got a lot of helpful information from her physician's office, but used the internet as a source of supplemental information, "The doctor's office is pretty good about providing information, but I got a lot of stuff off the internet and in books. I looked everywhere and then my husband would get worried and told me to stop because I would see the worst. I wanted to know what all of the possibilities were for me. I can deal with it." Like some of the other mothers, Stacy wanted to have as much information and knowledge as possible, even if the information was negative or frightened her. She did not want to be blindsided by any complications and the internet gave her access to all of the possible stories both good and bad. Her husband, however, did not fully appreciate her quest for knowledge as he felt that some of the extreme stories she found on the internet were not helping her to become prepared, but instead were unnecessarily scaring her and increasing her anxiety, which points to one of the potential downsides of consuming too much information.

Even though there was the potential to encounter information that would be upsetting or frightening, many women commented that one of the positives or benefits of using the internet and its information was that they were able to feel some control as they gathered information, read stories, and tried to assess the status of their pregnancies. Women could be selective in what types of information they searched for and had complete control over what sites they visited and what sites they did not. Michelle, mother of triplets, talked about why she preferred to gather information on the internet rather than watching TV, "I just kind of felt like it [television] was kind of outside my realm. It's not like online. Online you can choose what you read." If women started to read an article or story that frightened or disturbed them they could navigate away from the page with the click of a mouse button. Even though they could turn the TV off or stop reading once a story became upsetting, in the internet through searching and reading page titles, women felt like they had more control and could avoid a negative story entirely. Searches for successful pregnancy outcomes and positive stories of preemies were a great way to filter out some of the more negative information out there.

Having access to the internet also meant that women could be informed about their medical treatments and options and could do research on their own when trying to make health-related decisions. While pregnant with her triplets after previously losing her twin boys at 18 weeks, BethAnn used the internet to find any information she could that might help her continue her pregnancy and that would help her to be the best advocate for herself and her children. She laughs now to think about what her doctor must have thought as she was constantly suggesting different treatments and procedures to him. At one point he had to tell her that she needed to check the dates of what she was finding after she told him about a study that was over fifteen years old. For her though, the research and information seeking kept her mind busy and it helped her to feel a small amount of control over an incredibly uncertain situation. Even if her research simply confirmed her doctor's suggestions she felt better knowing that she had done her own investigation and she felt more confident in her doctor's treatment plan when it was backed up by the research she did.

Many of the women who had been pregnant within the past ten years mentioned internet forums as an important source of information and stories during their pregnancies. Women who had been pregnant more than ten years ago mentioned using forums as a source of information far less frequently than women who had been pregnant more recently. They explained that when they were pregnant the internet and forums were not as popular as they currently are. For example, Denise, whose triplets are now fifteen-years-old, explained that she did not even have internet access at her house until her triplets were a year old, so during her pregnancy when she was on strict bed rest the internet was not even an option. Similarly, Beth who spent over 20 weeks on bed rest and delivered her daughter in 1996, said that the internet was something she only used at work and the social aspect of the internet had not really started to take off, so she never even thought to go online and look for things like forums. As the prevalence of online forums grew, they gave women increased access to conversations and stories. Women were able to connect with women from all over the country and world, ask questions, and read about situations other women and children experienced, and perhaps most invaluably, and find women with similar experiences.

Donna, mother of twins and quadruplets, talked about how she came to appreciate and use forums when she was pregnant with her quadruplets. The forum she most often used was connected with the MOST (Mothers of Super Twins) organization. In order to access the forums, members had to enroll and pay a $20 membership fee. She initially balked at the cost until she spoke with another woman in her obstetrician's office who highly recommended joining the group. Donna followed her advice and remained an active member of MOST and even became a moderator for one of the forums. For her, the most helpful stories she found on the forums were one's that showed her that life with multiples was possible. She said what she read the most were stories that showed her, "there a lot of people who are surviving and thriving and loving it. There are people who have done this and survived. You know, this is what you are going to have to go through." Because members had to pay to comment she found that members were more dedicated and committed to belonging and supporting each other than other forums she had been on. The moderators here also seemed to do a good job of stopping any fighting or spreading of false information.

Another mother, Kiera, mother of surviving triplets described how message boards were an important way for her to learn about others' situations and how they dealt with the daily stresses of having multiples and preemies, "There are message boards I go on. One for same age triplets and quads which is all moms that have a 2 year-old and a two-and-a-half year old triplets and quads. And we're also really active, actually about four of the moms are here in Atlanta so I have actually met at least one of them in person through that. After Zoe died, that was also the first place I went was looking for a message board for bereaved mothers of multiples." At one point in the interview Kiera commented that her husband and grief counselor felt she spent too much time on the internet and were encouraging her to seek out more face-to-face relationships. For Kiera though, she preferred the internet as she was able to connect with so many people from all over the world and was easily able to connect with people who could relate to her life and experiences. Having triplets and then losing one after the first year is hardly a common experience, so she needed to go online to find people who had similar stories. She could also interact with others on her own time when she most needed it and when she was most feeling up to it. This part was critical for Kiera. Some days she woke up and did not have the time or mental energy to deal with others but when she was ready to engage and seek our support it was right at her fingertips.

Even though the internet offered a wealth of information and potential support, spending too much time on the internet and becoming upset by information they found was a common experience of many mothers. Jana is a mother of twins, but also has an adopted daughter who is only eight months older than her twins, so she often felt more like a triplet mom than a twin mom. She spoke highly of the message forum Triplet Connection, but also commented on some of the negative ramifications of her reading,

> So those [forums] are really helpful on some hands and of course you can't help but be gravitated to the grief stories or the stories of preemies that are born at different degrees. What constantly freaked me out was you would have stories of people's babies being born at 27 weeks and them doing great and then some being born at 30 weeks and having one or two pass away. So the variability in that information caused me a lot of anxiety. So finally my husband told me around 30 or 32 weeks, you are not allowed on the internet anymore because nothing good is coming of this and this is not helping you.

Her story points to one of the concerns the ability to access so much information presents. Having access to so many stories can be overwhelming to women, especially when as Jana pointed out, the stories contain so much variation. Stories with negative outcomes and complications existed next to hopeful and positive stories and trying to sort through all of those stories and figure out how they might apply or relate to one's own situation can be incredibly stressful and confusing. For women like Jana, the negative tales caused an overwhelming sense of fear as there was so little she could do to control her outcome and there was no way of knowing if her eventual story would be on the more positive or negative side.

Marie, mother of triplets, described using online forums to gather information about her pregnancy and raising triplets, "I probably went to the message boards at thebump.com the most. So there are the multiples board there and that is where I would say I got the majority of my information or they would direct me to other boards or other websites or books to read." She commented about the kinds of information and stories she sought out on forums,

> I think I used the message boards for you know materials, equipment, items that you need, schedule, kind of mommy things but as far as the pregnancy, I was really kind of a doctor's girl. I trusted my doctor totally and I listened to him. It

> is not that I didn't listen to the women on the boards but it's kind of like, but I definitely listened to my doctor about major, especially about activity level that I got really involved.

Like many women, she valued the opinion of her physician when it came to serious medical matters. Although she appreciated the stories she read on the message boards and found the general information about raising babies helpful as the advice was coming from women with actual experience, she deferred to her doctor when it came to setting guidelines for her pregnancy because she recognized and respected his expertise and authority.

One of the benefits of forums or message boards over just general web pages, is that women could ask specific questions or search for posts regarding the concerns or issues they had. Christine, mother of triplet girls, had concerns over her daughters being born prematurely and suffering from long-term disabilities. She used the internet to find the Triplet Connection forums and tried to find stories that would provide answers to her concerns. She explained, "I was specifically looking for like, okay, these people got through this, and even after they're born they're not, they seem like they're fine, but you're not sure, there could be delays down the road or whatever." Christine was very fearful that her daughter might have issues that she would not be aware of until they were older and starting school. She knew that preemies were at a higher risk for things like autism and learning disabilities, so when she came across women with older children who either were doing fine or had some issues she wanted to know things like, "How much did they weigh? How long were they in the NICU?" On forums, Christine was able to read the stories and get answers from women whose infants were older now and could speak personally about the issue of long-term complications. Stories about preterm infants and multiples who were healthy, happy children with no issues due to their prematurity gave her some hope and a reason to feel optimistic.

Searching for and reading the stories on forums was also a way for women to prepare themselves for potential outcomes and complications. Amy W., mother of twins, described how she enjoyed reading the posts on the different forums she visited and always paid attention to posts that described going into early labor. She often sought out threads by women who were further along in their pregnancies than herself to give her an idea of what was to come. She liked to follow their stories and find out facts about how their pregnancies progressed. In having a full background of the stories she was reading she felt like she could more accurately process the stories and determine which stories were the most relevant to her. These forums gave her access to pregnancy and delivery stories that she never would have heard or read because they were not the typical stories that her friends, family, and TV told.

More recently Facebook pages and groups have grown in popularity as a place where women can go to find information about high-risk pregnancy and different medical conditions. When I was pregnant with my triplets, Facebook existed, but at the time it was just starting to catch on with those not in college, so this was a resource I was not familiar with. One might consider Facebook to simply be a tool for connecting and keeping up with friends and family, but multiple women I spoke with whose preemies have been born in the last few years talked about the groups they found and joined for parents of preemies and parents of children with specific health issues. These groups provided information and support and helped many women to feel less alone. One of the benefits of Facebook groups is that women could find tailored groups for the specific condition they were dealing with, their children's gestational age or their children's medical conditions. Through Facebook women could find other families whose children had heart conditions, were multiples, had feeding issues, or had sensory problems. Samantha, mother of twins commented that Facebook seemed a little more controlled to her than just going to Google or a forum of parents of preemies because you could find a small group of people concerned with the same issue.

Another place women went for information and stories were blogs. Blogs are a relatively new phenomenon with their popularity taking off within the past decade. Some estimate that upward of 7000 new blogs are started each day (Glover 2006). With the invention of web software that allowed individuals with minimal skills and knowledge to start producing a blog, more and more individuals began to take up blogging as a hobby (Roush 2005). The proliferation of blogs has given numerous women the opportunity to write about and document their high-risk pregnancies, premature births, and their infants' lives. It has also given women experiencing these issues easy access to the stories of other women as many blogs are public and can easily be found through internet searches.

Kiera, mother of triplets, described one blog in particular that she enjoyed reading,

> Once the girls were born. I started, that's when I started to Google micropreemie and triplets and I would Google triplets and I would always go back to the very first post that the person made to try to figure out how early their kids were born so that I could find somebody that would know what I was going through and so I could see, like kay, are their kids okay, what are they dealing with?

Through her Googling, Kiera came across a blog from a mom of triplet boys in Kansas. She described her reading,

> I remember, her blog was the first I found where I could understand her. I felt like I am not alone because here is this woman who has this going on with her

> kids and they are 3 years old and look at what they are doing. I had read another blog with triplets, but not micropreemies, and I ended up asking that woman to do my blog banner and then she started to read my blog and said you need to talk to Kara and I was like, oh yeah, I read her blog all the time so she sent me because they are actually friends so she connected me with Kara so Kara and I, we have never talked on the phone, but we e-mail, Facebook and instant message all of the time.

The blog Kiera was referring to chronicles the lives of a family with triplet boys who were born at 24 weeks. Two of the boys are legally blind and each boy has a variety of issues related to his prematurity. Finding this blog gave Kiera a chance to read the stories of another family similar to hers. This is a prime example of how the internet can connect people and generate relationships between two people who might otherwise have never crossed paths. Kiera's blog reading led to the development of a friendship with another blog author as the two women shared many unfortunate similarities, yet also shared a sense of determination and hope.

An additional reason it seemed that the internet was mentioned so frequently was that being on bed rest gave a lot of the women the time to peruse the internet and find blogs to read and do web searches, and it was a way to cope with the boredom and tedium that accompanied their days. Michelle, mother of triplet boys, explained that she got her information, "mostly just online because I really couldn't do like anything else." She also described how much she enjoyed reading others' blogs. One of the best things about blogs versus articles she found or forums is that she could get a very in depth picture of what families lives were like and detailed accounts of their pregnancies, hospital stays, and life at home. It was not just a brief snapshot or a specific questions posted in a forum so she was able to have a background and context of these families' stories. She now wished that she had started a blog of her own to document her pregnancy and her sons' lives. "I mean, I loved reading people's blogs that were maybe a little bit ahead of me. I was so sick that I wasn't doing that [blogging]. Or like, I wish I had been doing that. What a great journal."

Some of the women commented that they had not been aware of the prevalence of blogs until they started looking for information about their high-risk pregnancy or premature infants. Astrid, mother of triplets, discovered a lot about the numerous resources available on the internet after she was placed on strict bed rest at 18 weeks. Prior to that, she was unaware of the popularity of blogs and how they worked. While on bed rest she started her own blog, survingtriplets.blogspot.com in 2007 and through this began to get connected to other mothers of triplets and higher order multiples and started keeping up with their blogs and reading their stories. As of January 2010, when we spoke, her blog has gotten over 25,000 hits, a testament to the popularity of blogs. As her triplets got older and she was able to get in and out of the house more and children's various health and developmental issues resolved, she did start to blog less and less, no longer needing the support network it gave her.

Other mothers' exposure to blogs began when they were dealing with their infertility and were undergoing fertility treatments. Many women, such as Christine, mother of triplets, made connections with other women experiencing similar fertility struggles and read blogs to see what kinds of treatments other women were using and to read about how they were coping with the emotional and physical stress. After she learned she was pregnant with triplets, Christine continued to read blogs, but now instead of focusing on infertility, she sought out blogs of fellow mothers with multiples. As she reflected on all of the reading she did during, before, and after her she pregnancy, she found that the information she gathered had an overall positive impact. Having prior exposure to stories with negative outcomes helped her to feel more prepared for her pregnancy experience. She explained, "but I guess I had done a lot of, I read a lot while I was going through the fertility treatments. I read a lot of blogs and stories and things and I kind of had read about some of the worst case scenarios out there. It wasn't like new information for me. You know, things can happen, like the worst possible scenario." Her exposure to blogs gave her an idea of what was to come in the form of very personal stories. Many of the negative things that arose in her pregnancy and her daughters' stay in the NICU did not surprise her because of her extensive blog reading. When asked if she ever tried to avoid reading blogs with negative outcomes she replied, "No, I just wanted to know what all of the possibilities were. I don't know, somehow that made me feel like I had some kind of control."

Blogs represented a unique way to access and read stories about other women's situations because of the format. Women were able to read what were essentially others' journal entries and could go back to when the blog was started and follow the stories from the beginning. Women also could keep up-to-date with the blogs they followed. Blogs were also unique in that they generally presented the story of one woman and her family in an incredible amount of detail. Another benefit to reading blogs was that they often inspired women to keep their own blogs as a journal of their pregnancy and NICU experience. This was a great way for women to keep both family and friends informed of what was happening and it also helped them to process what they were going through. After the NICU journey was over it was also a great way for women to look back at how far their children had come. Vicki's twin sons were born at 24 weeks and 4 days and spent 142 days in the NICU. She talked about how as time went on she and her husband reached a point where it was hard to keep going. She explained,

> We had a hit a wall. We started a blog after I found it was twins. I had no idea what was going on. It was therapeutic to write it and if I could help one person. I was 100% honest. I did not want to go to the hospital anymore. I remember feeling like, people talk about something that brought them to their knees, you just can't go on, but you do. You are mad and you are sad. We have a great family support. On the blog 100s of people read each post. That is what kept me writing. That is what kept me writing and it held me accountable.

The knowledge that so many people, both friends, family, and even strangers read what she wrote and cared so much about their family helped her to cope on her more difficult days.

EVALUATING INFORMATION

In looking at the information-seeking behaviors of women, it is important to understand how women evaluated the information they encountered. A website or book may present excellent and accurate information, but if the intended audience does not find the information or the source credible, it will not be well received or useful. On the flip side, someone may provide women with inaccurate or false information and if the information source is deemed credible, women may follow poor advice or suggestions. With so much information out there and with so much conflicting information a woman's ability to sift through and critically evaluate that information has serious implications for her mental well-being and potentially for her or her children's health. One important factor in assessing credibility for many women was medical expertise and experience. Women expressed their confidence in the advice of their physicians because of their experience of treating women with high-risk conditions such as multiple births. Christine described how she continued to see her regular obstetrician in conjunction with a maternal fetal specialist. She felt confident in her obstetrician's ability to effectively manage her pregnancy as he had handled triplets before and had years of experience so she did not feel that she needed to be exclusively seen by the high-risk doctor. Had her regular OB never handled a triplet pregnancy before, she most likely would have made a different decision.

When evaluating the stories and narratives they encountered either from friends or what they found online, a common factor that women used to evaluate they tended to accept the narratives of those similar to themselves and discount the narratives of those who were more dissimilar. When it came to seeking out stories, women often sought out stories from women that they saw as similar to themselves believing that similar women might have similar outcomes. In addition to similarity, women also valued personal experience with a high-risk pregnancy or a premature birth when it came to sharing information and offering advice. Often a source's experience trumped other credibility factors. Mandy, a mother with type I diabetes, tended to trust the stories and information she got from other mothers with diabetes over information she read or obtained from other sources,

> The general pregnancy books I read were fine, but I had a couple of diabetic books that well, they scared the bejeebies out of me. One of them said, well one of them said that the average diabetic person has at least one amniocentesis. And I was just like, why on earth would you? And then when I went to the diabetic clinic and went around the table, none of them had ever had one. And so I said, quite clearly, I think this book isn't what I would believe.

For Mandy, the other mothers' stories and experiences were more credible than the authors of the books she read. She privileged the lived experience of the diabetic mothers she talked to over the academic knowledge of the book authors who lacked firsthand experience with diabetes. Another common technique for assessing the validity of information found on the internet was to compare information on several sites to check for consistency (Lagan, Sinclair, and Kernohan 2011). If they found the same advice and numbers in several places they generally assumed that the information was accurate.

INFORMATION AVOIDERS

On the opposite end of the spectrum from the information seekers were women who avoided information and did not actively seek out additional information or stories beyond what their physicians told them. These women made a conscious effort to try not to read or hear stories that were upsetting to them and sometimes went out of their way to avoid coming across any upsetting or negative information. As one woman explained, stories could be even more upsetting than reading a list of complications, especially stories she heard from people she knew because the stories were personal and put a face to the statistics and medical issues. Nichole, mother of twins, described how she was glad that she had not been open to hearing a lot of negative stories because of their potentially upsetting nature. She explained, "Yeah, I think that if I had known or talked to more people who had twins, like if I had known all the stuff that happened to real people, I think I would have been more freaked out. But you know, reading that stuff, it's not so bad because it's like that's not so horrible, it's like, you know, that won't happen." When she read negative information on the internet or in a pamphlet, it was easier for her to minimize the seriousness of it or assume that it would not happen to her because the statistics and lists of facts were impersonal and did not hit her with the same emotional impact. She could distance herself from the information presented in lists and as facts in a way she could not when she heard or read a story about an actual family who had a bad experience.

After her twins were born at 34 weeks and 5 days and were small but healthy, she was more open to hearing negative stories from friends and family about other twin pregnancies and births. About a year after her twins were born, Nichole's cousin had twins who were born at 29 weeks. Unfortuantley, one of the twins passed away from complications related to prematurity. The loss was hard for the entire family, and especially Nichole. She said the experience made her even more greatful for the health of her twins. She is also thankful that she had not had too much exposure during her pregnancy to stories about the bad things that could happen. She had not heard stories like her cousins' that invovled loss so she did not spend a lot of time while she was pregnant worrying that one or both of her twins might not surivive. In some ways she was uniformed and naïve, but she sees this as a good thing as she feels that had she heard stories like this she would have been consumed with fear and unable to function throughout her pregnancy.

Jen, mother of twins who were born at 29 weeks, also explained how she tried to avoid exposing herself to stories that would upset her during her pregnancy, "I tried, I tried to cautiously use the internet, if there is such a thing. There are, there are a lot of stories out there of you know, 24 weekers who made it, and then there are a lot of stories of 24 weekers who didn't make it. And I tried for the longest time not to find information either way because I didn't, I felt like it wasn't my situation. It wasn't me and my babies." She avoided most stories because she felt like her sitaution was her own and there was no way to predict how her story would play out. There was no guarantee that her twins would have the same outcomes as those in the stories she heard, so she instead focused on herself and her situation.

Jen, like several other women was surprised by her avoidant tendencies as it went against her normal personality. She commented in general that she tried not to seek out too much information during her pregnancy, which surprised her. She commented that she tended to avoid a lot of stories and then went on to explain,

> Which is weird because of the controlling personality that I have. I guess that I would think that I would want to do that [search for information]. I would get enough information to know what to expect for the most part. You know, I talked to my OB all of the time about the difference of developing and stuff like that. But I really didn't spend hours upon hours researching because I think that would have freaked me out more with all the different things that could have happened. And I decided to focus on, you know, the positives, you know everybody's health and progressing the way they should and not court disaster.

Carla, mother of twins, also saw no reason to get extra information about things that could go wrong when everything was currently going well with her pregnancy. As she put it, looking up negative information would almost be like inviting problems in and she saw no reason to dwell on the negative until it was necessary.

Other women took a similar approach to negative stories and information, adopting the philosophy that increased knowledge of the negative things that could happen did not improve the situation because if bad things were going to happen they were going to happen. In some cases, ignorance was bliss, as women could keep their stress level as low and possible. Jessica, my sister-in-law who has type I diabetes, was diagnosed with Lupus in the first weeks of her second pregnancy. Because of her first pregnancy, she was very aware of the potential risks and complications related to diabetes, but knew almost nothing about the additional risks Lupus posed. For example, after her son was born, she learned that the risk of miscarriage is much higher for those with Lupus. The risk of miscarriage for a woman with Lupus is 10 percent due to related blood disorders (Alijotas-Reig, Palacio-Garcia, and Vilardell-Tarres 2009). She explained that she was glad she did not know this when she was pregnant as miscarriage was something completely out of her control, "I didn't know that at the beginning of the pregnancy, which I'm glad because I would have freaked out. Like I didn't, I honestly didn't try to read or look into Lupus that much." Instead of actively seeking out information about what could go wrong Jessica chose to focus on what she could control which was her diet and blood sugars during her pregnancy and otherwise she just listened to her doctor and avoided information or stories that would stress her out.

Other women described avoiding different stories because they did not feel as if the information applied to them or their situations. For example, many of the women who gave birth unexpectedly had not read a lot about premature birth and other complications because prior to their deliveries they were having a healthy pregnancy and did not see the need to read or seek out information about potential complications. There was a common belief among some of the women that seeking out stories about what could go wrong was in a way courting disaster and inviting bad things to happen. These women saw no value in preparing for the worst as the information would only be upsetting and most women believed it would be unnecessary. Their philosophy tended to be that there was no value in worrying about things that might never occur and if something bad did occur, they would then find the information they needed.

For example, several of the women who gave birth early due to preclampsia or other medical conditions had a sudden onset of symptoms and did not have much time to process what was happening. Prior to their symptoms they were having a typical pregnancy with only common symptoms and had few concerns about something going wrong, and therefore, they did not read a lot about premature labor and birth. Few ever anticipated that they would develop a complication like preeclampsia and many did not even know that complications such as PROM or IUGR even existed. This also meant that when their infants were born prematurely or they began to experience complications they felt completely unprepared for parenting a premature infant or having an infant in the NICU. Over and over women told me that they had always thought about having a preemie as something remote and abstract that happened to other people. Lisa's daughter was born at 28 weeks and 6 days after Lisa's bood pressure started to spike and could not be controlled. The experience was completely unexpected and Lisa who was 38 when she had her daughter told me that her primary concern had always been that she would have a hard time getting pregnant due to her age. Once she was pregnant she thought the hard part was over. After her daughter was born she remembered that two weeks before she was hospitalized she was at church and the congregation prayed for a member who had delievered her baby prematurely. "At the time it was like oh that is so sad," Lisa explained, but then she moved on and did not give it much thought, never thinking that she herself could end up in a similar sitaution.

Kiera, mother of triplets, avoided some of the more negative information because she did not see it applying to herself. When her daughters were born at 25 weeks, she felt incredibly unprepared. She explained that she had not read about the micropreemies and all of the complications because it was too frightening,

> I, at that time I avoided it. I didn't want to hear I didn't even want to think about that. And even knowing that I was high-risk, nobody talked to me about the fact that they very well could be born that early. They were talking to mc about 30 weeks, 32 weeks, 34 weeks, being the more common delivery. I definitely think I had the more positive kind of doctor. So I knew nothing about a micropreemie and I remember talking to people and them being like, oh my gosh, and I was like, yeah they'll be born early and they'll probably be in the NICU for a month, but then we will bring them home. I was very, very uninformed.

Kiera avoided these negative types of stories because of her confidence that her pregnancy would be fine as well as her lack of knowledge about just how complicated and dangerous a triplet pregnancy could be. Avoiding information was a way to protect herself from stress and worry, but when she was suddenly faced with the harsh reality of having critically ill children she had a hard time even comprehending what was happening.

After her daughters were born, Kiera had some regrets that she did not spend a little more time talking about and learning about potential complications. She described her reaction to a conversation with another triplet mother whose infants were born at 29 weeks,

> I remember the other mom that I talked to and I only talked to her once, but her kids were born at 29 weeks and when I talked to her I said, well I am never talking to her again because she was very much you know, here is what was bad. I wish now that I had talked to her more because her story was much more like my story. I mean her kids were born at 29 weeks and she was telling me all of the scary things that can happen and living in the NICU and bringing home medically fragile babies and I was just like, I am never talking to her again. She is so negative.

After their initial conversation, Kiera never spoke with the woman again as her negativity was off putting to Kiera who tried to maintain a hopeful attitude and was confident that she would deliver around 34 weeks. Later, when her daughters were born at 25 weeks she wished she had not avoided this woman as she saw how she could have been an excellent resource for both information and support.

Karen, mother of two sets of twins, also avoided looking up a lot of negative information about pregnancy and twin pregnancies as her pregnancies were relatively complication free. She explained that she didn't use the internet for much more than looking at gestational calendars. "I did [use the internet], but not too much. I was on the gestational calendars to just look, and I could look at my own calendar. They could make a calendar based on what you tell them. But since I didn't have too many complications, I didn't look up too much." She did have them make a calendar based on her due date that charted some of the expected milestones of her pregnancy, but other than that she just let her pregnancy progress and tried not to fill her mind with frightening possibilities. As long as things were going well, there was no reason to research or learn about all of the complications that could arise.

In looking at the stories of women who actively avoided information, the common theme was that women did so in order to protect themselves from anxiety and fear. Avoidance or escape is a coping techinique that does not directly try to deal with or better the problem but instead creates a space where the individual does not have to think about or deal with the problem (Folkman 1997). One avoidance technique is to deny something is occuring or to deny the seriousness of it. A mother experiencing preterm labor might refuse to accept that this could result in a preterm birth or a mother with a premature infant might tell herself and others that the infant is doing just fine despite serious health issues. Avoidance can also entail staying away from the topic or issue as in the case of narrative avoidance as a woman may change the channel when she hears a report about premature infants or change the subject when a friend starts telling a story about a premature infant. Some mothers may try to escape the problem by reading a book or going out shopping to get away from the stress. Other avoidance behaviors include sleeping, eating, avoiding others, and wishing things were different (Hamilton and Lobel 2008).

A study of coping mechanisms of parents in the NICU found that women were more likely than men to use avoidance as a coping strategy (Hughes et al. 1994). Avoidance strategies are more likely to be used when individuals feel a lack of control over situations or that situations cannot be changed. A study of the coping mechanisms of pregnant women found that as the pregnancy progressed, women were less likely to use avoidance as a coping strategy as the obvious physical changes and impending birth made it more difficult to avoid the reality of what was to come (Hamilton and Lobel 2008). The majority of studies have found that avoidance is less effective in handling and minimzing stress than problem approaching strategies such as finding a solution or gathering more information (Besser and Priel 2003; McIntosh, Stern, and Ferguson 2004; Miller, Stiff, and Ellis 1988; Reichman et al. 2000) which could indicate that if narrative avoidance is being used as a coping strategy, it may have some negative repercussions for women.

One of the outcomes of narrative avoidance was a lack of knowledge and awareness about what could go wrong and what it meant to have a premature baby. Depending on how a woman's pregnancy progressed, this lack of knowledge was either a blessing or a curse. Marie, mother of triplets, talked about how she had really had no idea of just how badly a triplet pregnancy could end. She actually had a friend who had twins who were born prematurely, but found she did not go to this friend for a lot for information during her pregnancy,

> I didn't talk to her a lot about the pregnancy. It was kind of weird, we're close friends but we did not and I think it is because, kind of like you just said, a little bit of that denial, I know they had a little bit of issues when they were born so I'm going to just pretend that this did not happen and I think my husband and I talk about this now, I don't think I realized how many risks there were when I was pregnant as I do now or I have now learned about or know about what could have happened or now I hear about some of these 23/24 weekers and I am like, oh my gosh. I didn't realize that at 24 weeks what that meant if they came out then.

Marie was fortunate to deliver her triplets at 35 weeks, so she did not feel as if the stories of her friend and others with very premature infants could have been helpful. She felt like her ignorance of the issues of very premature infants was positive. She explained, "I think it is a good thing because I think then you're not dwelling on it and then you're, I like information, but I don't need to be worrying about it because I don't think that's going to be good for the big picture."

A primary motivation for avoiding stories and seeking out additional information was to keep themselves from being paralyzed by fear. Denise, mother of triplets, explained how she thinks her avoidance of negative stories helped to keep her fear level down. She was assisted in her avoidance by the lack of internet access at home, but she also chose not to use the computer at work to look up information, "In a way I think it would have been more information, but in a way I think I would have been more frightened. Like I know when I went into my cerclage at 16 weeks, it never really occurred to me that something terrible could happen. It was kind of scary, but it's like, okay they're going to do this and then everything will be fine. It never really occurred to me that I was going to have my babies then." She felt that at the time, had she had access to more information about all of the potential outcomes of her pregnancy, she would not have been able to cope. For example, had she understood the acutely real risk of delivering at 16 weeks which would have ended her pregnancy, she would have been more frightened. This she explained would not have done her any good as knowing what could happen would not change what did happen. She went on to comment, "I wasn't that educated, but I guess that was a good thing for me because if I had had the internet, I probably would have just stressed myself out." Her avoidance arose partly out of her situation of having limited access to the internet but also out of a conscious effort to protect herself from anxiety.

Other women also found their situations helped or even forced them to avoid stories. Helene, mother of triplets born at 28 weeks, told a similar story. She found that while her triplets were in the NICU, she had limited time to be on the internet and look for stories of other preemies and their complications. Because most NICUs do not allow for cell phones to be the inside of the NICU many parents found they had far less opportunity to be online each day. Prior to her triplets' birth, Helene had avoided most stories about preemies and the NICU. She explained that because she avoided these stories she was very unprepared for the facts and reality of delivering her triplets so early. When they were born at 28 weeks she had not really considered what they would be like, what the NICU stay would entail, or what some of the common medical issues they face would be. She explained, "I didn't realize they were as medically fragile as they were. I don't know what I thought. I mean, it was probably great that I didn't know all these things because it probably protected me from being more scared." While in the NICU, her smallest triplet, CJ, contracted a MERSA infection in his eye. She described the situation,

> When they cultured the discharge it was MERSA and then when they cultured they had to give him a few blood transfusions, so he was struggling with that. Other than that he was fine. And it was probably just a good thing I was so busy with the other babies in the NICU and recovery. I didn't get a lot of computer time because if I had probably had more time to research and find out what MERSA really was, I would have freaked myself out. So it was a blessing that I was just sort of innocent and happy-go-lucky about the whole thing because it could have been really bad.

Sometimes women stopped searching for information because it was hard to find the type and quality of information they were looking for. For example, Jessica is a mother who started to experience major swelling around 20 weeks during her pregnancy with her daughter Quinn. After it was found that she did not have preclampsia, she was advised to take it easy, limit her salt, and put her feet up whenever possible. Her condition continued to worsen though and an ultrasound revealed there was stressed cord flow and her daughter was not getting all of the blood and nourishment she needed from the placenta. A few days later, a follow-up ultrasound showed that the stressed cordflow had progressed to reversed cordflow which caused doctors to deliver Quinn at 25 weeks. Because of her lack of nutrition, Quinn had severe IUGR and weighed just under a pound. Jessica recalled that when things first started going wrong with her pregnancy she was constantly on the computer searching for information, but a lot of what she found were message forums or individuals' pages and blog and for her this information was too anecdotal. She didn't want personal stories, she wanted hard facts and statistics as there was no way to know if an indivdiuals' experience would match hers. She also felt like most of the stories she found either presented a story with a terrible outcome or the best outcome possible. There were no middle of the road stories, and she had a hard time accepting that the best- and worst-case scenarios were the only possibilities. Once her daughter was born she and her husband made a conscious decision together not to go online and start Googling micropreemies and instead to put full faith and trust in Quinn's doctors and nurses. She wanted to avoid the horror stories as well as the stories where everything was perfect and by staying off of the internet she was able to focus on her daughter and her daily progress instead of getting caught up in all of the possibilities.

Sometimes women were unable to avoid stories they did not want to hear because the people around them insisted on sharing. My sister-in-law Jessica who has type I diabetes and Lupus worked as a billing specialist at an obstetrician's office during both of her pregnancies which meant she was confronted by stories from pregnant women all day long, every day she worked. Some of the stories were happy and typical, but many of the patients had major complications and almost every day she heard at least one story of something that could go wrong. She could not stop working, and she loved her job, but she had to develop a strategy that allowed her to ignore or block out the upsetting stories she encountered. She explained,

> I don't think you handle the negative stories. You just try to block them out. You try and put them in the back of somewhere. Because you can't, you can't. If you listen to all those stories, and let me say, I heard them every day, you know, the whole time I worked there, the whole time I was pregnant. And you know, I guess you try not to dwell on it. I mean, because I am an anxious person so I have to put that, you know back.

There was no way to avoid the stories because of her work at an obstetrician's office. Her best defense then was to try not to think too much about them after she heard them. As she acknowledged, she was by nature an anxious person and during her pregnancy she had to avoid thinking about or dwelling on stories that would add to her anxiety which meant only half-listening to the stories people told her and trying to put any of the unpleasant stories out of her mind.

Jessica was not alone in being in situations where she was presented with stories and information she did not want to hear, but had no way to avoid. Sometimes unwanted stories arose when women clicked on the wrong link while searching online or failed to change the station when a TV program had a storyline about premature birth, but more often than not, the unwanted stories came from other people including family and friends. This lead many women to question why people shared some of the stories they did and why people did not recognize that some stories would not be helpful or encouraging. Kelli, mother of twins, described a situation that occurred early in her pregnancy that still bothered her over a year later. One of her coworkers had been pregnant with twins and had lost one of them. Kelli had not known that her coworker's son had been a twin until her coworker shared this with her. She said when she was hearing the story she was thinking,

> I don't want to hear that. I mean like I guess it was good to know. But, you know it is always a concern. It is always a fear. It was always a concern with us. Like what would we do like if only one came out. And actually, the secretary where I worked had been pregnant with twins what was it 2 years 3 years? Before I got there. And ended up losing one really early on and then having the other one. So she had a 3 year old that should have been a twin but she lost the boy. So of course she told me that. And I'm like oh. And she told me right when I found out that it was a boy and a girl. And I asked when did you lose him? And she was like right about this time. And, it was like why would you tell someone that? Like at first I was a little offended.

Kelli did not want to hear this story because it represented one of her greatest fears, but she did not know how to ask her coworker to stop telling her story. She understood that this was a part of her coworker's story and she could see why her coworker felt compelled to talk about it, but she also felt that this story that she had never been told before had not been told at the best time.

Amy, mother of twins, was also surprised by some of the stories other people would tell her once they learned she was having twins. She explained "you know, people told me a lot of stories when I was pregnant about like twins who had died or whatever. So it was kind of the opposite and I thought, you know, what are they thinking, telling me that. So I heard more stories about times when things hadn't gone well." She was upset by these stories and could not understand why others thought they were appropriate to share with her. She was already upset and worried about what the future might be like and she wanted people to offer reassurance, not give her even more to be anxious about. These stories simply served to compound her worries.

Sometimes women were put into awkward situations as others wanted them to talk to other women who had been in similar situations and sometimes pushed women into a conversation they were not ready to have. When women were ready, they often were eager to meet other women who shared experiences and complications, but a forced conversation sometimes left women feeling uncomfortable. Kelly, mother of identical triplets, described an encounter like this,

> So there was one other triplet mom that I had met when I was just barely pregnant with mine and I was like 13, 14 weeks when I met her. So we were introduced through an acquaintance and the way it all happened I was just really kind of put off like I don't really want to talk to a stranger like suddenly I was face to face with this person that I did not know about her triplets. I think she had two boys and a girl or two girls and a boy and two kids.

Nothing the other mother talked about was horrible, but at the time, Kelly was not comfortable sitting down with a relative stranger to discuss many of the personal aspects of a triplet pregnancy. Being a more private person, Kelly was not one to just sit down and open up with a stranger because the stranger had triplets.

AVOIDING NORMAL AND POSITIVE

In discussing what types of information women sought out and avoided during a pregnancy it is easy to understand why information about risks, complications, and long-term outcomes could be both a source of comfort and distress. However, there was another type of information women sometimes found themselves avoiding while they were pregnant, while their babies were in the NICU, and even after their children were older which were stories about women with typical pregnancies and full-term babies or stories about other women who had high-risk pregnancies that had successful outcomes. As women struggled during their pregnancies and then watched their babies struggle during the first days and week of their lives, it could be painful to see the people around them having happy pregnancies or seeing women with similar complications who were able to deliver their babies full term. In the previous chapter, on comparison, we saw how comparing themselves to women who had better outcomes for their pregnancies or comparing their children to other preemies who had fewer medical issues could be disheartening for women when their own stories had not turned out as well. It might be logical to conclude that women tried to avoid stories about people who had normal pregnancies because in comparison they had not had the same outcomes, but as I talked with women it became clear that they avoided these stories not so much because they compared themselves to those women as there were often too many differences between them for comparisons to provide useful information, but because they made them angry, envious, and sad over what they had not experienced.

Kiera, mother of triplets, found herself avoiding stories of normal situations both when she was trying to get pregnant and then after her daughters were born at 25 weeks and suffered from severe complications and spent months in the NICU. She described her difficulty with hearing these kinds of stories on TV or from friends who had not shared her struggles,

> I remember, Britney Spears was pregnant when I was going through fertility treatments and that is what pissed me off. It was hard to talk to friends who had their healthy singletons and complaining about not getting any sleep and their baby was up all night or being tired of breastfeeding or breastfeeding for a week and deciding that they just couldn't do it and I thought, oh my gosh, I would give anything to be able to breastfeed my babies and I think that is why I retreated from the friends that I had for so long because they just couldn't relate to what my life was now.

Kiera had a hard time hearing about people such as Britney Spears who was pregnant and hadn't even planned it, and later had trouble listening to mothers talk about normal infant issues. Because of this, she chose to withdraw from most people and media so she would not be exposed to stories that upset her.

Sometimes the stories that bothered women were not even about difficult pregnancies or premature children. Donna R, mother of twins, often found her friends sharing stories with her describing their difficulties and stresses. She often was upset by the stories as she felt that her friends struggles were very minor compared to her own. She tried to be sympathetic when she heard her friends' stories, but she often found herself ignoring most of what they said. "I tried to listen to my friends. . . . They probably tried to share their stories or whatever. They act like what they are going through is just so darn awful or whatever. . ." Donna tried to listen to the stories of her friends and even to be sympathetic to their complaints, but she found she had to start ignoring the stories because she became too upset when she heard them. As a working mother of twins and another young daughter, her life was very challenging and she felt resentful of friends who complained about what Donna saw as relatively easy situations. She did not feel as if she could ask her friends not to share their stories, so while they were talking she just tried to ignore what they were saying or put it out of her mind.

One of the things that was very difficult for a lot of women was being on social media where they were often confronted by friends' and families' updates and photos about their pregnancies and newborns. Women wanted to be happy for their friends and family and they were, but at the same time, it could be very difficult to log in and see a picture of a friend showing off her 38-week belly or of her chubby-cheeked newborn getting his first bath at home when your own baby was born at 25 weeks and spent over four months in the hospital. Several women mentioned avoiding using social media or even blocking or unfollowing someone because it was too hard to see all of their happy pictures. Women often felt guilty for these feelings of envy and anger or believed that their feelings were somewhat irrational, but the pain they felt was real and not exposing themselves to stories and images was one of the easiest strategies for avoiding the pain.

Another situation that sometimes caused stress or discomfort was when good family or good friends had full-term healthy babies shortly after women's preemies were born. Even though women were happy that the baby was born and was healthy, many women described how going to the hospital to visit the mom and new baby was hard. Just being in the hospital itself could be difficult as it brought back a lot of memories. Sometimes women had not been back in a hospital since their children had been discharged from the NICU and the smells and sounds that are almost universal to the hospital atmosphere were too much for women to handle. Even if women were not too bothered by being in the hospital, the ritual of going to the postpartum room carrying presents and flowers was also a reminder of the visitors women never had and how different the first days of their babies' lives were. Again, they were happy for their friends or family and did not want anyone to have a bad pregnancy or an unhealthy child, but they also did not want to have to stare at what they had wanted and not gotten.

One woman shared with me how difficult it was for to cope with other people's pregnancies after her traumatic experiences. Stephanie's first son was stillborn and her second son was born at 29 weeks and spent over two months in the hospital. Shortly after her second son was born her best friend got pregnant with her first child and this was difficult for both Stephanie and her friend. She described the strain,

> It was hard for her to share her happiness. She invited me to the baby shower and she invited me and I couldn't go. When the baby was born she called my mom. It took me about a day but I was like I really need to go, she doesn't have anyone coming in and sharing her excitement. I felt like I had to go do that. I didn't hold him and I went and showed my support I didn't stay long, but I at least went, but it was hard.

Stephanie knew that it was not her friend's fault that her own pregnancies had gone so terribly, and she did not want to punish her friend for that, but it was a very emotional and painful process for Stephanie to provide the support she knew her friend needed and deserved.

TENSION BETWEEN KNOWING AND NOT KNOWING

Throughout the interviews women discussed the stories they tried to avoid in order to protect themselves from feelings of fear and anxiety. Many women tried not to consider the possibilities of having very premature or sick infants as they adopted a belief that a positive attitude was best and thinking about the negative possibilities would only invite trouble or harm. The avoidance of negative or upsetting stories seemed to be a protective mechanism. However, some women regretted their avoidance of certain stories and information after they gave birth prematurely. As they were struggling to deal with the NICU as well as their infants' various health issues they began to wish they had more exposure to stories like their own. Not having prior knowledge or stories to draw from made their situations feel even more confusing and overwhelming as women had no idea what was happening and could not rely on others' stories to give them a sense of how events would proceed. In essence, a tension exists between keeping women informed of the possibilities while respecting their desire to avoid upsetting stories.

For some women, their active avoidance of information about potential complications and the risks of prematurity meant that they were completely shocked when things cropped up and went wrong. Once they were in a critical situation, they often wished that they had more information so they could be more mentally prepared for what they were facing. On the opposite end of the spectrum were the information seekers who sought out, listened to, and read everything they could find. Some women described having an unhealthy compulsion to gather information about all of the possibilities no matter how rare or frightening. Women explained feeling more in control when they had information, but at times, the sense of control became a sense of panic as women were overwhelmed with all of the stories they consumed and the information they gathered. Women spoke of being almost paralyzed with fear as they imagined the worst and wishing they had not been so anxious to hear and read so many negative stories. Women eventually realized that even in hearing or reading the worst, there was no way to completely prepare themselves for what it was like to see their infants in the NICU for the first time as no matter how much they had read or researched, they were still shocked and taken aback by the sight of their own baby hooked up to wires and machines and struggling to breathe. In terms of preparation, it did seem as if women who had toured the NICU prior to the birth did tend to have a little easier time adjusting to the NICU. This could be because most of the women who had toured the NICU were those who were experiencing complications meaning that these women also had more time to adjust to the possibility that their infants might be born early and require NICU time.

This tension between the stories women wanted to hear and allowed themselves to access and what they later wished they had heard or read presents an interesting dilemma for both women and those trying to help assist and support them. Those who have prior experience with high-risk pregnancies and multiple births and medical personnel might see the value in providing women with accurate information and stories concerning the potential risks and complications. Those with previous experience with high-risk pregnancies and premature births have the advantage of first-hand experience and observation to recognize the benefit of exposure to a variety of stories can have, even those with negative or less than stellar outcomes. However, those wishing to help women during this difficult time also may need to understand the importance of respecting women's desires regarding information and stories. For some women, the desire to avoid certain stories and information is based on a desire to protect themselves from additional emotional distress. A story told to an unwilling listener may not have the intended impact and may even have the complete opposite effect. When women encountered stories they wanted to avoid they often tried to ignore or forget those stories. This creates a challenge for those trying to support women as they have to balance their desire to impart information with women's desire for controlling the types of stories they encounter.

Perhaps one way to approach women who want to avoid negative stories would be to present the negative information as lists of facts and statistics rather than in story format to lessen the emotional impact. Women also could be directed toward specific negative information at different points in their pregnancies or while their infants are in the NICU rather than providing women with an overwhelming amount of information at their first appointments. For example, when a woman starts to have early contractions at 26 weeks, her physicians or nurse could then describe some of the concerns with her contractions and explain the general outlook for infants born at 26 weeks, but wait to go into more specific detail when it becomes evident that doctors will be unable to stop the labor. Additionally, all women should be encouraged to visit the NICU once they are diagnosed with a high-risk pregnancy. This visit should not be presented as something that is frightening or negative, but instead as an important way to prepare for the birth, similar to the way many parents visit the maternity ward prior to delivery so they know what to expect. A visit to the NICU could then inspire questions and concerns that could be addressed by physicians or nurses. In some situations women will be able to deliver healthy babies that do not need an NICU stay, but even though this is a possibility, the benefits that women described having visited the NICU prior to giving birth seem to be overwhelming and outweigh any potential anxiety an NICU visit might produce in women who might not ever have a child in the NICU.

The tension between having too much and too little information was not just created by women themselves. Women sometimes found themselves in a dilemma as they were being told to stay away from the internet by physicians and family members because it was providing upsetting stories. However, they saw the internet as a valuable source of information and stories and in many cases as a source of comfort and support which made them reluctant to stop using the internet during their pregnancies. Studies have found many advantages of using the internet to help women cope with and learn about many aspects of pregnancy (Lowe et al. 2009; Malik and Coulson 2008). Therefore, a ban on the internet, may not be the best approach to assist women as they seek out stories pertaining to their experiences. Rather than recommending that women entirely avoid the internet, women should be advised to use the internet in ways that are beneficial to them. One practical suggestion might be to recommend women set a limit on the time they spend online each day, which would limit the amount of information they could access. Often women used the internet for several hours a day to combat the monotony of bed rest. Having access to other activities such as watching videos, reading, sewing, or talking on the phone with friends could help pass time. Women should also be encouraged to discuss what they find on the internet with their medical team or with family in order to get clarification on any confusing aspects of the information and also to help women process how the stories and information they found on the internet apply to themselves. Discussing their fears and concerns that arise from internet reading could assist women in coping with those fears. Another suggestion would be to encourage women to identify some specific websites they find informative or supportive and visit only those sites rather than conducting internet searches which pull up a wide variety of sites and stories. By following these suggestions, women can continue to use the internet but potentially avoid becoming overwhelmed by what they read.

Another concern with internet usage was the validity and accuracy of the stories women were finding. Although relevant and accurate health information does exist on the internet, there are no controls over what is posted which means that poor, misleading, and conflicting information also is available (Keane 2009; Walczak 2009). In terms of pregnancy-related information, there is a concern that websites contain false or misleading information, or fail to include important information about risks and long-term complications. For example, Brazilian researchers conducted an analysis of nearly 200 websites that came up after Googling cesarean and found that over 70 percent of the sites had a poor to moderate quality of information with websites either providing false or inaccurate information or failing to provide enough information for women to fully understand the procedure and their options (Fioretti et al. 2015). These findings were echoed by Jesper, former editor of *BJOG*, which is an international journal focused on obstetrics and gynecology; in an editorial he wrote calling for increased education of women so that they could more skillfully navigate and discern the vast amount of faulty information on the internet (Jesper 2015). When women choose to visit online forums, there is no control over who is participating and what kinds of information and advice are being provided. Women may have a difficult time sifting through the stories they find and evaluating the credibility and validity of what they read (Bates et al. 2006). A better strategy might be to identify websites that contain accurate and useful information and direct women toward these sites.

The overarching theme of this chapter is that information can be both an invaluable resource as well as an incredible burden. We live in an information-rich society. Women can turn to doctors, nurses, friends, family, books, and TV to gather information and stories about pregnancy, and with the advances in the internet accessing information is as easy as typing some key terms into a search engine. For women who are experiencing a high-risk pregnancy or have a preemie, this abundance of information can be extremely beneficial as information can help answer their questions, let them know what question they should ask, prepare them for future possibilities, and allows them to become a more informed and active participant as they make decisions about their own and their children's healthcare. Paradoxically, this abundance of information can also be a burden and a source of added stress and anxiety. The challenge for women and those who love and care for them in both the personal and healthcare realms is to find the right balance between educating women and not causing them undue anxiety.

Chapter 7

As Seen on TV

Earlier in the book we met Catt who had to terminate one of her triplets during her pregnancy to save the pregnancy and her other two triplets. Following the termination surgery she was placed on bed rest and had a lot of time on her hands to watch TV, but she quickly found that she could no longer watch the shows about pregnancy that she had previously loved. When she did turn them on she found herself getting angry when she watched. She explained, "And it made me sick, like sick to my stomach to watch them because they were all happy and wonderful, and they had the rainbow." She was upset that the shows only were showing the happy side of birth and she was mad that her own pregnancy experience had been so hard and she already suffered a huge loss in the loss of her daughter and she still was unsure of what would happen to her surviving triplets. Catt is a pediatric nurse and says that prior to having children one of her favorite things to watch were the specials on channels like TLC and Discovery Health that featured medical anomalies like "the smallest girl in the word," or "the boy with five legs." After she had her children she found that she couldn't even watch any kind of medical shows because it was now too frightening to her to think that something else could possibly go wrong with one of her children. Having lost one child in utero and having her surviving triplets born early it terrified her that there was still so much out in the world that could hurt them. What she had once found entertaining, interesting, and informative, was now a source of pain and anxiety as it just added to her ongoing mental list of what dangers could possibly lurk in her surviving twin's future.

Media is a pervasive entity in our lives and through media we are often exposed to messages and stories about pregnancy and birth. In fact, it is difficult to flip through the channels on the TV without encountering some sort of reference to pregnancy, childbirth, or babies. Even commercials play on our general love of cute and tiny babies. One of my favorite series of commercials ever are black and white 30-second commercials that feature mothers engaging in the most basic of mothering tasks such as bathing a chubby infant in the sink or rocking a yawning, curly-haired infant in the nursery. The sounds in the commercial are soft music combined with the sweet giggles and sighs of the adorable baby closing with the tag line, “Having a Baby Changes Everything.” This Johnson & Johnson commercial epitomizes what could be considered a cultural ideal of motherhood—that having a child changes your world and this change means a life full of tender and joyous moments. This commercial gets me every time even though I am keenly aware of all of the less than tender and joyous moments that motherhood entails. Who doesn’t want to sit and rock a sleeping baby or see a baby respond to your tickles with a gummy grin? This commercial reminds viewers, and especially female viewers what ideal motherhood is and should be like. Mothers and in the case of this series the occasional father is not only wholly in love with their baby, but is completely fulfilled by all of the small tasks of raising that baby. The commercials do acknowledge that having a baby does change your life, but only in the most positive ways. Obviously the end goal of the commercial is to sell a product, so the beautifully shot scenes designed to elicit a maternal urge are a highly successful tool in reaching that goal, but I mention these ads because even if they are just another commercial, they are also another story of having a baby that viewers consume and without even consciously realizing it, that story can influence viewers’ beliefs and understanding of what it means to have a baby.

Of course not all TV depictions of pregnancy and childbirth are designed to sell products, but many are designed to attract viewers so fictional accounts of pregnancy and childbirth are often told in dramatic or humorous ways. As was noted in chapter 3, prior to 1950, the word pregnancy was itself taboo and women’s pregnancies were considered something private that was not discussed in public. This meant that while babies appeared on TV programs, it was not until 1952 that a pregnant Lucille Ball not only appeared on the I Love Lucy show in her pregnant state, but her pregnancy became a storyline on the show. This was revolutionary at the time as unlike today, any mention of something close to sex on TV was scandalous. Keep in mind that married couples were depicted as sleeping in side by side twin beds and did nothing more physical than share a chaste kiss before saying goodnight. During the second season of the widely popular show the episode, “Lucy is Enciente” aired and danced around Lucy’s condition as she humorously tried to get her husband to understand that she was pregnant without saying the actual word. Even the episode title used the French word for pregnancy and throughout the show Lucy used a variety of euphemisms such as expecting and in the family way as she tried to get Ricky to catch on. The season continued to chronicle

Lucy's pregnancy in a light-hearted and comical way and on January 19, 1953, more than 44 million Americans tuned in to watch the episode when Little Ricky was born, which was over 70 percent of all households that had a TV ("'I Love Lucy,' 'Lucy Is Enceinte' More than 60 Years Later and More Talked about TV Pregnancies" 2013; Bor 2013).

From that point on, pregnancy and childbirth became a staple of entertainment programming and TV shows regularly featured storylines with pregnant characters and births. Even though pregnancy was now an open topic on TV shows, it did not portray women in the delivery room delivering a baby until the 1980s. Notable on screen pregnancies and deliveries include Elyse Keaton's pregnancies with Andrew of *Family Ties*, Rachel's delivery of Emma Gellar-Greene on *Friends,* and Murphy Brown's pregnancy as a single woman which drew national attention and criticism from Vice-President Dan Quayle. Even though these storylines and birth scenes were included in programs primarily for entertainment value, they were often the closest that most women got to witness a delivery until they were in the delivery room themselves. *New York Times* reporter Andrew Newman noted that the depiction of pregnancy and birth on TV has come a long way since the days of *I Love Lucy*, that the pregnancy test brand, First Response, was actually paying for product placement in popular programs like *Sex in the City* (Newman 2009).

In the late 1990s, a new genre of TV programming hit the public which was reality TV. Now, instead of watching scripted shows for entertainment, people tuned in to watch real people just living their lives. The first reality program is considered to be MTV's *Real World* which billed itself as the true story of seven strangers picked to live in a house. Viewers loved the unscripted show and TV producers loved the low production costs. Various programs soon hit the airways including the Learning Channel's *A Baby Story* which quickly became one of its highest rated programs when it was introduced in 1998. This was a spinoff of the networks highly popular program, *A Wedding Story,* which told the story of a couple and followed them on their wedding day. The premise of *A Baby Story* was simple. Each episode featured a couple who was expecting and gave a little background on the couple, their family, and the pregnancy. The highlight of the program was the actual delivery where viewers were given a very up close look at the labor and delivery process whether it was a home water birth or a scheduled C-section. The program always ended with a follow-up of the couple and new baby or a babies a few months later once they were home and adjusted and everyone was smiling and doing well.

The success of *A Baby Story* led to *Bringing Home Baby*, a similar program but instead of chronicling the pregnancy and birth, this program showed what life was like the first 48 hours after the baby or babies came home. The public, or at least women of childbearing age, continued to be fascinated by these shows as they provided an intimate glimpse into the process or labor and delivery, and experiences that most people do not have the opportunity to directly observe. There have been a variety of other reality programs focused on pregnancy and childbirth, many of which focus specifically on women experiencing high-risk pregnancies including the popular series on Discovery Health, *Deliver Me*, which chronicles a high-risk obstetrics practice. These programs focused on pregnancies and deliveries with complications and frequently featured examples of premature birth, but it is important to note that these shows never reached the popularity or viewership of TLC's original programming. Whether this was due to the content of the programs or the fact that there were so many similar programs to choose from is unknown.

Pregnancy and childbirth have also made their appearance in the movies. Following the same sorts of storylines as TV depictions, pregnancies and births are often included for their dramatic or comedic effects and the scenes frequently rely heavily on cliché representations of labor and birth. Again, images of a bumbling fathers, a screaming woman, water breaking and gushing everywhere, and a frantic ride to the hospital can easily be called to mind. Classic films such as *Father of the Bride II* and *Look Who's Talking* provide comic depictions of childbirth and all that can possibly go wrong before the delivery, but end with a happy mother, father, and newborn. When a movie presents a different picture of pregnancy or tells a different story about woman and her childbirth, it is often unsettling to audiences who are used to equating a child being born with happiness. Some notable exceptions to more traditional storylines include the critically acclaimed independent film *Juno* in which a teenage girl learns she is pregnant and opts to have the baby and give it up for adoption as well as the somewhat raunchy comedy *Knocked Up* where a single woman finds out she is pregnant after having a one night stand with a man she met in a bar. In both of these films the pregnancy itself is not a welcome event as both women are not ready to become mothers and much of the storyline focuses on the women's struggle to decide what to do and whether or not she is ready to be a mother.

One may wonder why accounts of pregnancy and childbirth both fictional and nonfictional draw so many viewers and make such good TV. Media commentator Zoe Williams (2012) explains that logically one might think that birth would turn viewers off as it is at times a gross and intimate process involving a large amount of body parts and bodily fluids, but she argues that the pull of storylines involving birth is that it is both dramatic and universal. Pregnancy and childbirth is something that is common to the human experience which means that audiences can relate at some level, even if they have not been pregnant themselves. Birth is dramatic in that it frequently involves pain, the full range of human emotions, and in the end a new life has entered the world.

WHY IT MATTERS

So we know that pregnancy and birth are shown on TV, appear in film, and are written about in books, but the question is why or does this even matter. How much of a role does the media, broadly define as entertainment and news programs, movies, books, and magazines, play in both educating the public about and shaping their perceptions of pregnancy and childbirth? When radio and TV were first gaining in popularity, media scholars argued that media was a magic bullet and the messages that were sent out were received by the audience. Over time this theory was mostly disproved as multiple people could hear or watch the same program and come away with differing ideas and opinions (Scheufele and Tewksbury 2007; Neuman and Guggenheim 2011). More modern research and thought on how media influences the public can be found in Gerbner's Cultivation Hypothesis which proposes that the messages sent by the mass media shape the public's perception and belief concerning reality. The basic idea of the Cultivation Hypothesis is that the images and messages the public see on TV work to shape the public's beliefs concerning the world. The more the audience sees something on TV, the more they believe that this is an accurate representation of reality. For example, studies have found that the more violent programs one watches, the more likely someone is to believe that the world around them is violent and the more likely they are to fear being the victim of a crime (Potter 1986; Gerbner 1998). It stands to reason then, that the images and stories of pregnancy and childbirth we see on TV shape our beliefs as to what pregnancy and childbirth are like and perhaps even more importantly what the experiences should be like.

It can also be argued that the media might be even more powerful in shaping perceptions of childbirth and pregnancy than it is shaping ideas about other phenomena due to the limited exposure the public has to the actual events and lack of personal experience with the events. Most people have not been in a delivery room unless they or their partner has given birth and until they have personally experienced it, the majority of women do not have a good idea of just what will go on during a delivery. Researchers Handfiled, Turnbull, and Bell (2006) explain that with the medicalization of childbirth and the modernization of the American family, few women have directly observed a birth and instead must rely on media representations to observe what occurs. The statistics and evidence certainly support this claim. In 2006, the Center for Childbirth released its report *Listening to Mothers II*, one of the most comprehensive surveys of women in the United States who had given birth during the previous year. Of the 1583 women interviewed, 68 percent reported that they regularly watched reality programs about pregnancy. Of women who were pregnant for the first time, 72 percent said the shows helped them to understand what birth might be like (Declercq et al. 2002).

In it more recent report from 2013, *Listening to Mothers* III, the Center reported that 65 percent of women still reported watching reality-based programs. Additional questions revealed that women said the programs got them excited about the upcoming birth, taught them about medical terminology, gave them information about delivery, and 25 percent said the shows actually contributed to their anxiety about the upcoming birth (Corry 2013). In terms of sexual health in general, TV programs, including fictional shows are a primary source of information for women under the age of 30. A 2009 study conducted by the The National Campaign to Prevent Teen Unwanted Pregnancy reported that 43 percent of women aged 18–29 use the media as the primary source of information to learn about their reproductive health and also named media as their preferred method for learning about sexual health over professional sources such as their physician or a nurse. This means that a large percentage of women of childbearing age are learning about pregnancy, pregnancy symptoms, and pregnancy complications from watching TV shows.

One may think that once a woman is pregnant, she might start to rely on more traditional sources, but some research indicates that this is not the case. Studies have found that there has been an increase in TV viewing specifically for the purpose of learning about pregnancy and delivery is taking place as the number of women attending birthing classes decreases. In 2002, 70 percent of first-time mothers reported taking a child birth preparation class whereas in 2012 only 59 percent reported taking a class (Declercq et al. 2002). Young (2010) argues that as women rely more and more on media for information, it becomes increasingly important to be aware of media content and how women use the media to inform their understanding of pregnancy and childbirth as well as their medical decisions. Even though pregnancy shows are billed as reality program, meaning they depict events as they occurred instead of reenacting something and following a script, there is still a large amount of editing that is done to condense what might have been a 15-hour labor into a neat 21-minute TV segment meaning viewers do not get the full story.

Because women are using TV as an information source, it is important to know then what is being portrayed on TV and in terms of high-risk pregnancies and premature birth and if these issues are being sufficiently addressed? A 2014 study of prime time TV and sexual and reproductive health found that there were several storylines featuring pregnancy and delivery complications as these topics made for good dramatic storytelling. Further analysis of the programs showed that only 42 percent on the shows had a moderate level of accurate informational content and that the storylines tended to focus on the life and death situations that arose from the complications rather than the symptoms and ways to prevent complications. The positive of their findings that there was some exposure to pregnancy complications and premature birth, but the storylines were not always entirely accurate and the information was portrayed in such a dramatic way that it would be easy for the audience to discount the possibility of something similar happening in their own lives (Pariera et al. 2014).

It is easy to be critical of media for their fictional depictions of labor and childbirth or for glossing over serious complications, but media can be an excellent way to spread awareness and educate the public about health issues and health issues specially related to pregnancy and premature birth. The field of Entertainment Education exists to insert key health messages and information into entertainment programming in the attempts to both educate the public and to influence them to engage in positive health behaviors. Medical dramas such as *ER* and *Grey's Anatomy* have been credited with raising awareness about multiple medical conditions and increasing audience member's desire to engage in preventative health behaviors. So it is important to recognize that not all education and information that comes from the media is bad, and often women and the general public learn a lot about medical conditions and treatment options from TV viewing. Studies have shown that after episodes of popular TV shows with a medical storyline air, there is often a large increase in the number of times that medical condition is searched on Google, indicating that the fictional stories are prompting viewers to seek out more information. In 2013, the widely popular British drama, *Downton Abbey*, featured a storyline where one of the main female characters, Lady Sybil, died following childbirth after her preeclampsia progressed so far that she suffered from seizures and her condition progressed to eclampsia, a condition for which there is no cure. The show was applauded for bringing attention to a serious medical issue that many women are unware of until they are diagnosed. After the program aired, audiences turned to Google to find out more making preeclampsia one of the most searched terms that day (Brown 2013).

Not only are TV shows, and specifically reality shows teaching women about the ins and outs of pregnancy, but media has also contributed to a societal narrative as to how pregnancy and birth should progress, what a woman should experience and feel, and how mothers should relate to their new infants. Certainly variations of this tale exist as women differ in their actual birth experience ranging from being assisted by a midwife at home or being admitted to the hospital for a scheduled C-section. However, there is a general script these stories follow which has given rise to several criticisms. The story begins with an overriding perception that motherhood is and should be a woman's ultimate goal. This promotes the ideal of the purely unselfish mother who would do anything and everything for her offspring as well as the notion that there is instantaneous bonding and joy upon the birth of an infant. The pain and agony of childbirth is almost always worth it and quickly forgotten once a woman holds her new baby in her arms. This narrative does not allow for a woman to be tired, stressed, or confused when their new infants enter the world.

Media scholars and the general public have mounted criticisms of both fictional and actual accounts of pregnancy and childbirth on TV and in the movies for what are inaccurate or cliché portrayals. One of the major criticisms is the reliance of medical interventions in the deliveries which reaffirms the idea that pregnancy is a condition that needs to be highly monitored and controlled by the medical field. The majority of the time, labor and delivery are portrayed as something urgent and requiring immediate medical attention. Think of fathers rushing to the hospital as their wives sit next to them screaming that the baby is about to come or a woman's water breaking and just a few minutes later she is on the delivery table ready to push. These depictions are generally for dramatic and a comedic effect, but critics argue that these create a general fear of labor and delivery as well as a belief that immediate medical intervention is needed (West 2010). Another critique is the equating of a fast delivery with a good delivery, and the inclusion of a happy ending despite any complications that present themselves. For as much drama and peril is shown, once a woman learns that her baby is coming, programs or birth scenes almost always end with a healthy baby and happy parents. Very rarely do we see babies born with complications or mothers and babies needing extensive medical intervention after the birth (Morris and McInerney 2010).

Sears and Godderis (2011), prominent media scholars, argue that we need to pay particular attention to the impacts of reality. They explain that one of the reasons reality is so powerful in shaping the audiences beliefs is that it is presented as true and factual rather than as a scripted drama. Even though there may just be a camera recording the scenes, there is a long editing process that selects which scenes to show and how to put those scenes together that shapes and molds the story that is told. In reviewing episodes of *A Baby Story*, they found that the show served to reinforce the medical model of childbirth and generally portrayed women as passive participants in the delivery process by showing them following doctors' and nurses' orders without question. In not showing women discussing different birth and pain management options, they felt there was a missed opportunity to educate the audience that women can be active participants in their labor and deliveries and have the right to ask questions and make choices. No matter what the praise or criticism of pregnancy and birth portrayals are, there is a general consensus that watching TV and other media is one of the general ways that women learn what pregnancy should be like and develop an idea of what childbirth will entail.

HIGH-RISK PREGNANCY ON TV

Although pregnancy and birth have become a staple of entertainment and reality programming, storylines featuring high-risk pregnancies and premature births are less common, and when these types of storylines are included, they are often depicted in less than accurate ways. Just a few weeks ago I was flipping through the TV looking for something mindless to lose myself in and I came across the episode of *Friends* when Phoebe, who acted as a surrogate for her brother, delivered a set of triplets. I stopped and watched the episode curious as to how the event would be depicted. The delivery was typical for a sitcom, and I probably would have enjoyed it if I was not so busy noting all of the incredible inaccuracies. The show never mentioned how far along Phoebe was, but the closing scene of the episode showed Phoebe alone in her recovery room holding three typical sized newborns, none of which were hooked up to any kind of machine or monitor which would make one assume they were pretty close to full term. Obviously *Friends* is a comedy and the purpose of the show is to entertain and make people laugh, but even comedies can contribute to the cultural narrative about birth and pregnancy.

The general consensus among the women I spoke with who had high-risk pregnancies or premature babies is that there is a lack of depictions of pregnancies with complications and when these types of storylines are included they are often full of inaccuracies and do not adequately portray the true risk involved with having a preemie. Many medical dramas such as *ER*, *Grey's Anatomy*, and *Private Practice* have included stories of different pregnancy and delivery complications and although one may argue that there are benefits in terms of raising awareness about the possibility or having a preemie, preemie moms themselves are often frustrated by the stories they see. In an ongoing discussion on a forum on The Bump, a social website for pregnant women and mothers, women wrote about the worst offenders of inaccurate portrayals of premature birth. One mother wrote, "My fav is the Grey's episode where Alex kangaroos a 27 weeker for like three days straight with no monitors, tubes, vents, IV. . .nothing! I actually stopped watching after that." In this episode the 27-week infant was given little chance of survival, so Alex who was a neonatal resident took it upon himself to kangaroo the baby who regained his strength and survived. The lack of tubes and the fact that most parents are only allowed to hold their

27 weekers for limited amounts of time made the program seem unbelievable. This gives rise to the concern that programs like this give the public and future preemie parents an unrealistic expectation of what it is like to have a preemie in the hospital.

The medical drama *Private Practice* which aired from 2007 to 2013 frequently had storylines where a woman's pregnancy was high risk or a baby was born early as one of the main characters on the show, Addison Sheppard, was a neonatologist. Even though women appreciated that there was some acknowledgment of the fact that not every pregnancy goes perfectly and results in a full-term healthy baby, they were highly critical of how those stories played out. For one thing, Addison was almost always able to save the mother and child. Even though she may have mentioned the risks of prematurity at some point to the parents, the episodes almost always ended with the forecasting of a bright future for the baby. The NICU was sometimes shown, but almost always things were not entirely medically accurate and the *Private Practice* medical staff were frequently able to work miracles. There was, also, very rarely a follow up on the cases so viewers had no idea of what issues a 24-week preemie faced a year or two later.

There have been some programs though, that have been recognized for accurately portraying medical issues related to pregnancy and early delivery and bringing much needed public attention to these medical issues. The first season of the popular medical drama *ER* included an episode titled "Love's Labor Lost" in which a woman 38 weeks pregnant came to the ER complaining of not feeling well and frequent urination. She was diagnosed with a urinary tract infection, given a prescription, and discharged. After she collapses in the hospital parking lot she is brought back into the ER and has a seizure caused by her high blood pressure. What doctors had missed when she was first in the ER was that she was in the late stages of preeclampsia and went on to develop full blown eclampsia. Her labor was immediately induced, but problems during the delivery forced doctors to perform an emergency C-section during which the woman had another seizure. Doctors were able to save the baby, but the mother passed away during surgery. Some may think this was just an overly dramatic portrayal of pregnancy to grab viewers, but the reality is that once a woman progresses to full blown eclampsia the risk of seizure, stroke, and even death is high. This episode brought attention to the condition as well as some of the early warning signs and also prompted pregnant women to ask their doctors about the condition. A *Chicago Tribune* article reported that obstetricians including Dr. Martin Hyman, chief of obstetrics at a New York City hospital received a deluge of calls from pregnant patients concerned about potential symptoms. While the majority of these patients were just fine, the episode was applauded for impelling women to pay attention to their bodies and symptoms as preeclampsia if closely monitored and appropriately treated can result a successful and healthy delivery for both the mother and baby (Condor 1995).

Even though it has been criticized, *Private Practice*, has been recognized for some of its storylines involving high-risk pregnancies and severe pregnancy complications. Perhaps one of the most heart wrenching storylines took place when one of the doctors on the program, Amelia Shepherd, learned that the baby she was carrying had anencephaly, a rare neural condition where parts of the baby's brain and skull do not grow. This condition is always fatal and the majority of infants with the condition live for just a few minutes after birth. Dr. Shepherd chose to carry her baby to term and planned to donate the baby's organs after birth. The storyline tracked her prenatal care as well as her mental and emotional struggles during the pregnancy and the storyline culminated with an episode titled, "Gone Baby Gone" which chronicled the doctor's labor and delivery. The show ended with Amelia holding her newborn daughter who let out a few squeaks before Amelia handed the baby off to the waiting medical team that would harvest the organs. This episode struck a chord with viewers as well as women who had similar experiences who appreciated the show telling the story.

In talking about the influence of media on perceptions of pregnancy and childbirth, it is important to look at the specific genre of reality TV shows that depict the lives of family with higher-order multiples. Even though these programs generally do not follow the family during the pregnancy, they often came up in the interviews where women had multiples. Most of the general audience sees these shows as an entertaining look at families with a lot of young children, but the fact is that these shows are also depicting children whose mother's underwent a high-risk pregnancy and children who due to their multiples status were sometimes born very prematurely. These shows have the opportunity to portray the ongoing struggles of families with preemies, something that is not generally seen on TV. The first show that grabbed America's attention was *Jon and Kate + 8* which chronicled the lives of Jon and Kate Gosselin and their eight children who were a set of twins and a set of sextuplets. The program originally aired on Discovery Health and in 2009 was picked up by TLC and became one of the station's highest rated programs ever. America was fascinated by the family and tuned in to see how the family navigated life with eight small children and the sextuplets who despite their prematurity were healthy and thriving. After six seasons Jon and Kate divorced and the show was renamed *Kate + 8* and after two seasons was cancelled.

Feeding off of the popularity of *Jon + Kate*, other shows about multiples soon followed including *Table for Twelve, Quints by Surprise*, *Make Room for Multiples*, and *Raising Sextuplets*. As the rate of multiple births in the country grew, so too did the public's fascination with what it is like to raise four, five, or six babies at once. In the majority of these programs the children were in good health and had few long-term complications due to their prematurity. The one exception was on *Table for Twelve* which aired for two seasons on TLC and followed the Hayes family, a New Jersey family with two sets of twins and a set of sextuplets. Born at 32, weeks five of the sextuplets have no health issues or delays, but one of the girls has cerebral palsy and is confined to a wheelchair. Her disability is a part of the show and the parents are very open about how her prematurity directly contributed to her medical issues.

When it comes to multiple births and the risks of prematurity, there has also been criticism of the ways that news media covers this topic. Charles and Shivas (2002) analyzed the ways that newspapers covered the issues of illegal drug use during pregnancy and the continuation of pregnancies with multiple fetuses. They reported that although both these health issues presented great risk to the infants, due to the threat of preterm birth and other complications, news coverage condemned the use of illegal drugs while portraying multiple births as miraculous occurrences. This is of course not to say that using illegal drugs is at all equivalent to having higher-order multiples, but instead they argued that the media's positive portrayal of multiple births was a contributing factor to the general belief that multiple pregnancies are fun and exciting and suggest a general lack of knowledge or concern about the risks involved. In not focusing on the risks of prematurity both in terms of infant survival and long-term complications, they argued that the media was doing a disservice to the public. In a critique of the way that the news sensationalizes multiple births, Australian media commentator Bettina Arndt argued that too much focus in the media is of cute photo ops of multiples wearing matching outfits and too little focus on the real hardships of having multiples. She wrote, "What we don't see are the parents torn apart by grief over lost babies. . . . We hear little about parents who spend months setting next to hospital incubators while premature babies fight to survive. And rarely are we told of the disabilities affecting many of these children including the increased risk for blindness, cerebral palsy, organ dysfunction, and learning disabilities" (Ardnt 2006).

The public and media's fascination with higher-order multiple births, the term used to denote pregnancies of triplets or more, led Mothers of Super Twins (MOST), super twins being another nickname for triplets or more, to issue a position statement on media exposure and multiple births. Some of the reasons families may participate in media interviews and other types of programming include their excitement and desire to share their children with the community as well as pressure from media who want a good story or other sources such as hospital administrators who desire positive press for their organizations. MOST also recognizes though that media coverage and participation in media projects can quickly go wrong for families as they open themselves up to intense scrutiny from the public for their choices, including the choice to proceed with a higher-order multiple pregnancy as well as their decisions about how to raise their children and manage their finances. Another critique of a majority of the media coverage is that it is very one sided and will often prevent either an overly pessimistic or optimistic view on multiples, births which serves to reinforce the positive and negative beliefs the public has and misses the opportunities to provide real education about the challenges that parents of multiple preemies face.

READ ALL ABOUT IT

Another popular way that women learn about pregnancy is by reading. Countless books have been written about pregnancy, childbirth, taking care of infants, and childrearing. A search on Amazon.com for pregnancy-related books bring up over 195,000 results to choose from. Purchasing pregnancy books is another rite of passage for many, akin to buying bridal magazines after getting engaged. In her book *Pregnancy in Practice*, Sallie Han (2013) describes how pregnancy in many ways becomes a literary event as women start to read up on pregnancy and delivery because the situation is so new and foreign to them. The purchasing of pregnancy and child-rearing books is similar to the ritual of buying maternity clothes. It is a behavior that is only done when one is pregnant and it marks a woman as an expectant mother. Of course women can talk to friends and family and other women, but as she notes in her book, a lot of women felt that the information they found in books was more accurate and more representative of women in general than the anecdotal tales they heard or read from individual women. For many, the printed word held more authority than advice from a friend or even what she could find online. Interestingly enough, not every popular pregnancy guide book is written by an obstetrician or even someone from the medical field, but in general there was a perception that if the book made it to the shelf it had some credibility.

After my positive pregnancy test with my first pregnancy, the first thing I did was have my husband take me to Barnes & Noble so I could purchase my own copy of *What to Expect When you are Expecting* written by Eisenberg, Murkoff, and Hathway. There were a lot of options on the shelves, but this was the book that I most connected to pregnancy and it was the book I had heard others talk about and had seen on relatives' and friends' shelves, so this was the book I got. It seemed to me that owning this book was not only a way to gather information, but it was also a symbolic way for me to declare to myself that I was pregnant and now could join the ranks of all of the other mothers I knew. I was not alone in my choice as this was the most commonly mentioned book when I spoke with women. The book is currently in its 4th edition, was on the *New York Times* bestseller list for over eight years, and was named one of the most influential books of the past 25 years by USA Today. Countless women have used this book to guide them through their pregnancies as it covers the changes a woman undergoes and the development of the baby from conception to birth.

This book is not without its critics though from both professionals and the women themselves who have read and own it. A 2005 article in the *New York Times* reported that Brigham Obstretrics and Gynecology, a practice affiliated with Brigham and Women's Hospital in Boston specifically advises its patients not to read *What to Expect* calling the book alarmist and creating unnecessary concern for women about potential complications (Kantor 2005). Many women have also complained about the book as they said it created worries that they never even knew they should have. The worries often came from the section of each chapter that in the first two editions was labeled "What you may be concerned about this month" which is a written as a Q&A and warns women about potential threats to a healthy pregnancy including a poor diet, chemical exposure, and excessive physical activity. Huffington Post contributor Lisa Belkin wrote about how reading the book during her first pregnancy cause her massive anxiety as she became obsessed with everything she ate and did, constantly worrying about things that could harm the baby. She also found herself panicking over every pregnancy symptom as she wondered if it could point to a more serious complication (Belkin 2012). In her book *The Rhetoric of Pregnancy*, Marika Seigel (2013) shared her experience of buying and leafing through her own copy of *What to Expect*, after she learned she was pregnant with her first child. Her excitement quickly turned to an underlying state of anxiety as she read about what she might be concerned about each month and discovered problems and complications that she never knew existed. The general critiques of Murkoff's books are not that she presents information about risks and complications with pregnancy, as this is critical information that women need, but instead her focus on relatively obscure risks such as a warning in an early edition to avoid oral sex during pregnancy as it could potentially cause an embolism that could be fatal for mother and child.

Even though *What to Expect* has been one of the best-selling pregnancy books of the past 30 years, countless pregnancy books provide an account of what happens during a pregnancy and childbirth from a medical standpoint. There have also been other popular books written from a lay person's perspective that promise to give women the truth about pregnancy and delivery such as *The Girlfriends Guide to Pregnancy* or Jenny McCarthy's *Belly Laughs*. In terms of books written specifically for high-risk pregnancies, fewer titles are available. For women pregnant with multiples, the book most commonly mentioned was *When You're Pregnant with Twins, Triplets, or Quads: Proven Guidelines for a Healthy Multiple Pregnancy* by Dr. Barbara Luke and Tamara Eberlein (2013), now in its 3rd edition. Some mothers also mentioned books about raising preemies and navigating the NICU as helpful resources.

Another written source of pregnancy-related information is newspapers and magazines. This source is different from pregnancy books as generally women do not go to the newspaper looking for specific pregnancy-related information, but will come across pregnancy-related articles and consume the information both when pregnant and when not pregnant. Women's Studies scholar, Katie Gentile documented an increase in the number of news items related to pregnancy after 2011, a fact she attributes to a cultural trend that places a high value on motherhood as one of women's penultimate achievements. What is interesting is not just that there are more news items about the topic, but what the content of those articles are. While a few articles reported on premature birth and pregnancy complications, the majority of articles focused on either celebrities' pregnancies or births, with a particular emphasis on women's weight loss after the birth, or on potential risks or dangers for pregnant women or on general ways to protect one's fertility. Now, the fact that risks were highlighted might seem like an encouraging finding, but a deeper look into the types of risks that were reported on shows that most of the reports focused on the potential hazards of not eating a healthy diet prior to conception and gaining too much weight during pregnancy. Few articles specifically addressed the symptoms, causes, or prevention of premature labor (Gentile 2011).

WOMEN'S EXPERIENCES WITH THE MEDIA

As women talked about what they had seen and read, it became apparent that TV and other media depictions of pregnancy, birth, and motherhood had given them expectations of what pregnancy and birth would be like. It was equally apparent that their own stories rarely looked like the stories they saw. This was a source of frustration and many times sadness. The interviews also revealed that some women sought out as much information as possible from the media while others preferred to take the less is more approach to their media consumption. Women were often critical of the media available to them and expressed the desire to have more options and more stories available. Finally the interviews showed that no matter how women felt about the media they consumed their own stories were greatly influenced by what they had watched and read about pregnancy.

As prior research has indicated, many women used media as a source of information. Almost every woman recalled at least one TV show or program she had watched about pregnancy and often women had watched multiple programs. Cynthia, mother of twins, described how she began watching *A Baby Story* and similar shows regularly once she was pregnant. She explained that she was most interested in watching programs about twins. Other mothers shared how they would search for TV programs about twins, triplets, and high-risk pregnancies, as these stories rang more true to their experiences than programs that depicted typical pregnancies. With the invention of digital recording devices women were able to enter search terms such as triplets or NICU to find and record programs with storylines similar to their own.

Amy, mother of twins, was a great example of how women actively sought out information by watching programs such as *A Baby Story*, and learning more about the birthing process,

> I think I found them more comforting than stressful. I don't know, just for me it seems, to think about how all of the birthing stuff goes down, it just gives me comfort. It's like, okay, I have seen it. It gives me just a little more insight on what's going to happen so that I wasn't in complete shock when, you know, I sort of could have, you know, an idea of what to expect, you know, if confronted with whatever. But usually they don't have the horrible ones of TV. You know, it's usually the regular, the normal. . . .

Amy initially watched the shows because it was her first pregnancy and she wanted some kind of idea of what was to come. When she experienced complications in her pregnancy and went into labor prematurely the programs no longer had prepared her and she had a difficult time comparing her experiences to those she had seen on TV.

In terms of books focused on high-risk pregnancy, the Dr. Luke book got mixed reviews as women expressed mixed feelings about the book. Some women believed it was an excellent guide, followed all the recommendations, and credited following the guidelines with their more positive outcomes. Some twin mothers told me they followed her advice as closely as possible and were able to carry their twins to at least 36 weeks. Other women disliked the book and felt as if some of her recommendations, such as eating 5000 calories a day, were unrealistic. Still other women were put off by the blunt discussion of the possible complications of a multiple pregnancy and felt the book placed tremendous pressure on them to have a great outcome such as those featured in the book because the they felt that the book implied that having a successful pregnancy with multiples was just a matter of following the book's suggestions.

Astrid, mother of triplets, was one of the women who liked Dr Luke's books. She explained, ". . .The Doctor Luke book was very informative. It opened my eyes quite a bit to what could be." For her, the stories of very premature infants with severe complications helped her to understand what the risks of early delivery were and strengthened her resolve to do anything in her power to ensure a good outcome. Another mother of triplets, Ambrosia, talked about one of the most powerful images in the book which was a page that featured the footprints of infants born at each week of gestation. "They show you these picture of the babies at 24 weeks, like their head size and their foot. And you are like, okay, I don't want that to be me." Several other women mentioned the foot image and the stories they read of extremely premature infants as a driving force to stay on strict bed rest and follow all of their doctors' orders in an attempt to prevent their own stories from featuring such tiny and premature infants.

For some of the women who experienced more rare complications or pregnancies with higher-order multiples, books, and TV were one of the few places where they could find stories about situations like their own. Christine spoke about watching the popular program, *Jon and Kate + 8*. As a parent of triplets she had an added interest in how this family tried to raise their two sets of multiples. She explained that although she did not particularly enjoy or admire the family, she did appreciate seeing a depiction of family life that more closely resembled her own. She explained, "I do watch *Jon and Kate + 8*, but sometimes get annoyed by it. Sometimes, I don't know, sometimes it kind of helps validate me sometimes." This show represented one of the few stories she saw on TV that somewhat mirrored her own life and experiences and even though she did not particularly like the show she still watched for the sense of connection and familiarity. The program normalized her own experiences as she observed another family whose life was even more crazy and chaotic than her own.

Another mother of triplets had a slightly different reaction to the reality program. Jenny, mother of triplets and a singleton, also talked about watching *Jon and Kate + 8*. "Like, I watch *Jon and Kate* and I just sit there and think, oh my god, how does she do it? Because I'm like, I'm ready to pull my hair out now. I cannot imagine. I cannot imagine having six and the two older." She was also in awe of the many trips and outings that they were able to take. "And then I see the places they take them and that was great. They live in a much bigger city and there is much more to do. But I'm thinking, I wouldn't be taking my three to any of those places. Because you think, there is too much to get into and they're going to get lost." In this case the program was setting up expectations for Jenny of what life with multiples should be like, but rather than identifying with what she saw, she compared her own experiences and found her story to be lacking. Further discussion did bring up the issue of the money the show generated and some of the help the family received that was not featured on air, which allowed the family to participate in so many opportunities.

Other mothers discussed how popular reality programs and news featuring multiples gave an inaccurate picture of the risks and challenges of having multiples. They pointed to shows such as *Jon + Kate Plus 8* or the national fascination with the Nadeya Suleman, dubbed the "octomom," a California woman who gave birth to octuplets in 2009, as examples of stories that did not characterize the true nature of having multiples and the risks associated with higher-order multiple births. Much of the focus of the programs was on what they described as the cute factor and crazy antics of several babies, but rarely did the issues of developmental delays, health conditions, and the stress of the experience on the mother and the family come up. They also complained that many of the programs did not detail the behind the scenes help families had such as nannies, cleaning services, volunteers, and financial assistance. More than one of the mothers of triplets who was interviewed mentioned that others assumed they were showered with free gifts from companies when, in reality, the most women reported getting was a case of free formula and a box or two of diapers.

AVOIDING MEDIA

Several of the women who gave birth to premature infants went through a period where they tried to avoid hearing or reading stories about other women who had given birth to full-term infants. The success or happy stories of others dredged up feelings of bitterness and envy. The happy stories often stood in stark contrast to the women's experiences, so they tried to avoid them altogether in order to minimize their bitter and envious reactions. For example, some of the women described turning off TV programs when a full-term infant was depicted, as it was too hard to see someone else's happiness, ideal delivery, or healthy infants. Women also avoided stories about infants who did not need time in the NICU because they were too hard to hear and watch, and the scenes of women cuddling with their babies after delivery and dredged up feelings of envy and grief.

Women also avoid media sometimes because it was too upsetting or scary. Michelle, a mother of triplets, described how she was selective in what kinds of TV programs she watched, such as *A Baby Story*. When asked if she watched these kinds of programs, she replied, "Not while I was pregnant, not like, and especially when it was something scary." Jenny, mother of triplets, explained, "I tried hard not to research it too well." Jenny actively tried to avoid information about all of the complications of a triplet pregnancy.

Nancy, mother of twins, also struggled with infertility and hated watching programs filled with pregnancies and infants. She found that even after she became pregnant, she still did not want to watch shows such as *A Baby Story*, "Yeah, I mean when I was in the hospital on bed rest for two weeks. The only channels they had were like the local TV channels and like the baby channels and I was like I don't want to see a C-section, I don't want to see—I'm pretty grossed out anyway. I don't like it and I had never watched those shows because of the whole infertility thing. I kind of just pushed that out of my mind."

Karen is the mother of two sets of twins, one boy-boy and one boy-girl. As we spoke, Karen struck me as an incredibly pragmatic person who focused on doing what she needed to do to raise her children successfully. She explained that during her first pregnancy she felt that she was obligated to watch shows about pregnancy and childbirth. She believed that watching the programs was part of what you did when you were pregnant similar to registering for baby items and reading pregnancy magazines. As her pregnancy progressed, she quit watching the programs, and even now she tends to isolate herself from a lot of media. She explained,

> I had to watch them when I was pregnant because I thought that I should. Then I was in pregnant mom mode, and now, I don't like to hear about people having problems. And I'm not just watching the news because I don't like hearing about it. Which makes me a little naïve to the world, but I found that it happen regardless of having to hear it, I don't feel like the world is bad. I just don't feel like hearing about child abductions. I don't feel like hearing about an accident or that a kid was killed.

For Karen, seeing, knowing, and hearing about the bad things that could happen did not change if they were going to happen, so she saw no reason to expose herself to the negative information.

Carla, mother of twins, found herself watching fewer programs specifically about pregnancy and childbirth as her pregnancy progressed. She explained, "I started to watch the Discovery Channel, *A Baby Story*, I watch the specials on TV. And everyone was having C-sections and they were still screaming in pain and it's just like, I'm like, I'm not watching that every night. So I stopped watching those shows because I don't want to see that every night. And I got enough of like, okay, that's what did happen." For both these women the reality of having a caesarean and potential complications were too real, and TV programs depicting painful and stressful deliveries were not entertaining or soothing, but instead just one more source of stress. This brings to light the interesting tension discussed at length in the previous chapter that many women found between wanting to be informed and being critical of media programs for not showing more pregnancies with complications, and also not wanting to be confronted with frightening story lines and images.

In addition to TV programs, women also talked to me about some of the different books they received as gifts or bought for themselves to read. In addition to pregnancy books, some women got books about life in the NICU after their babies were born. Sam was one of those moms. After her daughter was born she started reading a few books she got from the store, but quickly stopped. She explained that her thinking was along the lines of, "I am living this, I don't need to be reading this." She felt like each day she was living everything the book was talking about and describing, so there was no point in reading it. Cora was another mom who did not find books written specifically about prematurity to be helpful. Someone recommended that she get a book and she did, but only flipped through a few pages before she was so overwhelmed that she had to put it down. At this point she decided that she would rely on the doctors and nurses to tell her what issues her daughter had and what she needed to be worried about. The preemie book had too many bad possibilities for Cora to think about. A lot of mother's mentioned getting a book from the NICU from the March of Dimes that covered some of the basics of the premature babies and NICU terminology, but many said that they only glanced through it and instead tended to learn about the NICU and the different machines and terms from their nurses. Haley went out and bought a book about raising a preemie but she quickly quit reading it because as she said, "I didn't need to read the book. I was living the book."

Dissatisfaction with Media

As women's pregnancies progressed and they gave birth, many began to view media more critically. Christine, mother of triplets, talked about watching *Bringing Home Baby,* with her husband during her pregnancy and while her daughters were in the NICU. *Bringing Home Baby* is a program that follows families for the first 48 hours after their infants come home from the hospital. As Christine contemplated what it would be like to bring her three infants home she found herself examining the stories she saw with a critical eye, "Yeah I know, after the girls were born. I remember my husband, and I we were watching one show, it's *Bringing Home Baby*, and they had like the woman and husband and the woman's parents were there. And it was like, you people need four adults to care for one baby? You know, isn't that pathetic?" Other moms complained that when babies were born early the show skipped over the time in the NICU and jumped ahead to a few months later when the baby or babies were home from the hospital and doing well.

In this case, Christine's story differed from the norm she often saw on TV and, rather than making her feel bad about her own experience, it made her question the authenticity and accuracy of the programs on TV. She wondered if the shows made infants look so difficult to care for, for the drama effect rather than telling the true story. It also angered her that no TV programs were discussing how hard it is to have infants who are sick and in the NICU, unable to come home. The more she watched, the less she trusted the TV programs as a source of reliable information because the stories she was seeing did not ring true to her personal experience. A few of the triplet mothers I talked with mentioned how excited they were to see that episodes of *A Baby Story* and *Bringing Home Baby* were going to feature families with triplets. After viewing the programs they were disappointed because only a brief overview of the pregnancy was given and the time in the NICU was only mentioned in passing. Viewers who were not familiar with triplet pregnancies and the NICU would have no idea how high-risk the pregnancies actually were and when NICU time is reduced to a sentence stating the babies were in the hospital for five weeks, the general audience does not understand what those five weeks might have been like for the babies, mothers, and families.

Women were also critical of the books they read in terms of their discussion of birth and its complications. Many of the women spoke somewhat negatively about *What to Expect When You're Expecting*. Although the book has been criticized by many for being too alarmist in its coverage of the many possible complications of pregnancy/delivery and promoting paranoia, women who experienced complications found that the book lacked the detail they wanted and needed. Mary, mother of her son, Max, who was born at 32 weeks when her blood pressure spiked, remarked that only two pages at the back of the book discussed preeclampsia, rather than an entire chapter. After she was diagnosed with preeclampsia, the book was no longer useful to her. It is interesting to hear the criticisms of women who had pregnancy complications as compared to those with women who had typical pregnancies. Whereas many women thought that books such as *What to Expect* focused too much on what could go wrong, women who did have things go wrong found that there was not enough information. Women who did not have complications found all of the information on risks, many of which had a very low probability, was too much to take in and felt that it caused them undue worry. When women did have complications though, the brief one or two paragraph entries on the different conditions were hardly detailed enough to satisfy their informational needs. This points directly to the tension between being informed and protecting oneself from information that might be frightening or upsetting. So many women were blindsided when complications arose or when they went into premature labor as they had mostly skimmed over the complications section of the books they had or had simply not read them because they thought it did not pertain to themselves. For people and groups who are trying to educate women about premature birth and complications such as preeclampsia this presents a huge challenge. How does one keep women informed about risks and warning signs without scaring them so much that they stop reading or listening while providing enough information and education to assist women who are experiencing the risks?

When it came to pregnancies with multiples, some women complained about the lack of useful books as they had a hard time applying the information, advice, and stories to their own situations. Kelli, mother of twins, talked about her disappointment with the available books on twin pregnancies. She explained,

> I looked in the book *Pregnancy for Dummies* and I looked and there is like a page or a paragraph and they would just say the most idiotic things like, oh, it [having twins] is pretty much the same as having one. You just have two, and I am like, no, clearly whoever wrote that did not have multiple children. The *What to Expect When You are Expecting* book made me mad. It just would say it was just like having one but you have two, or three, or four. And I'm like no, honestly this is not helping, it is not just like having another.

Other mothers echoed the sentiment that the authors of these books who were giving them advice and information about raising multiples, raising preemies, or even coping with a high-risk pregnancy often had no direct experience and seemed out of touch.

Amy, mother of twin boys, also described her disappointment with the books she was able to find, "Well we didn't have the internet in our apartment then. You know we were just in a little apartment in Tampa. And I guess then, I mean, I read books, went to the library and got books about multiples. Um, a lot of this stuff does not seem to apply all of the sudden. Like it won't match stuff about multiples, so it's like, well shoot, well so that's not really helpful."

The authors' credibility were often questioned as women placed a much higher value on direct experience than on education or titles. If the author did not have firsthand experience with having or treating a high-risk pregnancy or multiples, women were more likely to reject the information.

The one notable exception to women's criticism of many of the books they found was their appreciation for biographies of other NICU moms. Most women did not read these until after they had delivered early and been through the NICU, but those who did remarked on how helpful it was to read a story that was so similar to their own. This was the first time that many women had heard another mother articulate some of the emotions they had felt and it was so reassuring to them. Because women had already been through the early delivery and NICU, the books were not frightening and upsetting, but instead were inspiring and reassuring. Women told me that sometimes when reading a book by a former preemie parent it was the first time that they ever felt like another person could articulate the thoughts and feelings they had during their pregnancies and while their children were in the NICU.

One of the primary functions of TV, movies, and books is to tell stories, so it of no surprise that media is a common source for women for pregnancy and birth narratives. Even when women are not actively seeking out such stories, they are often included within broader storylines and news reports about pregnancy and birth appear on a regular basis. Because media plays such a larger role in shaping the public's understanding about issues, the ways that pregnancy, birth, high-risk pregnancies, and premature birth are depicted by the media play a large role in both educating the public and forming their expectations of pregnancy and birth-related issues. For women actively seeking out pregnancy and birth narratives, there are a plethora of media sources women can turn to from reality TV programs to pregnancy guidebooks. It is important then to evaluate what stories and information the media is presenting, and even more importantly how women are using those stories to inform their own sense and decision-making. This chapter also points to the opportunity and need to provide multiple accounts of pregnancy and birth and to provide accurate depictions from trusted sources.

Chapter 8

Terrible Pregnancies and Traumatic Births

From the beginning of her pregnancy with her triplets, Julie's pregnancy was difficult. She was incredibly sick and was unable to keep anything down from almost the moment that she had a positive pregnancy test. When they saw three circles at her first ultrasound she started to cry and was on the verge of hysteria as she had no idea how she and her husband could possibly cope with three babies. Later that day as she continued to be violently ill and started to show signs of dehydration she was admitted to the hospital for IV fluids. As her pregnancy progressed her nausea continued to get worse and worse and she was both dehydrated and getting no nutrition which was presenting a threat to both her and the babies health. To treat her she got a home-health nurse who would come daily and administer IV fluids and Zofran, an anti-nausea medication. She also had a PICC line inserted so that she could get TPN, which is a nutritional supplement that bypasses the stomach. She continued to feel miserable but at least was able to get nutrition to her triplets.

Things continued to get worse as Julie's pregnancy progressed. She described just how bad things got.

> *I went in at 20 weeks for an ultrasound and that's when we saw that I was funneling with a bulging bag and I was having contractions that I thought were the babies moving. When the ultrasound tech got down to the bottom baby they were whispering and said see this, this where your cervix is supposed to be. My husband and I were just kind of quiet. The nurse came in and was like Julie I think you already know what is going on. And I just started crying and I thought I was going to lose all 3 of them. The doctor drew us a diagram and he said this is your little girl and her bag is bulging, we are going to try to do cerclage, but if we rupture her bag we might lose her, but we might be able to keep the boys in.*

They knew the procedure was risky, but there was nothing else to do. Julie was admitted to the hospital. Before the procedure they put her in the Trendelenburg position which is a reclined position where the feet are higher than the head to completely minimize the pressure on her cervix and gave her antibiotics to help prevent infection. Because her cervix was so dilated and bag or water was bulging so far that it took over two hours to get the stitches in and the entire time her husband was in the waiting room freaking out as he kept imaging that the worst had happened and they would lose all three babies.

After the procedure, she was in the hospital for a few more days with bleeding and was then sent home with orders to be on strict bed rest meaning that she even ate her meals lying down. The only time she left her bedroom was for a weekly appointment on Wednesdays and she was allowed to shower once a week. When she went for her appointment at 23 weeks they discovered that baby C had hardly any fluid in her sac. Because she was not yet 24 weeks there was nothing the hospital would or could do so they sent her home to wait and cry and hope for the best. When she made it to 24 weeks she was admitted to the hospital again and after the doctors made some changes to her medications enough fluid returned to her daughter's sac that she was sent home again on strict bed rest. At 25 weeks and 2 days she felt like she was leaking fluid, but when she called the OB's office the nurse told her that most likely one of the triplets was just lying on her bladder. The next day she started to have some terrible back pains and once they got too intense she called her husband at work and told him he needed to come home and take her to the hospital. She was having contractions one to two minutes apart and one of the baby's water had broken. At the hospital they immediately put her on an IV of magnesium sulfate to halt her labor.

Her contractions did slow and she continued with the pregnancy until 26 weeks and 3 days. On this day her contractions started to increase and the additional medications they gave her were not slowing anything down. The doctor came into her room and told her that they needed to deliver the babies that day. She was not at all ready for the babies to be born as it was still much too early. She described her reaction to learning that she was going in for delivery, "I was hysterically shaking, I was saying they are going to die they are going to die, it is too early. It took forever to get the spinal in. We thought they were not going to make it. I was only 8 pounds over my starting weight. When I laid down on the table I did not even look like I had a belly." When the first baby was born, a boy, they heard a small cry and his sister and brother quickly followed. All three babies were intubated in the operating room and then covered with plastic to keep their skin moist. She begged to be able to see them and the nurses moved the heating tables closer to her head so she was able to catch a quick glimpse of her children.

The triplets were then taken to the NICU and her husband followed the babies. She describes how frightening it all was, "I was so scared I did not know what to think. I was sure they would die before I got to see them. I did not want anyone seeing them before me. I was in recovery. I just kept crying. We've been through so much."

Full of medications, bed rest, isolation, and hospitalizations, her pregnancy and delivery were painful, stressful, and traumatic. Julie's pregnancy and delivery were hardly what Julie had ever imagined. For many women, who start to experience complications or are diagnosed with a high-risk pregnancy early in their pregnancy, they have a similar story. While the specifics as far as what complications women had differed, with Julie's case being on the more extreme end, the common denominator was weeks and even months of fear and anxiety as women endured everything from restricted physical activity to invasive medical treatments to prolong their pregnancy and give their children the best chance at survival and a healthy life.

One of the most common complications that leads to a high-risk pregnancy is premature labor which is defined as contractions experienced prior to 37 weeks. Not much is known about how to prevent preterm labor and birth, which makes it a difficult problem to address. Basic recommendations include getting prompt and adequate prenatal care, maintaining proper nutrition, consuming the recommended amount of folic acid, and avoiding smoking or drinking alcohol ("March of Dimes Peristats" 2014). It also is essential that women recognize the signs of preterm labor so they can seek prompt treatment. A common treatment for preterm labor is some type of bedrest so that pressure on the cervix is lessened. Physicians also can treat women with tocolytic drugs (i.e., medications that postpone labor) such as terbutaline, magnesium sulfate, and indocin. Unfortunately, in general, these drugs only postpone labor for one or two days and some have serious side effects for mothers. The lack of certainty about how to treat and prevent preterm labor and delivery leaves women in a difficult position as they are forced to make sense of their situation and make decisions in the midst of conflicting information. As almost all of the women I spoke with told me though, when they were experiencing preterm labor they would pretty much do anything and would have been willing to try whatever their doctors suggested if they thought that it would give them a chance of stopping their labor and carry their babies further.

In talking about the challenges of coping with premature labor and a high-risk pregnancy, the topic of bed rest and its impact on women and pregnancies is central as this is one of the most commonly prescribed treatments. In the past ten years, more and more research has looked at the practice of prescribing bed rest for pregnant women both in terms of its physical and psychological impacts. The evidence of whether bed rest is beneficial in preventing preterm birth is not entirely conclusive and a growing amount of evidence suggests that prolonged bed rest and particularly strict bed rest where women must lie down all day or are hospitalized can have detrimental effects on women's physical and mental health (Bigelow and Stone 2011; McCarty-Singleton and Sciscione 2014; Goldenberg et al. 1994; Noble and Sorger 2004). The general consensus seems to be that bed rest cannot be harmful even if it may not be proven to be helpful. There are some serious concerns and difficulties that go along with bed rest though including the difficulty of ceasing all activities, the strain on other family members, physical deterioration due to lack of movement, psychological impact, and it takes away a woman's ability to participate in many of the social rites of pregnancy such as wearing maternity clothes or preparing the nursery (McDermott-Perez 2007; Noble and Sorger 2004).

Women who were on bed rest felt that it was very misunderstood by the general public. More than once women recounted stories of friends or family making comments to them about how nice it would be to have some time to rest before the baby or babies came or told women how much they wished they could be on bed rest so they could get a break from their job and household responsibilities. These comments were often infuriating, as bed rest was rarely something women described as pleasant or even relaxing. Astrid, mother of triplets born at 34 weeks, explained that the first day or two it was nice to just lie in bed and watch TV, but after that the days were long, tedious, and hard. Her husband worked all day, so she was alone except for an occasional visitor. She could read and go on the computer, but after a while even those activities grew wearisome. On top of that she was physically uncomfortable and could not change positions in a way that relieved much of the pressure her triplets were placing on her body.

Shelley was put on strict bed rest after she had surgery at 11 weeks to remove her twin son who planted in her fallopian tube instead of the uterus. His twin sister survived the surgery and doctors did everything they could do to keep Shelly pregnant which included home monitoring of her daughter's heartbeat every day and weekly doctor's appointments. Shelly is a high-school teacher, and she was not used to not being constantly busy and interacting with her students and the staff and the days of not doing anything other than search the web and watch TV quickly started to wear on her sanity. "It was grueling and horrible," she said, "I begged for them to send homework home for me to grade and I wanted to talk to the sub every day." Her doctor kept telling her that it was important for her to take it easy and stay calm, and while she followed her doctor's order as far as her physical activity, she was miserable almost the entire time. Few people understood just how hard it was to just lie there every day hoping for the best. With so little to do she there was nothing to distract her from constant thoughts of the son she had lost and her worry that she would lose her daughter as well.

Like Julie, Ashley's pregnancy was difficult and full of complications from almost the very beginning. She and her husband were unable to conceive on their own and had done a series of IUIs and IVF treatments. She had gotten pregnant multiple times but these pregnancies always ended after just a few weeks in a miscarriage. When she and her husband learned that the latest round of IVF had worked and two of the embryos had implanted, they tried to prepare themselves for the worst. Ashley had three embryos implanted and while the third did not implant, while it was dissolving, it caused a tear in the placenta between the twins which caused Ashley to bleed throughout her entire pregnancy, which was a constant source of anxiety as she constantly thought she was losing the pregnancy. Her doctors suggested they terminate the pregnancy as they did not think it was viable and were concerned about the amount of blood Ashely was losing, but she refused. She had never gotten this far in a pregnancy before, and she was unwilling to not give her twins and the pregnancy a chance. Because of the blood loss, Ashely became severely anemic and her husband became very concerned and she told him that if there ever was a time when there was a choice between saving her or saving the babies, she wanted him to save the babies. It was a terrible conversation to have at any time during a pregnancy, but given their circumstances, it was a conversation that needed to be had.

As her pregnancy progressed, it seemed like each week there was a new crisis. At 16 weeks she was admitted for the first time to the hospital for bed rest. She then let her work know that she was going to take a leave of absence and would not be able to return until after the twins were born. After a few days she was discharged and sent home with orders to be on strict bed rest and to see her high-risk doctor weekly. Each week she had an ultrasound and each week she dealt with bleeding and intermittent contractions. She was in and out of the hospital as she would go in for an IV of magnesium sulfate and once her contractions were under control she would be sent back home with a prescription of terbutaline until the next scare. As all of this was happening, as dire as things were, Ashley clung to her belief that the babies will be okay and she would make it to the point of viability. Looking back she sees that she was living in a state of denial because to acknowledge the very real risk of both of her babies dying was just too much.

At 23 weeks, the doctor told her that she needed to make it to at least 24 weeks for the pregnancy to be viable, but they had a lot of concerns about her daughter. The ultrasounds showed that her daughter had a consistently low level of amniotic fluid and they could not see her kidneys which lead doctors to believe that she possibly had a birth defect and would not survive either to delivery or for long after. This was devastating news to hear and Ashley spent the next few weeks trying to come to terms with the fact that her daughter would not live and began to plan her memorial service. Even though she was still pregnant she was already starting to say good-bye. Her daughter continued to live though, and around 26 weeks Ashley decided that she was tired of people constantly telling her that she would not take home her twins and adopted the attitude that her twins would live. She knew there was a high likelihood that her daughter would have some kind of syndrome and major health issues, but as far as she was concerned, they would deal with the issues as they came, but she was only going to focus on her children being born and living.

At 27 weeks Ashley was admitted to the hospital for the last time. Each time the doctor tried to wean her off of the magnesium her contractions would start up again, so she was unable to return home. Although the days were long and boring, Ashley coped by setting small milestones for herself such as making it another week or making it to her shower. She was determined to make it to at least 34 weeks, but her body did not cooperate. On September 11 she was exactly 29 weeks and she remembered thinking that this was definitely not the day she wanted her twins to be born, but on that day she started profusely bleeding from a placental abruption. When she stood up she felt like all of the blood of was rushing out of her body and yelled for help as she honestly thought that she might be dying. When her doctor came she looked at her and simply said, "game over" and called for the team to prep her for surgery. Luckily Ashley's husband was able to make it to the hospital in time to go into the delivery with her and both were able to breathe a small sigh of relief when they heard each of their babies cry.

Unlike Ashley, Vicki's pregnancy was progressing normally and at 20 weeks she was excited to go in for her first ultrasound to see her baby for the first time. Her birthday was the next week and as the ultrasound technician started, she looked at Vicki and told her that she had an early birthday present for her. It turned out that Vicki was pregnant with twins. Vicki who had never even thought that it might be twins was understandably shocked. As she tried to absorb the idea of having not just one but two babies, she also learned that her cervix was already shortening. Because she was pregnant with twins and now considered high risk she was scheduled to come in for weekly visits. The next week they found that her cervix had drastically shortened so she was admitted to the hospital for an emergency cerclage. In general the best time for a preventative cerclage is between 12 and 14 weeks, but in cases like Vicki's, physicians may opt to try a cerclage to sustain a pregnancy. Although cerclages placed at later weeks in the pregnancy are not as effective as preventative cerclages, they have been shown to be successful in prolonging a pregnancy and allowing the pregnancy to continue at least to the point of viability (Gupta, Emary, and Impey 2010; Abo-Yaqoub, Mohammed, and Saleh 2012). Following the procedure Vicki was discharged with orders to be on strict bed rest. When Vicki went in the following week she and her husband were encouraged to see that there had been no change in her cervical length and they took this as a sign that the cerclage was working.

Vicki spent the next two weeks lying in bed concentrating on staying pregnant and everything seemed to be going fine until she woke up in the middle of the night bleeding heavily. Her husband rushed her to the hospital and a quick examination revealed that she had gone into labor and the bleeding was caused by the stiches ripping out of her cervix. Because she was only 24 weeks and 3 days pregnant they did everything they could to stop her labor. She was given shots of terbutaline and put on an IV of magnesium sulfate to slow her contractions and was given steroid shots to mature the babies' lungs. A neonatologist came down to talk to her and her husband, and basically he warned them that if they delivered this early there was a good chance that they might not survive, and if they did, they could have serious medical and cognitive issues. Vicki so badly wanted to stay pregnant and she just kept thinking that she just had to stay as still as possible and she willed her body to work with her. She described what was going through her head, "You lay as still as you can. You pray for the best at that point. They had strong heartbeats what was going to happen when they get out." Unfortunately her body would not cooperate and even with all of the medication she was on, her contractions continued. Her doctor came and in and told her that he wanted to deliver the twins because he was afraid that she would start to deliver on her own and because of their size, the twins might not make it.

As she was taken into surgery she remembers the doctor telling her not to be alarmed if she did not hear the babies cry. She also vividly remembers the anesthesiologist who kept her calm during the surgery. At one point she started shaking whether from cold or nerves she does not know, but her anesthesiologist kept talking to her while rubbing her arms, and she says that without his calming presence she doesn't think she would have made it through the delivery without having a complete breakdown. As each baby was delivered Vicki and her husband Damon learned that they had two sons whom they named Ethan and Sawyer. Damon was able to go over and see the boys before they were taken to the NICU and they were both encouraged when one of the tiny babies was strong enough to grasp Damon's finger. From that point on Vicki says her memory is spotty, but she does remember being wheeled through the NICU after recovery so she was able to see her sons for the first time.

Like Vicki, Elaine's pregnancy was difficult because she was carrying twins. She actually did not know she was carrying twins though until problems started. At her first ultrasound which was very early in her pregnancy to confirm her due date, only one baby was detected. Shortly after this she started to have some bleeding so she went back for another scan and the ultrasound showed there was a second baby. Both heartbeats were strong, so they determined she was not having a miscarriage and sent her home. She continued to have intermittent bleeding and after a few weeks, a strange fluid came out with the blood. Her doctor did not know what it was, but she was still pregnant, so she just went day by day, hoping for the best. About six weeks later she started to bleed heavily. Because she was not far enough along for the pregnancy to be viable she was told to go to the ER, rather than the women's clinic. The OB on call saw that the babies, two girls, were doing fine, diagnosed her with a possible subchorionic bleed, which is bleeding caused during pregnancy when blood accumulates in the chorionic membrane or in the folds of the placenta which cause the placenta to pull away from the uterine wall. These types of bleeds occur in 20 percent of all pregnancies, and there is no way to tell if the bleeding will resolve itself or result in a miscarriage. The doctor told her there was nothing more they could do and sent them home to wait and hope for the best.

From there, things continued to go downhill. The same day she went to the ER her husband lost his job. She continued to have a lot of unexplained bleeding and was placed on modified bed rest, meaning she was allowed to get up and get things for herself, but she was restricted from lifting things or engaging in any vigorous activity. She started to grow increasingly uncomfortable and was unable to sit in the same position for long. She started to have contractions she could feel, but each time she went into the labor and delivery unit they found that the length of her cervix had not changed and determined they were just Braxton Hick's contractions. One day she passed what looked like a clot to her. She was being seen at a high-risk practice, but her doctor did not test the clot to determine what it was and because she was not in active labor told her not to worry about it. Unsatisfied with this response, she told him that she just felt like something was off and he told her that if she ever had reason to think that something was wrong to head straight to labor and delivery. She continued to pass what almost looked like tissue, but otherwise she detected no changes until at 27 weeks she started to have painful contractions. She drank water to see if that would help her contractions subside, and when they did not she and her husband returned to the labor and delivery unit and found out that her cervix was dilated to 2 cm. She was immediately admitted to the hospital for full bad rest and close monitoring. The girls continued to do fine and even though she was still passing some kind of tissues, her contractions started to slow. She got her first steroid shot, and the plan was to send her home after she got the second shot.

After getting the second shot they did another scan to check on the babies before Elaine was discharged and one the babies, Lydia, was not doing her practice breathing, an indication that the baby could be in some kind of distress. Elaine was told she would stay another night and they would check the babies again in the morning. Around 6:00 the next morning Elaine went into hard labor. The doctor on call ordered pain medication and an IV of magnesium sulfate to slow her contractions. When he went to check her cervix he announced that there had been a massive rupture of her membranes and she was fully dilated. At that point there was race to get the babies delivered. They worked to get the spinal block in while her husband put on his scrubs. Elaine's IV then popped and Lydia's head was starting to come out of the birth canal as a nurse tried to push it back in. They had no time to spare, so Elaine was put under for the surgery and her husband was not allowed into the OR to watch. Following the delivery, things continued to be rough for Elaine and her girls, she explained, "Amazingly they survived the initial things and nothing went wrong. Carol's cord was draped down and had Lydia come out, Carol would not have lived. They took them to a NICU and my recovery was terrible. No one was able to tell the night nurse that I did not have an epidural and I was in so much pain. I finally said you've got to call the doctor. It took me about a month before I felt human again."

While many people consider having twins routine as they seem to be more and more common as the current rate of twin births in the United States is up to about 3 percent of all births, these stories as well as the statistics show that a twin pregnancy is hardly routine. Only 40 percent of twins are born full term and more than 12 percent of twins are born prior to 32 weeks (Martin et al. 2013). Samantha's pregnancy with twins was high risk, not only because she was carrying twins, but she had also delivered her first son at only 19 weeks after her water broke early. Doctors told her that it could have just been a fluke thing and she could very likely have no issues with her second pregnancy, but she was unwilling to just let things progress. Prior to getting pregnant again she requested that she also be seen by a high-risk obstetrician and got a referral from her regular obstetrician. After getting the referral she met with the high-risk doctor and talked to him about how he would manage her pregnancy. His plan included checking her cervix every week, starting weekly B-12 shots at 16 weeks, and putting in a cerclage if he detected any change in her cervical length. She was given the go ahead to try to get pregnant again and was cautiously excited when she learned she was pregnant with twin girls.

At 15 weeks she had her first cervical check and everything looked good. Two weeks later she returned for an ultrasound to see how the girls were growing and they found out that her cervix was only 0.2 centimeters. She could not believe this was happening again and she looked right at her doctor and told him that she could not lose this pregnancy. He then scheduled her for an emergency cerclage. The procedure which was supposed to take only 15 minutes ended up taking over two hours. It turned out that Samantha has an unusually narrow pelvic bone and the doctor was having trouble getting to her cervix to insert the stitch. Following the procedure she went home and put herself on bed rest. Her doctor told her it was not necessary, but she was going to try everything she could to keep her pregnancy going. At her 25-week appointment she was 2 centimeters dilated and the doctor told her to go home and pack a bag and return as she was going to be admitted to the hospital for the duration of her pregnancy.

After she was there for five days she woke up with some pain in her abdomen. It was not a horrible pain and almost felt like gas pain, but she let her nurse know that something was happening. The nurse hooked her up to the contraction monitor and it did not show any activity. She continued to feel like something was wrong and could not get comfortable. Her husband was getting ready to leave and she told him that she was going to get up and use the bathroom before he left and as she stood up there was a gush of blood. They paged the nurse who came in, checked her, and explained that she would be headed in for a C-section immediately because her water had broken, she was in labor, and the twins were breach. The prep and surgery went very quickly and both girls came out crying, but quickly had to be put on ventilators and were taken to the NICU where Samantha did not see them until the following day. After all Samantha had been through with the loss of her son and then doing everything she could to have a healthy pregnancy, her delivery and her daughter's birth were nothing like what she had hoped for.

Jacque was pregnant with only one baby, but also had complications from almost the beginning of her pregnancy. Around 10 weeks she suffered from a subchorionic hemotoma and assumed she was having a miscarriage as she was passing fist-sized clots. She went in to the hospital to be checked and the ultrasound showed that the baby's heartbeat was still strong and she was sent home with the reassurance that this happens sometimes and does not mean that the pregnancy will end. Over the next few weeks this happened several more times and the bleeding continued to be very heavy, but suddenly the episodes stopped and Jacque assumed that the rest of her pregnancy would be fine. At 26 weeks and 4 days Jacque was doing some packing to get ready for their upcoming move when she noticed some strange looking mucus when she went to the bathroom. She texted a friend to ask if this was normal and her friend texted back an emphatic no, so Jacque called her doctor's office and the doctor on call asked her if she was having any contractions. Jacque responded that she did not know what a contraction felt like. The doctor reassured her that if she was not feeling any pain she was fine and without painful contractions she would not be dilating. Jacque still felt like something was wrong, but she trusted the doctor.

Throughout the night there was more mucus and toward the morning there was also some blood. Jacque called the doctor again and this time she recommended that Jacque head to the hospital just to have everything checked out.

Jacque was still not panicked at this point and went ahead and drove herself to the hospital, not thinking that this was serious enough that her husband needed to go with her. As the ultrasound technician was doing the scan she got very quiet and would not make eye contact with Jacque. Shortly after her doctor came in and explained that Jacque was almost fully dilated and there was nothing they could do to stop the labor and that she was going to deliver her daughter that day. She was given a steroid shot to at least mature the lungs a little bit and during that time her husband and their families were able to get to the hospital. At this point Jacque was almost hysterical. She was so afraid of the delivery that she asked if she could just be put under, but they explained that it was better for her if she was not put under general anesthesia. So many thoughts were swirling through her mind that she had a hard time processing everything that was happening.

She described what she was going through as she went into for the delivery.

> I was horrified. They had put me on mag, I was dry heaving and vomiting I was sweating, I was out of it I was distraught the anesthesiologist and OB kept talking with me, they were there with me. When she was born she let a little mewl. I knew a little, I didn't know a lot, so I wondered, will she be born alive? What is even going to happen? How big will she be? She let a tiny little cry and we took that as a good sign. They brought her over to me for actually quite a while and then they whisked her away. She weighed 2 pounds 7 ounces bigger than they thought we took that as a good sign.

As terrifying and upsetting as the delivery was, Jacque quickly forced herself to come to terms with what had happened so that she could be there for her daughter. She explained, "For me, in this situation, the train is leaving and the quicker you get on board the easier it is going to be for you. This is your reality. The faster you embrace this reality and move forward, the easier it is going to be."

Nicole's pregnancy was also high-risk and full of complications from almost the moment she conceived her daughter Kennedy. Nicole and her husband were actually shocked when they found out she was pregnant. A few months prior to learning she was pregnant, her gynecologist had diagnosed her with large uterine fibroids and told her she would most likely have a difficult time getting pregnant and sent her to a reproductive endocrinologist. A uterine fibroid is a benign tumor that grows in the uterus and while they are often asymptomatic, fibroids can grow large enough that they become painful and can interfere with normal menstruation. Nicole consulted with the reproductive endocrinologist who recommended that she have the fibroids surgically removed and once she recovered, she could start trying for a baby; so Nicole went ahead and scheduled her surgery for the next month. Unbeknownst to Nicole or her doctors was that she was already pregnant. After a few weeks of feeling slightly off and kind of crampy, Nicole took a home pregnancy test and it was positive. This was in May and at that point she was about eight weeks pregnant. She immediately called the doctor who told her to come in immediately. When a woman with fibroids gets pregnant, the biggest concern is where the baby implants in the uterus. An ultrasound showed that the baby had implanted away from the fibroids which was positive, but her reproductive endocrinologist warned her that he had seen these types of pregnancies before and there was no way to predict how it would go. Some women went on to have successful, normal pregnancies while others went on to miscarry.

At this point, Nicole's care was transferred back to her regular OB and also planned to consult with a maternal fetal specialist. Despite her fibroids she was feeling great and she and her husband were very excited as they had always wanted to have kids. A few days before her first appointment with the maternal fetal specialist at the end of May, she was at work sitting at her desk and felt a gush of fluid and thought maybe she had lost control of her bladder and wet herself. When she looked down though, she was not sitting in a pile of urine, but instead a pile of blood. She went to the bathroom and was convinced that she was having a miscarriage as she kept bleeding and large clots containing what looked like clumps of tissue started to come out. She was in no pain, but the bleeding would not stop, so a friend at work drove her to the hospital. She was quickly seen in the ER and to her surprise, they quickly found a heartbeat and found that her cervix was still closed. They were not sure what had happened. They said that possibly she had been pregnant with twins and lost one of them or it was something else and she would just have to wait until she saw her maternal fetal specialist.

At that appointment, the doctor informed her that the bleeding had been caused by a suchorionic hemorrhage. Her fibroids were rapidly growing and weakening the uterine walls and the placenta was starting to pull away which was causing her bleeding and there was a fifty-fifty chance that she would lose the pregnancy. There was nothing she could do other than go home, drink a lot of water, and try to take it easy. Her doctor told her that if she could make it to 23 weeks then they would have some options and the baby might be viable. If she could make it to 28 weeks that would be even better, and if she made it all of the way to 32 weeks he would go ahead and deliver her then. Nicole was of course heartbroken and anxious and went home feeling like she was going to spend the next few weeks just sitting around waiting to lose her baby. As time went on though she continued to feel fine and stayed pregnant, so she started to breathe a little more easily. Toward the end of June she started to feel some pain in her abdomen that quickly went from painful to excruciating. She quickly went into her regular OB who explained that her fibroids were actually necrotizing or dying from lack of blood. Although this in itself was not dangerous, she was in so much pain that her heart rate was elevating so the doctor sent her home with a prescription for Percocet to help take the edge of her agony and told her that once the fibroids were completely dead the pain would stop.

The following Monday she had an appointment with her high-risk doctor for an ultrasound where they would be able to find out the sex of the baby. The Percocet was not doing much to alleviate her pain and she could hardly lie still during the scan due to the pain. They found out that she was having a girl and then she was admitted to the hospital for the next week so she could be on IV pain medication as the rest of her fibroids died off. After she was discharged the pain was gone and she went back to feeling fine for a couple of weeks and then she started to have some back pain. Every time she went to the doctor there was still a heartbeat so she just tried to cope with the pain. The last few days of July the pain changed though, and it was now radiating throughout her back. She told her husband that she thought she was having contractions and needed to go to the OR. At the hospital she was monitored and the machine was not picking up contractions. The doctor on call was about to send her home with another prescription for pain medication when he decided to quickly check her cervix before she went. When he checked her she was completely effaced and had no cervical length. They quickly admitted her and sent her up to labor and delivery and explained that this was where she would stay until she delivered. She was still in a lot of pain but the monitor was still not picking up any uterine activity. Nicole took the belt and moved it to the side of her stomach where there were no fibroids and the monitor showed she was contracting every one to two minutes and was in the middle of hard labor. The nurses immediately started her on an IV of magnesium and her contractions started to slow. The neonatologist came in to talk to them and explained that at 24 weeks the outcomes if she delivered were most likely not very good. They gave her the steroid shots for the lungs and inserted a vaginal pessary, which is a device used to treat a prolapsed uterus to help hold her uterus up since here cervix was not there and told her that they would work to keep her daughter in for as long as possible as each hour would help.

Amazingly the treatments worked and Nicole's labor was stopped. A few days later she was up using the bathroom she felt a gush of water. She called for her nurse who determined that her water had broken and she had gone into labor again and restarted the magnesium IV. The neonatoglogist came up again and discussed how even though she was further along, it was still very early and the risks to the baby were high. Her regular OB was out of town and the doctor on call also talked about the risks of delivery. Because of the fibroids, the doctor would be unable to do cut across her lower abdomen for the C-section, which meant that she would need a classical incision and because she was so early, her uterine walls were still very thick which made the surgery more difficult and could possibly be fatal for the baby. Because they had stopped her contractions they could keep her pregnancy going, but because her water had broken, there was a very large risk of infection. Now Nicole was on complete bed rest and was not even allowed to get up to use the bathroom.

At 26 weeks, Nicole was using a bedpan when she felt like she was pushing out a clot. She buzzed for a nurse who rushed in to check her. The next thing Nicole knew there were four doctors in the room. It turns out that Nicole was fully dilated, was in labor, and the baby's foot was in the birth canal. One of the doctors explained that they were going to deliver the baby now, but instead of going in for a C-section they were going to do a vaginal delivery right there. They started Pitocin to get her contractions to kick in, but it was not working. The doctor looked at Nicole and told her that she was just going to have to start pushing because they needed to get the baby out. After four strong pushes, Kennedy was born. The NICU team quickly grabbed her and went to work on her, and Nicole kept asking if she was breathing. After a few moments they heard a tiny cry and the doctor gave her a thumbs up and she knew that at least her daughter was alive. The NICU team quickly left and Nicole was put under and taken to surgery so they could remove the placenta and it was not until the next day that she was able to go up and see her daughter in the NICU and start the NICU journey.

Sam's experience with a traumatic high-risk pregnancy began just after her first trimester when some of her prenatal testing came back indicating that something was wrong with the baby and potentially the baby had Trisomy 18 which is a chromosomal abnormality in which children have 3 copies of the 18th chromosome which leads to serious deformities of the child's organs and body. Because of these serious defects the majority of infants with Trisomy 18 are stillborn and of those who do survive past birth, only 10 percent survive the first year (Boghossian et al. 2014). At 16 weeks Sam returned for a scan and again the doctors found that something was wrong with the baby, but they were not sure what it was. They knew it was a girl and that her measurement was off, but they were not sure what was causing it. The next step was to go to a specialist to have amniocentesis which revealed that her daughter did not have Trisomy 18, but something was wrong with the baby, they just could not determine exactly what it was. The next week when she was 19 weeks pregnant, Sam went in for another scan with the specialist and this time he thought that the abnormal measurements were possibly because the baby had a skeletal dysplasia, more commonly known as dwarfism. The doctor went on to tell Sam and her husband that cases of skeletal dysplasia are rarely detected so early in a pregnancy and because of this, her daughter probably had one of the most severe forms which would most likely be fatal. The doctor showed them pictures of other babies who had been stillborn with the condition and discussed with them the option of terminating the pregnancy. Before making that decision though, he recommended that they go to see another specialist who might be able to give them a more specific diagnosis, but he made it very clear in his opinion that their daughter had a lethal condition and would not be born alive. Sam remembers how cold and blunt he was the entire time he was talking to them and she and her husband left the appointment feeling devastated.

As they struggled to come to terms with what the specialist had told them, Sam went in for one of her routine prenatal appoints with her regular OB. At that appointment her OB informed her that she could no longer be Sam's doctor as her pregnancy was too high-risk and there was no NICU at the hospital where her OB practiced. It took some time before Sam could find an OB that was willing to take her on as patient as most told her that her case was too complicated. She finally found a doctor who agreed to oversee her case and deliver the baby, but he asked for her to go see another specialist that he thought might be able to give them a more accurate diagnosis. At 23 weeks she had an appointment with the specialist and the first thing he did was another scan. As he was looking at the images, Sam waited with her arm across her face, dreading hearing this doctor's opinion and more bad news. To her complete surprise this doctor told them that although their daughter's measurements were all small, they were all in proportion, so he thought she was possibly just a small baby and nothing was wrong. He told her to return in six weeks for another scan to see how the baby was growing. While this doctor's opinion was somewhat a relief, Sam was still not convinced that everything was fine as each doctor that she had talked with had told them something different.

At 28 weeks Sam went to her regular OB for a checkup and after seeing how flat Sam's stomach still looked he told her he was sending her immediately for another ultrasound. Sam had barely gained any weight at that point even though she was not having morning sickness and she was still wearing her regular clothes and she explained that if she did not tell someone they would have no idea that she was pregnant. He also warned her that if the ultrasound showed anything funny he would might have to deliver her daughter that day so she needed to get ready for the hospital. Sam was not ready for her daughter to be born and could not believe that she might be born so early. The scan showed that something was wrong with the umbilical cord and her daughter was not getting all of the nutrition she needed which was contributing to her small size. The initial plan was to deliver within the next 48 hours, but even though the flow of the umbilical card was restricted, the baby was still doing well as far as her movements and heart rate and she passed her nonstress test. So at that point her doctor decided to admit her for the remainder of the pregnancy for close monitoring. Sam started to mentally prepare herself to be in the hospital for the next ten weeks or so, convinced that she could hold out until at least 37 weeks.

Sam got her first round of the steroid shots, but what she did not know was that the monitors were picking up decelerations in her daughter's heart rate. Early the next day she had another ultrasound and this showed continued issues with the baby's heart rate and additional signs of fetal distress. After having only one round of steroid shots Sam was taken in for a C-section at 29 weeks and her daughter Kyla was born weighing just 1 pound 13 ounces and was only the size of a 24- or 25-week baby. Sam described what it was like during the delivery, "I was absolutely terrified. I was just beyond terrified. I was in the room and they were giving me the epidural and I just couldn't stop checking the heart monitor. The absolute fear you know someone is right, the first is right and she is going to die or the second is right and she did not get the nutrients." The next morning the neonatologist came down to her room and told Sam and her husband that they did not think Kyla had dwarfism but instead had restricted growth throughout the pregnancy because she was not properly nourished. Even though she was premature and very tiny, the joy that Sam felt was overwhelming. Even though the second specialist had told them that it was most likely not dwarfism, there was no way to tell for sure until her daughter was born and throughout the pregnancy Sam had carried with her the constant fear that her baby would not live, which was a horrible way to go through a pregnancy.

Unlike Sam, other than bad morning sickness until 18 weeks, Heather also was having a complication-free pregnancy up until she went in for a routine ultrasound at 20 weeks and learned that her cervix was already starting to thin. This was surprising as she had not felt any contractions or had any indication that something was wrong. Her doctors felt that it was too late to have a cerclage, so Heather instead opted to go on full bed rest at home with the hopes that limiting the pressure on her cervix would stop it from thinning any more. At 25 weeks she started to have some bad back pain and her husband insisted that she go in to the hospital to have it checked. At the hospital she learned that the pain was due to back labor. Her blood pressure was running a little high and there was some protein in her urine so they admitted her overnight for observation and her blood pressure remained high throughout the night. The next morning the medical staff informed her that she would need to stay at the hospital until she delivered. Heather started to mentally prepare herself for another three months on hospital bed rest. After a few days, her condition continued to worsen and the doctor told her that she would not carry her baby full term, but they would try to keep her pregnant as long as possible. Even though she was on magnesium sulfate and having terrible side effects including nausea, double vision, and hot flashes, the medication was not working to bring her blood pressure down. As her blood pressure climbed her brain started to swell and her doctors determined that she was at risk for having a stroke and needed to deliver her immediately. They broke her water and started her on Pitocin and told her that she needed to deliver within the next 24 hours or she would need to go in for a C-section. During her labor they put a lead on the baby's head to monitor her heart rate. As she was nearing the 24-hour mark the baby's heart rate started to drop and was not going back up into normal ranges.

The next thing Heather knew a team of doctors and nurses came to the room and they started to prep her for surgery. They got the epidural in easily, but it was only numbing her right side so they put her under for the surgery and her husband was not allowed in to see the delivery. Just a few minutes later, their daughter Megan was born weighing just 1 pound 9 ounces and was only 14 inches long. She was much smaller than the doctors had anticipated, but they later discovered that the baby had IUGR, because Heather's placenta had not been providing enough nutrition. Megan's initial APGAR scores were two at one minute and not much higher a few minutes later and she was black and blue from birth trauma. She was not breathing or moving when she was born and immediately needed to put on the ventilator and was rushed to the NICU. Heather was so traumatized by the delivery that she does not even remember the first time she was wheeled down to the NICU to see her daughter, which was when she was already three-days old, but her husband has told her that she became hysterical at the sight of her struggling daughter and had to be taken back to her room.

Heather's first pregnancy and birth was so traumatic that it took her a long time before she was ready to get pregnant again, but six years later after consulting with her OB, she was ready to try again. Her OB explained that most women do not have preeclampsia with subsequent deliveries so this was not something she needed to be overly concerned about. There was some concern with possible IUGR and early delivery, but her doctor encouraged to go ahead and try again and they would just monitor her pregnancy more closely. She and her husband finally decided they were ready and she got pregnant right away. She had very bad morning sickness, but otherwise things seemed to be okay until 19 weeks when she started to have terrible pains that felt like contractions and she was sure she was starting to miscarry. She went straight to her OB who determined she was not in labor, but had a kidney stone that was trying to pass. This was the best news Heather could have hoped for and she went home and a few days later passed the stone. The doctor continued to monitor her very closely both because of her prior early delivery and to make sure that the baby was growing properly and getting the needed nutrition from the placenta. Her blood pressure tended to be toward the high side, but Heather stuck to a strict low-salt diet and was able to keep her numbers within normal range.

At 30 weeks everything was looking good and at her regular checkup her doctor told her that he thought she would carry this baby full term. That weekend she had a baby shower, something she was not able to do before her daughter was born, and throughout the day she was having terrible back pain. She did not say anything until the shower was over and then had her husband drive her to the hospital where they confirmed she was having contractions. After three rounds of trebutaline shots her contractions subsided and she was sent home with a prescription of the pill form of terbutaline. The next week when she went to her doctor for a weekly checkup everything was looking good when Heather felt a dull pain in her belly which quickly intensified until Heather was in so much pain that she could not get off of the table. Her doctor did not think the pain was from contractions but instructed Heather's mother who had come to the appointment with her to take her across to the hospital to have things checked out further in the ER. As Heather was being wheeled across to the hospital every bump and turn sent a searing pain through her abdomen that made her feel as if she was being ripped in half. At the hospital they ran a full battery of tests, but could not determine the cause of her pain. They thought that she could possibly have the shingles virus, so she was not allowed to be admitted to labor and delivery unit as shingles can be very harmful to pregnant women and infants.

None of the pain medications they tried did anything to stop the pain which was so excruciating that Heather was put into a medically induced coma so that she would be unaware of the pain. During that time she had three MRIs, none of which found anything to explain what was wrong. They brought Heather out of the coma and explained to her and her husband that the next step was to do exploratory surgery, but they could not do that until she delivered the baby. Her pain was at least bearable now so she was discharged from the hospital. At her next appointment, when she was 32 weeks, they did an amniocentesis which showed that the baby's lungs were developed and because of this the doctor decided to do a C-section that day. Her son John was born breathing on his own and weighed 3 pounds and 14 ounces. Everything looked great with him, which was a huge relief. Shortly after he was delivered the doctor came around the side of the curtain and said that he had found a problem and needed her to sign some forms because he needed to remove her uterus. She told him to do whatever he needed to do, and that day she had a full hysterectomy and had her appendix removed. What the doctor had found was a placental accretea which is a condition where the placenta attaches abnormally to the uterine wall. Although this condition was not the cause of her pain, it was something her doctor had not detected and had she had a vaginal delivery she could have experienced life-threatening hemorrhaging. The doctors never did find the source of her pain, but Heather credits it with saving her life. Placental accretea is most often found in women who have had multiple C-sections as the uterine scarring causes the abnormal attachment. Having had only one prior surgical delivery, Heather was not at high risk for the condition, so it was not something her doctor was looking for and had it gone undetected it could have cost her and her son their lives.

Like Heather, Tracey had two high-risk pregnancies. Her first pregnancy was a triplet pregnancy that she delivered at 25 weeks and 6 days. When she discovered she was pregnant again with a singleton at age 39 she was surprised, but thrilled as she had never been able to conceive on her own. Even though things were going well with her pregnancy she had a nagging feeling that something was not right. She assumed that her anxiety was just due to the complications of her last pregnancy, but the feeling would not go away and she had an amniocentesis done to determine if there were any genetic issues. The test came back normal and when she went home she was able to relax a little until she got a very bad case of the influenza virus and a reoccurring urinary tract infection. Even though she was having no cramping or contractions she still felt like something was off. When she was around 22 weeks she was outside raking leaves when she started to feel some contractions. She went inside to lie down and drink some water and the contractions subsided. She went to work and once there she started to feel the contractions again. She called her doctor who instructed her to go to the hospital for an ultrasound which detected that her amniotic sac was leaking and there was hardly any fluid around the baby. All Tracey could think was that it was happening again and they were facing another premature birth and long NICU stay.

What the doctor told her next completely shocked her though. Because she was not even 23 weeks pregnant which was considered previable, there was nothing the hospital would do. If she got to 24 weeks they would intervene, but because the fluid levels were so low and she was still leaking they assumed that the baby would die in the next few days. She begged them to do something, but they kept explaining that there was nothing to do and worked on getting her papers ready for discharge. As this was happening there was a shift change and a new OB came on duty. She was new to the hospital and came to talk to Heather. After hearing her story and checking over her charts she told Heather that she was a strong Christian and would fight for this baby. If the hospital she was in would not keep her, she would find another hospital that would. After calling around she found a doctor who worked at Creighton medical center who was willing to take Heather on as a patient so Heather was transported by ambulance to Omaha which was about an hour away from where she lived, where she went on to spend the rest of her pregnancy.

On the day she was 23 weeks pregnant they came in and gave her the first steroid shot and 24 hours later she got the second. Shortly after getting the second shot she went into heavy labor with painful contractions. When the OB checked to see if she was dilated he found that her membranes had ruptured and the baby's foot was hanging in the birth canal. Even though she was only 23 weeks and 2 days pregnant she was going to have the baby that day. Heather was alone in Omaha and she called her husband and her sister and told them they needed to come now. She was terrified at this point and is very thankful to the anesthesiologist who acted as her support person and tried to keep her calm. Her sister was able to get there just moments before Heather's daughter Carly was born. Heather remembers that as they held her up all she could think of was just how small she was as she weighed only 1 pound and 2 ounces. Despite the fact that she was so early, she did great from the beginning and after 111 days came home from the NICU without any type of oxygen, monitors, or feeding tube. Heather is quick to highlight how amazing Carly's story is and she likes to share Carly's story as it is an excellent example of how there is no way to accurately predict what a preemie's journey will be like.

In some cases women's pregnancies were high risk and because of that, their babies were born too early to survive. One of the women who experienced this was Kari. She and her husband had been unable to get pregnant on their own so they were referred to a fertility specialist. Prior to getting pregnant with the triplets she had five miscarriages. When she and her husband learned she was carrying triplets her doctors offered the option to reduce the pregnancy to one or two, but Kari and her husband were against this and went ahead with the pregnancy and were thrilled when she made it past her first trimester. Around 18 weeks Kari started to have contractions. Because it was so early, the doctors said there was not anything they could do. At 21 weeks Kari started to dilate and she went in for an emergency cerclage and was admitted to the hospital on full bed rest in the hopes that she would be able to stay pregnant until she reached the point of viability. She continued to contract though, and in addition to the strain on her cervix when she had the cerclage put in, bacteria was introduced into her cervix and she developed an infection that passed to the lowest triplet. In attempt to save the other two triplets doctors decided to deliver the first baby in the hopes that by removing the infection Kari could stay pregnant for a few weeks longer. This was a few days before Kari was 24 weeks pregnant and the policy at the hospital for infants born that early was to assess the baby and if they were under a pound they would generally let the baby go. They delivered her daughter vaginally and she lived for only a few minutes. Kari was able to hold her before she said good-bye and although she was grieving the loss of her daughter she tried to focus on keeping herself pregnant.

After she delivered her daughter, the next challenge was for her to deliver her daughter's placenta without going into full labor and delivering the other babies. The next morning when her doctor came to check on her, he felt her to see if the placenta was loose and he felt a foot. The second triplet's water had broken and after just a few pushes she delivered her son who also lived for only a few minutes. Luckily her husband was in the room at the time as it all happened so quickly. At this point, the doctor told her that they were going to try and keep the third baby in, but he was concerned that the infection in the uterus was too wide-spread, but they would wait and see. As the day went on Kari continued to feel worse, and worse and her blood pressure continued to drop which made her light headed and at several points she almost started to blackout. At one point she asked a nurse if she was going to die. The nurse assured her that she wouldn't, but as Kari's health continued to deteriorate her doctor came in and said that they were going to stop using the preventative medications and let nature take its course. The next morning Kari delivered her daughter at exactly 24 weeks and this time the NICU team was there and immediately took her and started to perform life-saving measures. Kari's daughter lived for two months before she succumbed to an infection. Looking back, Kari knows it was for the best as her daughter had severe brain bleeds, but she still mourns for her triplets. Shortly after losing her triplets she became pregnant again, this time with twins. This pregnancy was also very high risk and she went on full bed rest at 24 weeks. This time around things were so much harder for her emotionally. When she was pregnant with the triplets she was just so excited that her pregnancy lasted past her first trimester and she was very unaware of how many complications there could be. Now that she had seen just how badly things could end she was even more anxious. Luckily she went on to deliver her twins at 36 weeks, and although they were early they were healthy and survived.

While many women who deliver early have a lot of complications and know that there is a possibility that they will go into labor early, other women suddenly go into labor without any warning. Some women were having perfectly normal pregnancies so their early labor and deliveries were completely unexpected and therefore were often even more traumatic as they had no mental preparation. For example, Jamie was having a completely normal pregnancy until she delivered her daughter at just 27 weeks. Jamie had decided they were ready to start trying to have a baby and just six weeks after she went off of her birth control she found out she was pregnant. She did have terrible morning sickness throughout her pregnancy, but other than that she just experienced typical symptoms. Around 26 weeks she noticed some light spotting over the weekend. She called her OB's office and they told that since the bleeding was not heavy she should just take it easy and try to put her feet up. On Tuesday she woke up with a headache. Jamie had a history of migraines and this was not even close to the worst headache she ever had, so she went ahead to work figuring it would eventually go away. The pain did not go away and she just felt like something was wrong. At 3:30 she called her doctor's office and told the nurse that her headaches would not go away. The nurse recommended that she take some pain reliever and see if that worked. An hour later her head was still throbbing so the nurse told her to drive to the hospital where she was going to deliver to have some blood work done.

The hospital was fairly close to her work, so Jamie got there quickly. While they were checking her vitals they found that her blood pressure was 230 over 115 and there was a high amount of protein in her urine. At that point Jamie was told she was going to be transfered to another hospital because the hospital where she was did not have an NICU. At that point Jamie could barely understand what was happening. She kept telling the doctors and nurses that she was only 27 weeks pregnant, so she was not ready to deliver. They went ahead and started an IV and a catheter at the first hospital and Jamie called her husband and told him to meet her at the next hospital. As soon as she arrived at the second hospital they started prepping her for surgery. When her husband arrived he found her room, and as he walked in, a nurse handed him a pair of scrubs and told him his baby was going to be born that day. Jamie and her husband did not know the sex of the baby and Jamie remembers them announcing that it was a girl and her husband hearing a tiny cry. Their daughter Aubry was born weighing only 1 pound 8 ounces and she was the size of a 24 weeker. After the delivery, Jamie learned that she had a severe case of preeclampsia that had progressed very rapidly, and her liver and kidneys had both started to shut down. Doctors told her that given how serious her case was, it was a miracle that she had not started to have seizures or had a stroke. Jamie still remembers how terrifying and surreal the entire experience was and says she and her husband are on the fence about having another baby as they do not think they could handle another traumatic birth.

Even though Angi was pregnant with twins during her first pregnancy, she was having no complications up until her routine appointment at 28 weeks when the doctor found that her cervix was starting to funnel so they told her to go home and be on modified bed rest for the next two weeks when they would check her cervix again. She had not seen her regular OB at the appointment and later that day she got a call from her doctor who wanted her to come back in two days just to be careful. Two days later she returned to her OB's office and her cervix was not just funneling, but she was 3 centimeters dilated. She was immediately admitted to the hospital and started to get terbutaline injections to slow her contractions. The shots were working so she just stayed in the hospital for the next two weeks. After two weeks she started to feel some painful contractions, but the contraction monitor was not picking up any uterine activity. When she complained the nurse on duty told her it was probably indigestion, but as the day went on the pains continued. When the shift changed, Angi's new nurse moved the contraction monitor, and much to the medical staff's surprise, Angi was having contractions every five minutes, so they started to prep her to start a magnesium drip. While they were working on getting the IV in a nurse checked Angi and she was dilated to 7 centimeters. The bottom twin was breach, so the nurses informed Angi that she would be going in for a C-section as soon as she was prepped. Angi and her husband, who was luckily there with her visiting at the time, could not believe what the nurses were telling them. It went from the relative calm of we are going to try a new medication to, you are delivering now. Angi's husband asked the nurses if they could just have a minute to think about things, and the nurse told him no, that they needed to get her delivered as quickly as possible, so at 30 weeks and 4 days her son and daughter were born weighing 3 pound 7 ounces and 3 pound 2 ounces. Angi says that even though she had been in the hospital for two weeks she was completely unprepared for her twins' emergency delivery. She and her husband both assumed that she would be on hospital bed rest for several more weeks, and did not think much about the possibility of having the twins so early and needing to spend an extended time in the NICU with them.

When the twins were two, Angi got pregnant again. She was nervous that it was twins again and could hardly wait for her appointment at 12 weeks to find out. Her husband went with her that day and as soon as two circles appeared on the screen she started to cry and cried throughout the rest of the scan. Her husband tried to reassure her that it was going to be fine and the babies were both healthy, but she was worried that she would have complications again and that if they were born too early they might have serious medical issues. Because of her history of premature delivery, Angi went in the next morning for a preventative cerclage. She had some activity restrictions and also was unable to lift her toddlers which was very challenging. Everything was going fine until she woke up at 29 weeks and felt like she was having contractions. She went into the hospital to get checked and the monitor showed that she was having contractions every five minutes Because of the cerclage her cervix looked fine, so she was started on a magnesium drip and her doctor told her that optimistically she could stay pregnant until at least 35 weeks.

After a few days, her contractions seemed to be under control so she was taken off of the magnesium and spent the next six weeks in the hospital on strict bed rest. This time was incredibly hard on Angi and her husband as they had their twins at home, but also wanted someone to be with her at the hospital in case something happened and she had to deliver immediately. Between her parents and her husband they managed to have someone with the kids and at the hospital, but it put a strain on everyone. Angi also fought feelings of intense boredom and restlessness, but knew that staying in bed was the best thing she could do. When she was around 32 weeks a nurse offered to let her take a ride in a wheelchair around the hospital just to get out, but Angi declined because she thought that if she got out of her room once it would be hard to go back in. As the weeks went on and Angi stayed pregnant, her doctor scheduled a C-section at 35 weeks. While in the hospital Angi was on a blood thinner to help prevent clots. Three days before her scheduled delivery the pharmacy was late in sending up her blood thinner. This was going to be her last dose as she needed to be off of the blood thinners for the delivery. She asked the nurse if she could just skip the final dose, but the nurse insisted that she have it. About four hours later Angi's water broke and she started to bleed profusely because her cerclage ripped out and she was still on blood thinners. The nurses gave her a shot of trebuatline to slow the contractions while they were getting her ready for surgery, but she continued to have painful contractions and was losing a large amount of blood.

What happened next Angi actually has no memory of, but she has pieced together a general idea of what happened from what people have told her. After the C-section, the surgeon attempted to repair the tear in her cervix, but due to the blood thinners could not get the stitch to hold. She was sent to recovery where she started to experience some shoulder pain which can be an indicator of internal bleeding. She started to code and was transferred to the ICU where she was closely monitored and given a blood transfusion. The next morning her blood counts were still dangerously low so she was taken back to surgery to see if they could repair her cervix. In the end, Angi received 17 units of blood, plasma, and platelets to replace the blood she had lost. She had a central line put in and her arms and legs were covered with bruises. She was unable to get up to go to the NICU, so once the twins were stable nurses would bring the babies down to her room a few times a day so she could see them until she was discharged from the hospital. For the next two years Angi suffered from posttraumatic stress from the delivery and coming so close to dying while delivering her twins. Angi and her husband had always wanted five children, but after two very difficult pregnancies, they are unwilling to take the risk of another high-risk twin pregnancy.

Monica, who was pregnant with just one baby had absolutely no reason to suspect that her daughter might be born early. She did have a clotting disorder, but that was treated with twice daily shots of a blood thinner and otherwise she was having a typical pregnancy until she was 27 weeks and 6 days pregnant and woke up with a pounding headache. She went to work and worked her entire shift, but her headache continued to get worse. She called her OB who told her to go into the hospital to get checked out. Unbeknownst to Monica, she had a rapidly developing preeclampsia and as her blood pressure continued to rise, her kidneys were starting to shut down. She did not realize when she was admitted that she would not be discharged until after her son was born. The magnesium she was on was making her incredibly ill and she noticed that her son was not moving nearly as much as he had been, which nurses told her was a side effect of the medication. Unfortunately, her body continued to shut down, and just two days after she was admitted, her doctor came in to tell her that they were taking her to deliver the baby right then.

A team came in to prep her for surgery and she was rushed to the OR and the surgery itself was very traumatic for Monica. Because her son was so small the doctor was having a hard time pulling him and out and she could overhear doctors and nurses shouting out tense orders. When her son came out there was silence and she waited for what felt like forever until she finally heard a small cry and knew he was breathing on his own. She asked to see him and a nurse briefly lifted him up, but all she could see was his tiny foot. Around this time her epidural started to wear off and she screamed and tried to sit up as she started to be able to feel the doctors working on her. The anesthesiologist immediately put her under and the next thing she remembers is waking up in recovery. Because she was still on an IV of magnesium sulfate she was not allowed to go down to the NICU until the next day, so some nurses came down to let her know that her son Colt was doing well. When she was finally able to get up and walk around she got into a wheelchair and wheeled herself to the NICU. A nurse helped her to scrub in and then took her over to her son's isolete. She was overcome by guilt, sadness, and fear and sat next to him quietly crying as she whispered over and over to him how sorry she was. It was one of the hardest moments for her of his entire NICU stay. "Having a baby is supposed to be so happy," she told me, "and this was just so sad."

For Kelli, her pregnancy experience was very similar. She was pregnant with her first child, and she and her husband were so happy and excited. Other than some mild morning sickness and fatigue everything was going very well. When she was 24 weeks she was at work as usual and just was not feeling well and started having some cramps. She decided to go home thinking that she just needed to drink some water and put her feet up. As she was driving home she started to have more painful cramps and she wondered if they were contractions, but she remembers thinking that she had not even read the section of her *What to Expect* Book yet about labor, so she just tried to keep telling herself that it was too early and that she would be fine. There was a lot of traffic that day and as she approached each exit she considered getting off and driving herself to the hospital, but then would talk herself out of it, wanting just to be home. After an hour she finally made it home and went inside to say hello to her husband. She knew he had plans to go out with his friends that night so she almost didn't tell him she wasn't feeling well because she did not want him to feel like he had to stay home with her. The cramping continued to get worse though so she told him she felt sick and wanted to rest. Her next step was to call her mom who did not answer and then she called her mother-in-law who started to ask her a series of questions including if she was bleeding. Kelli had not thought to check and went into the bathroom where she discovered that she was in fact bleeding. Her mother-in-law told her to lie down and have her husband call 911. When the ambulance got there the paramedics quickly assessed her and the baby and told them that they thought she was fine and it was probably just a bad bladder infection and she should follow-up with her doctor. Kelli's husband insisted that they take her into the hospital and they agreed, but as they were driving they did not put on the sirens or rush there. The contractions continued to feel stronger and Kelli told the paramedics she thought she was having a contraction so they told her to lie on her side and take some deep breaths. There was no urgency in their actions and Kellie wondered if she was overreacting but soon she was having trouble talking during the pains and the paramedic suddenly began to look more concerned and told Kellie that she might be in labor.

At that point the paramedic started her on an IV and within a few minutes they were at the hospital, but for some reason the ambulance was parked at the wrong entrance so they were at the opposite end of the hospital, away from the labor and delivery unit. As they were wheeling her through the hospital Kellie's water broke and she felt a gush of water. At this point her husband was starting to lose it. Up until this point he had not realized just how serious this was and he did not understand what was happening. She was wheeled into a room and the nurse told them that at this point her labor was so far progressed that there was nothing that could be done and she would be delivering her baby that day. Kellie's husband responded that he wanted someone in the room that knew what could be done immediately, and the OB on call quickly came in and ordered that Kellie be taken to the OR for the delivery. At that point there was some debate over just how far along she was. Her due date had been changed at least once and they were not sure if she was 24 weeks yet and therefore did not know if the baby was viable and were trying to decide if they would have her deliver vaginally or surgically.

As this discussion was going on, Kellie had a million thoughts going through her head, some of which she looks back on and can hardly believe that this was what she was thinking about given the gravity of the situation. She was very worried that they would lose her clothing and shoes and she also worried that her husband had not called the insurance company yet. In the back of her mind she had a thought that they would need to be preapproved for the delivery and if they did not call, their insurance would not cover it. At this points she honestly thought that she had already lost the baby because it was just too early and she did not even consider the fact that it is possible for a baby born that early to live. Her anxiety was more about the impacts of the surgery on her at that point as she thought that she would be delivering her baby who either already have passed away or would die shortly after. He anxiety continued to grow as the discussion about how to deliver her intensified. She told the doctor that she did not know how to push because she had not taken her childbirth preparation class yet and she didn't think she would know how to deliver her baby. She thought that the doctors were concerned not because they were trying to save the baby, but because they were worried about her and trying to save her life. She kept apologizing to her husband, feeling so terrible that she had gone into labor and their baby had died. When they finally made the decision to put her under for the surgery she was almost relieved because then she did not have to think or make any decisions and the responsibility was entirely taken out of her hands.

When she woke up later in the recovery room, her brother-in-law was sitting next to her and she could not understand why he was there and not her husband. He told her that her husband was in the NICU with her son and she could not believe it. Her son had lived, he was alive, something she had not even thought was possible. Her son was delivered around 7:00 at night and around 3:00 in the morning her doctor determined she was well enough to go up to the NICU and see him for the first time. This was also a traumatic experience. She was still disoriented, in a tremendous amount of pain, and she did not know that the NICU would be full of babies in a large room. They wheeled her up to her son who weighed just 1 pound and in her mind he did not even look like a real baby and she could not come to terms with the fact that this tiny creature in front of her was in fact her son. Despite his early birth, her son survived and now is a healthy teenager, but she has never forgotten the trauma and fear of his delivery.

The experience of having complications during a pregnancy or during a birth can be incredibly traumatic. Even years later when their children were grown and healthy, women could still easily recall the feelings of fear, sadness, and exhaustion that often consumed them as they struggled to stay pregnant, cope with the mental and physical pain, and to come to terms with what was happening. A tension often arises as women try to balance their own well-being with that of their unborn child which can result in increased feelings of stress and trauma. Examining the lived experience of high-risk pregnancy and births can shed light on not just the physical but emotional and mental challenges women face. For some women who were able to successfully carry their baby or babies to term, much of the stress and trauma ended after the birth, but for the majority of women I spoke with, the stress and trauma was just beginning as the next step in their journey was the NICU.

Chapter 9

Life in the NICU

After having a relatively uncomplicated pregnancy, Kelli's twins were born at 34 weeks. She had gone in for a routine ultrasound, and the technician saw Kellie's daughter Kyle had stopped growing, which meant that she had to go in that day to deliver the babies. After they were born they went to the NICU where they spent about three weeks growing and learning how to eat. Even though they did not have serious health issues Kelli describes how difficult it was to have them in the NICU after she was discharged from the hospital. She described what a strange experience it was,

> *Like even our family and friends, people didn't know how to handle that. Like at all. They, people didn't, they didn't want to see them or see me. People were not comfortable with going to see them in the NICU and didn't even want to ask how things were going. It was really just a weird kind of limbo kind of time. And it was really kind of weird because, you are pumping. You are up every 3 hours and you are pumping, and there are no babies. So it was just really weird.*

Kelli is quick to tell people that overall her NICU experience was generally positive as her twins did very well and she felt like the staff did an excellent job of caring for her children and keeping her and the husband informed about how they were doing when they could not be there, but it was still a strange experience and one she would never like to repeat. After the twins were about a week old, some of their family who lived out of town came down to meet the twins and after a quick stop at the hospital to see the babies, the group went out to lunch at AppleBee's. Being there with them just felt strange to Kelli. Here she was out "celebrating" the birth of her twins, but they were not with them, but instead were back in the hospital. This was not at all how Kellie had imagined her babies meeting their relatives would be like.

> *The environment of the NICU itself felt strange and sterile to Kelli. She further explained, "And I still felt like it was a zoo in there. I mean they were in their little boxes. Their little cages. I felt like they were in baby cages. So the whole NICU experience I felt it was very positive but it was very bitter sweet. I felt like I needed to be there all the time. I was going back and forth, I mean at least once a day to give milk. But I wanted to go more. But I still couldn't drive because of the c-section."*

Kelli wanted to be with her children and be a mom to them in whatever ways she could, but her husband had to return to work and she had limited transportation. This made the adjustment to her new role as a mother more difficult as she could not always be with her children. She was also exhausted both physically and mentally. When she was home she was pumping every three hours to establish her milk supply and to be able to provide her twins with breast milk, so she was still sleep deprived, but found it sad to wake up in the middle of the night to pump for babies that she could not hold. Her daughter came home two days before her son, which made those two days even more of a balancing act as Kelli tried to take care of both of her children. Her stories illustrate that even when infants are not in critical condition, the NICU experience is still challenging, sad, and stressful for parents.

As almost any parent whose child or children have spent time in the NICU can tell you, the NICU can feel like its own little world, and a bizarre one at that. To enter, people often have to be buzzed in as it is frequently a locked unit. Once admitted they need to carefully scrub in before being able to go in where the babies are, and then, there are numerous plastic beds and incubators holding incredibly small babies who are hooked up to a variety of machines that are constantly dinging, beeping, and flashing. People often refer to the NICU roller coaster which refers to both the progress of the NICU patients who rapidly shift from doing great to having major setbacks as well as the emotions parents experience from being terrified that a child might die to being elated that a baby gained an ounce since his last weigh in. Almost every NICU parent will tell you that you cannot truly understand what it is like for your baby to be born and then need intensive medical care to survive until you have been there. This can be frustrating for many parents and presents an interesting tension as they would not wish premature birth or an NICU experience on anyone, but they also wish that other people could have more understanding of their experiences.

The previous chapter addressed the issue of unmet expectation when it came to pregnancy, childbirth, and the first moments of parenthood. Most women did not get to hold their children immediately after birth and many did not even see them for between 12 to 24 hours after the delivery. When women did get to see them for the first time in the NICU, the experience was often overwhelming and emotional as they were shocked and saddened to see such tiny babies hooked up to what seemed like a hundred tubes, monitors, and wires. For some women, when they first see their children there is still a question of if the baby will survive making the experience even more traumatic. Even if the baby is far enough along to not be worried about survival, there are still questions of just how sick the babies are, what long-term health complications they might have, and how long they will be in the hospital.

For DeeAnne, watching her daughter Kendra the first few days in the NICU after she was born at 26 weeks weighing just 1 pound 4 ounces and being only 12 inches long was the worst thing she has ever been through. She had never thought that she would ever be in a situation where she would have to watch her daughter fight for her life. She explained,

> If you have never experienced this, people think you are speaking a foreign language that they cannot wrap their brain around. You can't fathom watching your child fight for its life until you are standing there. They were bagging her and I was standing there watching and a nurse came up to me and asked, 'are you ok?' I never need to see that again for the rest of my life.

Even once her daughter was fairly stable, the NICU remained a scary and surreal place for her. In describing how she reacted to the NICU she said, "For that first month I was probably like a deer in headlights. I felt like I just went through the motions that first month." She said the one way she was able to cope was to treat it like a job. She got up every morning went to the NICU, sat with Kendra, participated as much as she could in her care and then at night she would go home and the next day she would start all over again.

After the initial shock and disorientation faded, women began to come to terms with the fact that their baby or babies were born early. It was then that they began the sometimes grueling process of learning about the health issues of their children, learning how to parent a preemie, and how to navigate life in the NICU. In an article in *Pediatric Nursing* magazine (Heermann, Wilson, and Wilhelm, 2005) traced the journey of women as they transitioned from being an outsider in the NICU environment to that of feeling like the mother of their infants who were in the NICU. At first, many mothers were overwhelmed by the NICU environment and it took time for women to become comfortable enough with the environment to be able to place a primary focus on their infants. During the first days of their infants' stays, they reported feeling as if they were simply a visitor rather than a parent as they had not really had time to bond yet or get to know their baby. With time, women became more secure in their role as the mother of their infants and many eventually became comfortable enough with the situation to become an active agent in the situation by contributing to the baby's care and engaging with the medical staff to learn more about their child and their child's conditions. Some even took their agency as far as becoming an advocate for their infants, although others never felt they took on their parent role entirely until their infants were discharged.

Tracey whose triplets were born just prior to 26 weeks, was not given much hope after they were born. Tracey had gone in for an emergency cerclage at 24 weeks and during the procedure *E. coli* bacteria was introduced into her uterus. The triplet closest to her cervix, Conner, developed an inuterine *E. coli* infection which eventually caused his heart rate to plummet, which necessitated an emergency delivery. Tracey was not awake for the delivery and when she came into the recovery room, her husband had brought down Polaroid pictures of the babies and told her that the babies were not doing well, especially Conner, whose plummeting heart rate had necessitated the delivery, as he weighed barely more than a pound and was covered in bruises from the efforts of the medical team to resuscitate him. The neonatologist was painting a very bleak picture and wanted Tracey to come in and see Conner as soon as she was out of recovery, because he did not think that Connor would survive. Connor did survive, but he and his brother and sister continued to have a rough time. The next round of bad news came after they had their first head ultrasounds and they learned that Connor had bilateral grade four brain bleeds, their son Caden had a grade two on one side and a grade four on the other, and their daughter Cheynne had a grade three and four. Unsure of what exactly this meant, Tracey turned to Google and quickly surmised this was not good at all, and there was a very good chance that there could be permanent brain damage. Tracey and her husband had a meeting with the pediatric neurologist and they were immediately put off by her somewhat cold and condescending manner. She gave them little hope for the long-term outcomes of their children given the severity of their brain bleeds and suggested that they withdraw life-support measures because they were not as she put it, "prolonging their lives, but only delaying their deaths."

Tracey and her husband felt, however, that they needed to leave their children's fate in God's hands and even though they were approached several times about stopping all respiratory and feeding assistance, they repeatedly told the doctors no and eventually asked them to stop asking because it simply was not an option for them. At this point the doctors respected their wishes and this allowed Tracey and her husband to focus their mental energies on surviving the daily ups and downs of the NICU. As all of this was happening, Tracey was not only emotionally pushed to the edge, but she was physically struggling as well. *E. coli* bacteria got into her incision and it quickly became infected and was red, swollen, leaking pus, and incredibly painful. As the infection got worse her temperature started to spike and she was readmitted to the hospital and treated with IV antibiotics which meant that she was unable to visit the NICU for ten days. Slowly Tracey began to heal and her children started to make progress as well, and after several long months, her triplets came home, but she has never forgotten how terrible it was to have someone tell them that her children would be better off if she let them go.

One of the peculiar phenomenon of many premature infants is that when they are born they will often do fairly well for the first 24 to 48 hours, but as their bodies begin to tire from working so hard to breathe, digest food, and maintain their body temperature, they begin to struggle more and have more complications which can be alarming and difficult for parents. Christine's twins were born at 30 weeks after she experienced a placental abruption. The first 24 hours did not seem that bad to her, but on the second day things really hit her in terms of what the severity of the situation truly was. She explained,

> That first day they said everything was fine. You know, "everybody's doing great." And then it was on the second day they realized that there were digestive issues. I walk in there and they are putting an IV in his head, trying to find a good spot. Just you know, he's screaming and no one had told me anything like, they just didn't do a lot of communicating between the floor. And I had to get in a wheel chair be wheeled all the way down. With the C-section. So I was at, you know, like everyone else's mercy where somebody wanted to take me down there.

She described how she was worried about the twins when she went back to her room, but she was unable to move and get around as freely as she would like so she felt a real disconnect between herself and her twins.

WHAT CRISIS NOW?

Perhaps one of the most challenging things of being in the NICU is never knowing when something will go wrong. The earlier a baby is, the more likely they are to have setbacks and medical issues but any preemie often will follow the model of one step forward, two steps back. Jessica's daughter Quinn was born at 25 weeks after Jessica's blood pressure kept spiking. For the first two weeks, things were very touch and go with Quinn. Jessica and her husband were allowed to touch Quinn in her incubator, but not hold her as she was too fragile and unstable. Things had started to stabilize and the doctors were even talking about moving Quinn off the ventilator onto a C-PAP machine, which represented a huge step forward. Around this time, Jessica went for a follow-up visit with her doctor for her high blood pressure and when she and her husband returned to the hospital they were greeted at the NICU door by three social workers. While they were gone Quinn had crashed, gone completely gray, and had to be resuscitated. Tests revealed that Quinn had gotten an infection that went into her lungs and had made it almost impossible for her to breathe. The doctor's told them that Quinn's lungs were some of the worst they had ever seen. Luckily antibiotics were able to get rid of the infection, but it was still an uphill battle from there as the infection had caused so much damage. Four weeks after Quinn was born, Jessica was finally able to hold her daughter. Even though she was still on the ventilator and unstable, she had been without human touch and contact for too long and her doctors felt that the benefits of kangaroo care outweighed the risks. After 140 days, Quinn was finally able to come home.

Sometimes the crises comes not at the beginning, but after preemies have appeared to stabilize and are close to coming home. Sam's daughter Kyla was born at 29 weeks when Kyla's heart rate kept decelerating. During her pregnancy Kyla had always been measuring small and Sam was sent to several specialists who speculated that she might have dwarfism or that she was just small. She was terrified that her daughter would not be born alive, so even though she was born 11 weeks early and was only 1 pound 13 ounces, Sam was relieved and thankful that she was alive. Kyla did really well for a baby her size and started to consistently gain weight and came off of all breathing support fairly quickly, surprising both her medical team and her parents. She was transferred to the step down unit and one of the night nurses told Sam and her husband they needed to begin to prepare for her to come home. The very next day Kyla developed stage one necrotizing enterocolities (NEC). She had to go back on oxygen and even though she recovered from the infection without needing surgery, she was unable to eat for a week, which was a huge set back. At that point she quit growing and not only did she stop gaining weight, but she started to lose weight. She went back into the isolette because her body temperature kept dropping, and it was heartbreaking for Sam and her husband who had thought they were finally out of the woods. Eventually doctors discovered that Kyla had a stroke shortly after she was born and had a low level of IGG (immunoglobulin G) in her blood which was contributing to her lack of progression and growth. After a blood transfusion Kyla started to grow again and was discharged from the hospital

Another family who was greatly impacted by NEC was Stephanie and her husband whose twin boys Seamus and Morgen were born at 28 weeks and 1 day after her cervix started to shorten and her doctors were unable to stop her contractions. Stephanie said the first few days after the boys were born were a blur as she and her husband who were both exhausted and shocked as they struggled to comprehend what was happening and what issues their sons were facing. When the boys were four days old, Stephanie was able to hold Seamus for the first time and doctors attempted to feed both boys for the first time through an NG tube. When they checked to see if there was any residual in Morgen's stomach after the feeding, the fluid they retrieved had a green tinge, a sign of infection and most like the potentially fatal NEC. The NICU where the boys were did not have the capabilities to perform surgery if it was needed, so the decision was made to transport Morgen to Yale hospital which had an advanced neonatal surgical unit. Stephanie and her husband said good-bye to Seamus, got into the car and drove the 30 minutes to Yale so they could meet Morgen there who was being transported by ambulance. As Stephanie sat in the waiting room until the doctor was ready to speak to them, the entire situation seemed incredibly surreal. She had not taken her pain medication since the morning so she was in a lot of pain and was feeling completely overwhelmed. When a resident came out to talk to them, he asked who the mom was and it took Stephanie a moment to register that he was talking about her. Stephanie had not even held Morgen yet and did not really feel like she was his mom. The resident explained that their tiny son did have NEC and was being taken back to surgery immediately to remove the infected bowel. As the resident was talking, Stephanie had the terrible thought that if he did not survive the surgery it would be almost like he had never even been here and she never really would get the chance to be his mother.

Fortunately, Morgen survived the surgery and the doctors were able to remove all of the infected intestine. He came out of the surgery with an ostomy bag and the doctors explained that prior to being discharged from the hospital he would have another surgery to reconnect his intestines. At that point Stephanie and her husband needed to make a decision about Seamus and whether or not to have him transferred to Yale so that the babies would be at the same hospital. Ultimately they decided not to transfer him as he was doing well at the other NICU and they did not want to disrupt or stress him with a transfer. For the next 85 days, Stephanie and husband shuttled back and forth between the two hospitals as well as returned to work which meant that they were running literally every second of the day. When asked if she was exhausted during that time, Stephanie admitted that she was, but she had no choice and each day she just woke up and did what she had to do. After 85 days Seamus was discharged, and three weeks later Morgen was able to come home to join his brother.

Sometimes the crisis families experienced came in the form of bad or unwanted test results. Jacque who described the traumatic birth of her daughter Quinn in the previous chapter suffered through an equally traumatic NICU experience. A few days after she was born, Quinn was doing surprising well and Jacque was feeling cautiously optimistic until a nurse came and told her that the doctor was on the phone and wanted to discuss Quinn's head ultrasound with her. Jacque immediately began to panic and asked if the doctor had seen brain bleeds. The nurse shook her head no as the doctor's voice told her that the scan indicated that Quinn had abnormal brain structures. At that point Jacque started to shut down mentally and emotionally. She was already trying to cope with the aftermath of a traumatic birth and daily life with a micropreemie and now the doctor was telling her that there was something wrong with her daughter's brain. The next step was to get a CAT scan to get better images of the brain structure. The doctors and nurses asked her several times if she wanted to talk about it, and she refused, she did not want to think or talk about it at all and instead just waited for the results of the next test.

What doctors told them next was absolutely devastating. Quinn was diagnosed with probable holoprosencephaly which is a neurological condition where during fetal development the brain does not fully separate into the right and left hemispheres which leads to facial and cranial deformities as well as cognitive impairment. There are different levels of the condition and doctors thought she had one of the more mild forms, but even with a mild form there was a very high chance that she would never walk, and her cognitive capacity would be minimal, only slightly higher than a child in a persistent vegetative state. As Jacque described it, "the word devastation doesn't even really fit the way that we felt about it." They were being told that their daughter would basically have a very low quality of life and Jacque and her husband went to the hospital and asked if they could remove all forms of life support. Jacque explained what she and her husband were thinking, "My husband and I have no, we are not equipped mentally or emotionally to handle a severely disabled child. Had we known during the pregnancy we would have terminated immediately. If she is going to be a vegetable that is not going to be a life for her." Quality of life was important to Jacque and her husband and the thought of a child who would never be able to walk or run or communicate with them was not what they considered a full and happy life. Quinn did not meet the legal criteria for this to be an option though, so they continued to live day in and day out in the NICU. At this point Jacque said that she had to change her thinking, "I can't hope that my baby gets sick so we can turn off the vent and let her die." She knew that her daughter was here and she was just going to have to be the best mother she could be, "As a mom you just have got to love your kid, and it's your kid. It is hard and is not the way you would like it to be, but you have to do it."

Unhappy with their current neurologist, they consulted with another pediatric neurologist to get a second opinion. He told them that Quinn might actually have a condition called lissencephaly, another rare condition in which the brain is smooth instead of having folds. This was actually a better diagnosis, but their daughter would still have extreme developmental delays and most likely would have only the mental capacity of a young child. This doctor recommended that she have another MRI done around 38 weeks gestation and then they might be able to make a more definitive diagnosis. During the next weeks Jacque struggled to accept that her daughter's brain damage was as severe as they said and tried to imagine what the future might be like. Quinn's behavior made her wonder about the diagnosis though. Her daughter was starting to look around the room and would grasp onto her parents' fingers when they held them out. Some nurses commented that she seemed to be behaving like a neurotypical baby, but the doctors told her that these were just reflexes and no indication of advanced cerebral activity. Several times Jacque and her husband considered having their daughter transferred as they felt that the chief neonatologist had given up on their daughter because of her diagnosis, and therefore did not always treat her conditions as aggressively as they would have liked. For example, the doctor rarely adjusted her settings on her ventilator which is what is done when medical teams work to get preemies off of respiratory support. In the end though, it was not logistically possible to move her, so they just tried to advocate for their daughter as best they could.

When they got to 38 weeks Quinn went in for her MRI and Jacque and her husband nervously awaited the results. What happened next was something they never had even conceived of as possible. The neurologist called them in and explained that the latest images indicated that Quinn's brain was perfectly normal and she had no brain abnormalities. While many of their friends and family suggested that it was a miracle and that Quinn's brain had been healed, Jacque dismisses this and believes that the earlier tests were either not done correctly or the results were misread. Whatever the reason, they were obviously relieved and excited, but it took some time for them to transition from thinking that their daughter might never walk and would be mentally retarded to having a child that was a preemie, but otherwise completely normal. Although the experience was traumatic Jacque and her husband did go on to have another baby who was delivered full term and spent no time in the NICU.

THE DAILY GRIND

More than one women I spoke with referred to the time their infants were in the NICU as grueling and exhausting. Often parents had to take a deep breath before entering the NICU, because they never knew what new issue might have cropped up while they were gone or what kind of day their child would be having. Johanna's son Thomas was born at 30 weeks after she went into labor and the doctors were unable to stop it. He spent 65 days in the NICU and had a lot of setbacks and issues with his feeding that made their time in the NICU very difficult and draining. Johanna described what it was like for her,

> He was at our regional hospital and then he had to be transferred because he had hernia repair surgery. He had really persistent apnea. His first month he was making some progress and then at three and a half weeks old we got a call that he had had several episodes and needed a lumbar puncture. He needed oxygen support for the first seven weeks. He did not get his feeding tube out for a long time. It was a long two months. It was what setback is he going to have today? What feeding issues is he having? It was really tough.

For the first two months she could never really relax and it became almost routine to hear more bad news, which made the days seem even longer.

One of the primary issues for parents and mothers in terms of the day-to-day life in the NICU is how they will spend time with their infants once the women themselves are discharged from the hospital. The answer to this question is as varied as the women who must find an answer to it. Some hospitals have a rooming in program where parents are able to sleep in empty hospital rooms free of charge so that they do not have to leave the hospital if they do not want to. Mothers who had the option and used it were very thankful that they were able to "live" near their babies and spend as much time as they wanted in the NICU with them. Jolee was one of the women who stayed at the hospital until her son Noah was discharged. Noah was born at 24 weeks after Jolee's water broke at 20 weeks and he spent four months in the NICU. The hospital where he was born gave Jolee an empty room on the top floor where she slept and went when she was not with her son. In the four months she was there she only left the hospital three times to go to a movie with her daughter who was nine and had come to visit. At one point she was invited to a friend's shower and at the last minute decided not to go because it did not feel right to her to be at a party having fun while her son was still not stable. That morning she was actually called down to the NICU from her room because her son was crashing due to a case of NEC. She was so thankful that she had not left and could be there immediately to be with her son. Being able to be there constantly was one of the ways that Jolee was able to cope with his prematurity because she felt slightly more in control when she was nearby.

For many women though, rooming in was not an option at the hospital, or even if it was, they had other obligations such as returning to work or other children at home that did not allow them to be at the hospital 24 hours a day. This meant that parents had to figure out a way to negotiate how they spent their time between the hospital and their other responsibilities. Some women described treating visiting the NICU like it was a job. They would wake up, arrive at the NICU in time for morning rounds, spend the day in the NICU, taking breaks to eat lunch and pump and then would go home in the evening after evening rounds. Other families took shifts with one parent going in the morning and one going in the afternoon or evening. The NICU often became parents' entire world as they spent any time they were not sleeping or working visiting the hospital, talking with nurses and doctors, and caring for their child.

When Julie thinks about her triplets' time in the NICU, she recalls how tired she was as she tried to make sure that her three babies who were born at 25 weeks were doing okay. After she was released from the hospital she quickly fell into a routine which involved waking up early in the morning, pumping, getting ready, and then heading to the hospital where she would stay until ten or eleven that night. During the day she would pump, do kangaroo care when she could, be present for rounds, and go from room to room to spend time with each of her children. For the first few weeks when her triplets were more critical they were in an open unit, but once they were less critical they were moved to private rooms, so Julie had to go from room to room to be with them and found herself constantly running back and forth to talk to nurses and participate in their care. Because she was so busy going from baby to baby she says she had little time to meet and connect with other mothers so she mostly talked with the nursing staff and leaned on them for emotional support.

Lisa was another woman who found the long days in the NICU to be exhausting. She was thirty-eight when she got married and she and her husband started trying to have a baby right away. While she was in the process of getting started on fertility treatments she got pregnant on her own and she was overjoyed with what she called her miraculous pregnancy. Everything was going great until her blood pressure spiked at 28 weeks and she delivered her daughter at 28 weeks and 6 days. She found her daughter's time in the NICU to be one of the hardest things she had ever done. She described how she spent her time after her daughter was born,

> When I got discharged I had a nesting room and could stay there for a couple of days. I finally realized I could not just stay there. I felt lonelier. I would come home at 7, eat, pump, my husband would call in the middle of the night to check on her, I would get up and get ready to be there for her 11 am care. As I started feeling better, I would go and be there 12 hours a day. When she had her own room that was a lot easier, they would not kick you out. I would go home and pretend that nights were not happening.

Once Lisa left the hospital she just did what she had to do until she could go back again.

After Lisa's maternity leave ran out she had to return to work. This was hard for Lisa, especially because this meant that she missed morning rounds, which meant that she was not involved in a lot of the decisions regarding the care of her daughter and she felt out of the loop. She started using her vacation time because it was too stressful not to be at the hospital. This extremely challenging situation was not something I had considered prior to embarking on this project as I was able to take a break from my school and teaching for as long as I needed. For many women whose children had extended NICU stays, their maternity leave ran out and they had to return to work before their child or children were discharged from the hospital. After meeting so many women who had to go back to work because they needed the income and sometimes even more importantly needed the health insurance I gained a new appreciation for the struggles and sacrifices so many families have to deal with and make when babies are born too soon.

When I asked Monica, whose son was born prematurely if there is anything that could have made her NICU experience any better or any less stressful her answer was that she wishes her work would have been more accommodating and flexible with her scheduling. One thing that was extra challenging for Monica was that she and her husband lived about 90 miles away from the hospital so a trip to visit him took anywhere from 90 minutes to two hours each way depending on the traffic. Both she and her husband worked for the sheriff's department. She worked as the overnight dispatcher and her husband worked days. After her six weeks of maternity leave were up, she had to return to work full-time and there was no option for part-time work and quitting her job was not an option as they needed the income. Because of their work schedules, they were unable to visit the hospital every day, something that was incredibly difficult for her. There was even a day when Colt was having surgery and she was unable to get the day off to be there. Because she really had no options, she just tried to make the most of the time she had when she was able to visit and counted down the days until he could come home.

Women's decisions about how much time to be in the NICU and their actual ability to be in the NICU were often a source of stress and anxiety as women felt guilt over not being with their infants or guilt with not spending more time with their other family members. Johanna who earlier described how difficult it was to have her son Thomas in the NICU also delivered her second child, a daughter named Theresa early when her cervix started thinning and she went into labor. Her daughter received surfactant when she was born and only had to be intubated for a week, so overall she was much healthier than her brother was. People kept telling her that her NICU time seemed to be going so much better this time, but Johanna felt the complete opposite. For her it was almost harder to leave a healthier baby in the NICU each day because when Thomas was really sick and could not breathe on his own she knew he was in the only place where he would be kept alive. For her daughter, it was harder to accept that she needed to be there just so she could grow and learn to eat. She also struggled with feeling like she was not spending enough time at the hospital or at home. She explained the difficulty,

"When you only have one kid you can spend hours in the NICU, once you have another kid you can't. Thomas is a very attached kid. He was in early intervention services until he was two and he is very sensitive. I felt so torn, and I just couldn't be there all of the time. Either way, one of my kids was missing out."

Women, who cannot stay near the hospital because of obligations at home, may feel guilt over the limited time they can spend with their infants in the NICU or they may feel that can never leave the NICU and put their own health and mental welling at risk. Medical staff should work to relieve this guilt and assure mothers that their infants will be well taken care of and it is appropriate for mothers to leave the NICU and have some time away. Many mothers had the story ingrained in their minds that good mothers would constantly be by their infants' bedsides and failure to do so meant women were not being good mothers or that they were selfish for going home to nap or going out to eat. Women may need assistance to appreciate the unique nature of their situations and to recognize various ways that the mother role can be fulfilled. Hearing the stories of other mothers in the NICU and how they balanced their time could help women feel more comfortable with the situation and provide reassurance that their experiences and emotions are normal. These stories could be shared through support groups facilitated by women who had infants in the NICU. NICU nurses also could encourage mothers to leave and get rest when they are tired. If women express a reluctance to leave, nurses could provide reassurance that their infants are well taken care of in their absence and share stories of other mothers who balanced their time between the NICU and home.

One thing that women talked about they seemed almost embarrassed to admit was that there were times when the long days seemed tedious and even boring. There was a sense of it being like the movie *Ground Hog Day*, as each day seemed eerily similar to the previous one and the days just seemed to blend together. These types of feelings often came when their infants were more stable, so there were no daily medical dramas and issues, just days of babies sleeping, perfecting their breathing, and learning how to eat. In 2011, National Public Radio did a year-long series called the baby project where individuals presented brief audio diaries over the course of their pregnancy and beginning months of their babies' lives. Contributor Loriani Eckerle delivered her daughter at 34 weeks after developing HELLP syndrome which caused her liver to fail. In one of her segments Eckerle described what life was like for her in the NICU with somewhat brutal honesty. She said, "So what can I say about life in the neonatal intensive care unit? It sucks. Every day, I drag myself out of bed to go sit in an uncomfortable glider for a few hours and play mom under the eyes of yet another nurse. They try to loop me into her care by letting me do things like take her temperature and change her diaper. But what I really want to do is yank off the little security device around her ankle and make a run for it." She went on in the report to say that it might have been easier if her daughter was truly ill and needed constant medical attention, but instead they were just waiting for her daughter to be able to take all of her feedings by mouth and to get her weight up to 4 pounds 8 ounces so she could be discharged (Eckerle 2011).

In addition to the toll that the NICU can take on parents' emotions and time, there is often a very real economic toll that comes from having an infant with an extended NICU stay. A 2007 report released by the Institutes of Medicine stated that the average medical costs for a premature infant were $51,600, but that number can go much higher for infants born very early and some will rack up medical bills close to a million dollars (Birth et al. 2007). In addition to these medical bills and copays, there is the potential lost income from taking an extended leave from work. The same report estimates that the average woman who has a premature infant loses about $1500 more in income than a woman who has a full-term delivery. There are also a lot of small costs that can quickly add up such as the costs of getting to and from the NICU including gas and in some areas road tolls, eating multiple meals away from home, paying for sitters for other children, and parking fees. When parents live far from the hospital, which is often the case when people live in smaller towns as most small towns do not have a large NICU, these costs are multiplied. While insurance can help with the astronomical medical bills, insurance does not cover the additional living costs that many parents accrue. Some hospitals have programs to provide meal vouchers and gas cards to help alleviate costs and some parents are able to stay at the Ronald McDonald House, but many parents have to bear the costs on their own creating additional stress and anxiety.

LEARNING A NEW LANGUAGE

Part of the getting used to the NICU was becoming familiar with the unique terminology and phrases that pervade the NICU. Women learned the vocabulary from the medical staff, but they also learned it from listening and reading stories about high-risk pregnancies and NICU babies. As women began to learn the language of high-risk pregnancies and premature birth and began integrating the terminology into their own vocabularies, they began the process of transforming their identities into that of an NICU parent. The process of learning and using this unique language often was subconscious. Women who navigated the complexities of a high-risk pregnancy became very fluent in medical terminology in terms of medications, procedures, and tests. Several times preemie moms found themselves using medical terms and NICU jargon with others, forgetting that the general public is not well versed in such specific medical terminology. For example, some of the common tests or procedures women experienced during their high-risk pregnancies were nonstress tests (NSTs), high-resolution ultrasounds, and biophysical profiles (BBPs). In the interviews women made references to NSTs, high-res, and BBPs. Women also talked about their peri, a shortened name for a perinatologist which is a physician who specializes in high-risk pregnancies. One of the differences in a high-risk pregnancy compared to a typical pregnancy is the increased medical surveillance and interventions. As women became immersed in the medical arena they began to learn and use medical jargon which conveyed their knowledge of the situation. Becoming fluent in the language of the NICU was one of the ways that women felt more at ease as they were able to understand and communicate with the hospital workers.

Some of the language of the NICU was less formal than medical procedures and conditions and arose out of the unique situations and circumstances of the unit. Providing nutrition for small and sick infants was a primary concern in the NICU. Many of the women's infants were too small or weak to nurse, so women pumped their breast milk. Women talked about their need to pump and provide the "liquid gold" that their infants so desperately needed. Liquid gold was a term that conveyed the value of their breast milk and helped motivate them to keep up a rigorous pumping schedule. Some of the women referred to a special room where mothers in the NICU pumped with a name such as the "Mommy Express."

One trend in NICUs is for Caucasian male infants to struggle more than female infants or infants of other races. This phenomena is referred to by those with an intimate knowledge of the NICU as "wimpy white boy syndrome." This is not an actual medical condition and was used most often in a kind way to explain why white infant males were struggling in the NICU. Some women expressed gratitude over having girls as they did not need to be concerned with wimpy white boy syndrome. For example, Marie, mother of triplet girls, talked about her friend who had twins, "I did have a good friend who had twins, one boy and one girl, and the boy once again had wimpy white boy syndrome." Although the term sounds somewhat negative, many of the women I spoke with that had white sons used the term almost fondly as it was a way to explain why their sons sometimes struggled more than other babies in the unit born at the same gestational age.

Another common term women used freely was As and Bs. This referred to episodes of apnea (e.g., cessation of breathing) and brachycardia (e.g., slow heart rate) that are common to premature infants, but must be closely monitored. As and Bs was an easy way to refer to episodes infants had that required interventions. Some of the women even seemed to use the term in a way that suggested they did not fully understand what As and Bs were, but knew that they were common in premature infants and the reason for some of the constant monitoring. For example, Christina described some of the complications her daughter who was born at 33 weeks experienced, "well, she had some of those A's and B's and she came home on a monitor." Abbreviating a rather serious condition made it seem less threatening and scary for some parents.

Women also talked about their infants being tubed to describe when a gavage or an NG tube was inserted in infants' nostrils in order to feed them. At first, seeing their infants with tubes in their nose, unable to suck from a bottle was very upsetting for parents, but as time passed, tube feedings became part of life in the NICU. Women frequently talked about tube feedings as normal and viewed the time when their infants no longer needed the tubes as a great milestone. For example, Kiera, described taking two of her triplets home while still using NG tubes,

> they came home on NG tubes and would take four feedings by mouth in the day and then tube feedings at night. Even with their oral feedings, they wouldn't take their whole volume at any feeding. They would just get so tired and Lily had a hard time with her suction, she just wasn't an effective sucker. So a lot of times they would take what they could by mouth, and then we would tube feed the rest for their full feeding.

Again, having a shorthand way to refer to this medical procedure made it seem less intimidating and more normal.

Women also made references to their infants being "feeders and growers." Feeders and growers is the phrase used to describe infants in the NICU who have no issues other than not being able to take all of their feedings by mouth and needing to gain weight and grow. Being a feeder and grower was a desired state as it indicated that the infants had no serious complications or issues such as breathing or temperature problems. Jessica, mother or premature twins, talked about how well her sons did in the NICU, "one of them had the bradycardia, but they were just feeders and growers other than that." At larger hospitals with more than one NICU unit, being labeled a feeder and grower meant infants were able to be in the step-down unit meaning they were closer to going home.

Knowing and using the medical terminology and shorthand of the NICU helped women communicate, but it was also a way that identified them as a mother whose infant had been born with medical complications. Laura explained how she did not recognize her new language as unique until she took her triplets to the pediatrician's office,

> I took my kids to their pediatrician and their nurse is a former NICU nurse. She was asking me a question and I kept answering her with medical terms that

> I had picked up during our stay at the NICU. She looked at me and said, 'A new mom should not know those terms.' I looked back at her and said, 'You are so right.'

In addition to medical terminology, some of the common phrases women had heard or read became integrated into their stories. For example, many had repeatedly heard or read that for every day an infant stayed in the mother, it was two less days in the NICU. This became a mantra for some women as they repeated this phrase whenever their pregnancies became especially uncomfortable. Other women frequently talked about cooking their infants or keeping their infants cooking when discussing their attempts to stay pregnant and avoid early delivery. Women incorporated these phrases into their stories as they tried to stay emotionally focused on the difficult task of following a strict bed rest regimen or dealing with uncomfortable side effects from medications. For example, Astrid, mother of triplets, described how she reflected each day on how keeping her infants inside her would result in a shorter NICU stay. Whenever she was tempted to get up from bed rest or she was tired of her long and boring days she thought about the benefits of what she was doing for her triplets which strengthened her resolve. As women heard or read others' stories they learned a new language that allowed them to communicate more easily with others who were involved in similar situations. Familiarity with the lingo of high-risk pregnancies and premature birth also marked women as a member of that community and women found comfort in talking with others who shared their language because if someone understood the lingo and shorthand, it meant that they also understood what it was like to spend time in the NICU.

COMMUNICATION IN THE NICU

Another major factor in women's NICU experiences was the communication between themselves and the medical and support staff. This communication whether positive or negative, influenced women's perceptions of the NICU experience and the stories they subsequently told about it. While women shared with me countless stories of the invaluable source of information and communication, the NICU staff also shared stories where communication was strained, difficult, or confusing. The communication with medical staff was particularly important because many women struggled to understand and define their roles as mothers while their infants were in the NICU. Prior to giving birth, most women imagined what it would be like to be with their infants, and few of those stories included extended hospital stays or 2-pound infants who could only be fed through tubes in their noses. Women found the environment of the NICU overwhelming as they struggled to understand the different treatments and procedures their infants were undergoing. If their children's medical conditions were not fully explained and questions were left unanswered, women's anxiety was heightened. Additionally, many women found that it was difficult to understand their role as mother when their infants were under the care of medical staff and women had to seek permission to perform even the most basic childcare tasks such as changing diapers or bathing. The ways that the medical team communicated with them about taking on the parenting role had a large impact on how comfortable they felt in participating in their child's care.

Women who negotiated their identities as mothers and became the most comfortable with the NICU were those who felt they understood most of what was going on with their infants. This helped them to both make sense of the situation as well as feel that they could be better advocates for their infants. Understanding the procedures, tests, equipment, and examinations also helped them feel more in control of their situations. Having a sense of control and knowing what was happening to their infants helped them feel more like mothers rather than helpless observers. For example, almost all infants in the NICU are attached to a series of machines that monitor their breathing and heart rate in order to detect any difficulties with either function such as a slow or fast heartbeat or cessation in breathing. Times when infants struggle with their heart rate or breathing are labeled episodes and require intervention. Often the monitors sound when leads which are attached to the infants' skin become loose leading to false alarms. Educating mothers about how to determine if an alarm is false or truly indicative of a problem enables them to better care for their infants and alleviate some of their stress and concern that hearing frequent alarms can arouse. Parents reported feeling more confident and more like a parent once they could identify when an alarm was real by looking at the monitors and their child.

Traditionally, the education of parents in the NICU is the responsibility of the nurses who have the most direct contact with the infants and families. Although physicians provide information regarding diagnosis and treatment, they often are busy and rushed so further explanation and education becomes the responsibility of nurses (Jones, Woodhouse, and Rowe 2007). The informational needs of parents in the NICU are high because most infants in the NICU undergo an array of treatments, tests, and procedures (Rouck and Leys 2012). However, mothers varied in terms of how much information they wanted and how they wanted to receive that information. This was very similar to how women consumed and avoided information during their pregnancies. Again, the differences in needs and desires for information among NICU mothers is a critical point that needs to be addressed. While the general consensus is that knowledge is power, there are mothers who are not ready emotionally or mentally to hear all of the details, and too much information rather than being helpful can be detrimental. Mothers' needs also may vary over time as they make the transition from being overwhelmed by the birth of their infants to more active participants in their infants' care (Heermann, Wilson, and Wilhelm 2005). Some mothers preferred being more passive recipients of information than others, so medical staff needs to be sensitive to the informational needs of each mother. Some mothers want more detailed and complete information and others want only basic explanations. Medical staff should not have a set way of addressing mothers, but instead adjust their explanations based on the verbal and nonverbal cues mothers provide.

The best way to determine the informational needs of mothers is to ask what they would like to know and what questions they have. During explanations of medical procedures, staff needs to watch for nonverbal cues such as nodding that indicates mothers' interest in the topic. If mothers do not respond to explanations or their gaze starts to drift off, this is an indication that they might not want such a detailed explanation. Some women may have a lot of questions, but will struggle to articulate them or not want to bother nurses or other personnel who they assume are busy. Taking the time to chat with parents during care times and not appearing overly rushed may allow more quiet and passive parents to feel more comfortable in asking their questions and voicing concerns. When trying to educate mothers about the care of their infants, medical staff needs to recognize the knowledge and experience of mothers. Those mothers with older children may feel as if their parental abilities are being questioned if they are given explicit instructions in terms of bathing or diapering their infants. Parental identity can be further threatened when education and direction is done in a way that belittles a woman's capabilities.

One concern that some women raised about communication in the NICU is the tone in which parents are addressed by medical staff. Women want to feel they are the mothers of their infants and desire communication styles that do not threaten or question their maternal abilities. Some women shared stories about nurses who came across as controlling and paternalistic. Women felt that the nurses they had the most problems with were the nurses who had a lot of experience and therefore felt that there was only one way for things to be done and only one way for stories to be told. Many women were frustrated by the feeling that the nurses in the NICU were in charge and were telling them how to perform even the most basic tasks. Mothers recognized how medically fragile their infants were, but also desired the autonomy to be able to change and feed their child the way they wanted to. Meghan described her NICU experience with her twin sons by saying, "I was very naïve for a long time. It took me a while to come to terms with, you know not doing everything. You know, changing the diapers. I mean they were so fragile and I wasn't that eager to, you know let the nurse do it. And they are like, No! You need to stop doing this because you don't know what you are doing."

Donna who enjoyed and valued the relationship she had with the NICU nurses when her twin sons were born, had a few more negative interactions with the staff the second time she was in the NICU with her quadruplet daughters. She spoke of how she did not enjoy bathing her quadruplet daughters in the NICU, something that concerned the nurses in the unit. "They need to make sure you change the diaper, give the bath, and all that stuff. Well, it's like; this is the way I do stuff. And OK, I've got my stuff all over the place. And the nurse is like; well I do stuff that way. OK. And I got to the point where I hated doing the bath." The nurses worried that she was not connecting to her daughters, when the actual problem was that she resented being told how to do everything and not being able to bathe her daughters the way she wanted to. She already had a surviving twin who was born prematurely at home and felt capable of bathing infants. In these situations the ways that the nurses were sharing information was not in a way the women were receptive to. Obviously, the primary concern of medical staff is and should be the health and safety of their patients. Whenever medically safe and appropriate though, medical staff should try to involve mothers in their infants' care, which is often the case in the NICU, but care must also be taken to involve parents without coming across as overly paternalistic.

Additionally, staff needs to respect time when mothers may not want to be involved with the care and prefer to observe. If mothers decline requests to participate in care, staff should accept their response and not try to pressure mothers to participate when they are not ready or do not want to or take more time to show parents how things can be done and to reassure them that parents will not harm their child by doing things like changing diapers or feeding them. Other communication strategies that would benefit mothers are engaging in relational talk, being more informal, and expressing emotional concern. Communicative strategies to avoid are being overly formal, being demanding, and trying to be controlling (Jones, Woodhouse, and Rowe 2007).

Despite some of the negative experiences of some women, other women referred to their relationships with the medical staff and particularly their nurses as invaluable both because of the information they learned and the emotional support. Women who spent an extended amount of time in the hospital prior to giving birth or spent an extended amount of time with their infants in the NICU were the most likely to talk about hearing stories from hospital and medical staff as they had the most interaction with them. One of Donna's twin sons spent five months in the NICU due to a variety of birth defects. During this time she developed a relationship with many of her son's nurses and learned about former and current patients in the NICU. "I was at Children's Hospital for a good five months and because I had seen a lot and had really gotten to know the staff, they would always tell me things about other people's babies." Hearing the stories of other infants in the NICU helped Donna to put her son's challenges into perspective and reminded her that she was not the only mother who had experienced such trauma. She had access to these stories because of her prolonged interaction with the NICU staff.

Many women made connections with either the labor and delivery nurses or the NICU nurses. For infants who were in the NICU for an extended time, one of the important things that several hospitals allowed parents to do was to pick a team of primary nurses who would comprise the core medical team that would treat their children. Several women were surprised to learn that many of their nurses had themselves been through a high-risk or difficult pregnancy and had experience with being on bed rest or having an infant in the NICU. Hearing these stories was reassuring to the women as they felt both a connection to their nurses and felt that their nurses had an intimate knowledge of what they were going through. It was also encouraging to women to hear some of the nurses' stories and then hear about how well their children were now doing.

Medical staff also need to recognize that although they have witnessed and heard countless stories over their careers, for the majority of parents in the NICU their stories are new and unique. This uniqueness needs to be respected. Even though parents can learn a lot from the stories of other infants and families who have been through the NICU there are times when mothers just want to have their own experiences and create their own stories. Again, medical staff needs to be sensitive to mothers' verbal and nonverbal cues when deciding what stories to share. Adequate training on all aspects of communication including nonverbal cues could assist staff in better responding to mothers (Cegala and Broz 2003; Cegala and Broz 2002). One of the mothers I spoke with also works as an NICU nurse. She explained that she rarely shared her own story of a high-risk pregnancy because she wanted to respect the right of each family in the NICU to have their own experiences and the opportunity to create their own stories. When families asked about her experiences she was open with them and shared stories of other women as well, but she did not volunteer this information. For her, a family's time in the NICU was highly personal and she wanted to allow each family to have their own experiences. She also did not want patients to feel bad for her or compare their situations.

PARENTING IN THE NICU

As the introduction to this chapter mentioned, one of the more challenging things for many parents was to figure out to be a parent when their baby or babies were in the NICU and under the medical care of the NICU staff.

For extremely critical infants, parents could often do little more than sit by the bed side and occasionally reach in to rest their hand on their baby. Even the gentle act of stroking or rubbing, an almost instinctual movement when holding a newborn, can be overstimulating and almost painful for a preemie. Parents' ability to parent for their child was often reduced to changing a diaper every three hours and lifting their fragile baby to be weighed once a day. One thing that some parents did was to try to make their space and time in the NICU as "normal" as possible. This could be done by doing even the smallest things like bringing photos to tape to the side of the isolette or putting small toys or blankets into the bed. A lot of parents talked about celebrating holidays in the NICU and doing things like putting up small decorations, bringing gifts for their babies and the staff, and dressing their babies up in cute outfits.

Ashley's twins Quinn and James were born at 29 weeks and 2 days, after a very difficult pregnancy that ended on September 11 when she suffered from a placental abruption. She tried to make the NICU as much like a normal home for her children as she could. The NICU her twins were in had private rooms, so she and her husband decorated and brought books to read to them. She dressed them up for their first Halloween and brought candy to pass out to the nurses. She described her twins' first Thanksgiving which they spent in the NICU. Ashley and her husband opted to spend the day at the hospital celebrating with their babies as their own small family rather than attending a dinner with their extended family. She admits that it was somewhat lonely, but it also felt right to be with her children. The hospital cafeteria had a special Thanksgiving menu for the employees so she and her husband went down and got plates and sat next to their twins to enjoy their turkey and pumpkin pie.

Becoming an Advocate

Another important way that parents tried to actively parent their child was to be at the hospital each morning during rounds so that they could be aware of what was going on and hear from the doctors. One of the interesting things that many women spoke about when reflecting on their NICU experience was the process of finding their voices and becoming an advocate for their child. At the beginning of the NICU experience many parents are in shock and almost numb and often have no idea what their role is as far as making medical and care decisions for their child. Some parents are intimated by the medical staff and often lack even basic medical knowledge, making it difficult for them to be an active participant in making care decisions for their child. Parents may have concerns about upsetting or offending the medical staff, making them reluctant to be too aggressive in asking questions or pushing for different options. At larger hospitals there are often multiple nurses, doctors, and medical students who care for children in the NICU, so parents may not be able to form a relationship with the staff as there are constantly new people assigned to their child's case. Due to the lack of relationship and lack of medical knowledge, many parents had trouble voicing their opinions or asking questions. For many parents being present for rounds at the beginning was mostly so that they could stay informed about their child's progress and treatment plan, but as time went on, some parents began to participate in rounds more actively by asking questions and making suggestions.

Despite these difficulties, many mothers I met talked about how they slowly began to be more vocal after they realized that their child or children had no voice, and as a mother, it was their duty to fight for the best possible treatment for their children. Nicole's daughter Kennedy was born prematurely after Nicole suffered from fibroids and an incompetent cervix. While she was in the NICU, Nicole took it upon herself to become as informed as possible about Kennedy's condition after she noticed the lack of continuity of care. Kennedy was born at a large teaching hospital where the physician's rotated cases every two weeks and there were always different nurses. Nicole often felt frustrated when a new nurse was on the case who did not know her daughter or when a new physician came on to Kennedy's case because they did not know her daughter and her particular quirks. It would take a few days for the new caretakers to learn what was normal for Kennedy and this made Nicole feel as if the quality of care dropped during those times.

Nicole described herself as having a strong personality, but she said that when it came to her daughter she became even stronger. She was relentless and refused to back down when it came to getting the best treatment and care for her daughter. One of the things that Nicole did when she came each morning was to read through Kennedy's chart before rounds. She recalled one time when her father was visiting Kennedy while Nicole was at home and he texted her a picture of her daughter. The picture made Nicole think something was wrong as Kennedy just didn't look right so she went to the hospital and from her chart Nicole saw that Kennedy was having more apnea and brady episodes than normal. The nurse on Kennedy's care that day told Nicole not to worry because this was just what preemies do and they often have setbacks. Nicole refused to accept this answer though, so she went above the nurse to the physician on duty who determined that Kennedy had a severe upper respiratory infection and was in the beginning stages of pneumonia. After being treated with antibiotics she bounced back to her previous state. After this incident, Nicole requested to have that nurse removed from her daughter's care. In retrospect Nicole wishes she had been more active from the beginning in identifying primary nurses who would do the bulk of Kennedy's care. She saw that to have consistent care from nursing staff who knew her daughter and could sense even minor changes was invaluable in getting her daughter well enough to come home.

Another mom who found herself stepping into the advocate's role was Cindy whose daughter Zoey was born at 27 weeks and 1 day. Her daughter was in the NICU for six months and Cindy came every single day and sat by her bedside. Zoey was born at a large teaching hospital and one of the first things Cindy did was to establish who would be on Zoey's care team. She insisted that no medical students were assigned to Zoey's case and only would allow senior-level nurses on her team. Whenever Cindy observed a nurse doing something that bothered her such as not following doctors' orders or not following proper hygiene protocol Cindy had them removed from her daughter's care. At one point doctors wanted to do a surgical procedure on Zoey's stomach to help with her feeding issues. Cindy resisted the procedure and insisted that additional tests be done before she would agree to sign off on the surgery. As it turns out, Zoey did not need the procedure and instead had a G-tube inserted and was put on Zantac to help with her severe reflux. Cindy acknowledges that there were some nurses and medical staff who did not like her, but she also got very close to some nurses and staff who respected her efforts to be the best possible advocate for her daughter. After Zoey was discharged from the NICU Cindy ran into one of the residents at a Easter Seals function and he came up to tell Cindy how impressed he was with how far she fought to get the best care for her daughter.

Melissa says that her assertive and protective nature came after one of her twins, Isabella passed away at 11 days old. Meslissa's twins Isabella and Elijah were born at 23 weeks and 4 days, at the very edge of viability. The doctors warned Melissa of all of the risks, but they promised that they would do everything they could for her children. Both her babies were incredibly small and sick, and as she put it, the sickest babies in the unit. Isabella had grade two bilateral brain bleeds, her PDA was open, a collapsed lung, and her bowel perforated. Doctors wanted to let her go, but Melissa and her husband wanted to keep fighting. Doctors inserted a tube in her bowel to help drain off some of the infection, but two days later her lung collapsed again and the doctors told them it was time to let her go because her body was starting to shut down. They knew that there was nothing more that could be done, but they really were not ready to say good-bye. Melissa was furious with the nurses and doctors because she so desperately wanted just one of them to be on her side and tell her that there was still a chance. There were no other options though, so Isabella was taken off the ventilator and Melissa held her for the very first time as she passed away.

Meanwhile, Elijah, her surviving twin continued to struggle. He was switched back and forth from the ventilator to the oscillator, and the hole in his heart did not respond to the medication to close it. Even though he weighed under a pound, a surgical team from the UMass hospital agreed to perform the very risky surgery to close the hole as the medical team determined that this was his only chance at survival. Elijah survived the surgery and after his heart was fixed he turned the corner and began to grow and gain his strength. Melissa and her husband went to rounds every day so that they could be active members of the team and be as involved as possible with his care. Melissa explained that after losing her daughter she felt like her "mother bear" came out. She spoke with the nurse manager often and requested that her son had a consistent rotation of nurses on his case. She also insisted that his nurses always wore masks and any visitors properly scrubbed in and sanitized as she did not want to risk an infection setting him back on his progress. Melissa and her husband were overjoyed when Elijah got to come home the day before his due date after nearly four months in the NICU.

Sometimes it took some time for women to find their voice and feel comfortable speaking up and frequently women mentioned that it was the nurses who helped them to gain their confidence. When Ashley's twins James and Quinn were born at 29 weeks and 2 days, she spent the next 11 weeks almost entirely at the hospital. In the beginning she just listened during rounds, trying to understand what was going on with her children as far as medical treatments, but eventually she began to take a more active role in making decisions for her children. She gives all of the credit to the amazing nurses who took care of her twins and encouraged Ashley to ask the doctors questions and to speak up during rounds. She described how hard it was for her at first, "The nurse helped give me my voice. You really lose that because it is scary and you push down your mom gut feelings. It felt like they weren't really mine. I had to ask if I wanted to hold my kids. The nurses told me, you are their mom, you have to be able to advocate for them. Without them I think I would have been really scared." One of the things that Ashley fought for was to breastfeed her twins and to keep working with feeding therapy rather than rely solely on feeding tubes. She felt like the doctors were not even giving her twins a chance, but thanks to her constant pushing she did work on breastfeeding and her twins came home with no feeding tubes.

LOSS IN THE NICU

Due to medical and technological advancements, many premature infants survive and are able to go home from the hospital, but sometimes babies are born too soon or have severe complications and they pass away before they are ever released from the NICU. Melissa was not the only woman I met and spoke with who had lost a child after they were born. I was connected with Callista through one of my cousins. I had actually heard a little of her story before from my cousin, but only that she had delivered her twins very early. I never knew the details of her story and when I did connect with her I was both overwhelmed and amazed by what she told me. When Callista first learned she was pregnant with twins at 10 weeks her excitement quickly turned to fear when the ultrasound technician was unable to find a membrane between the two girls and it was discovered that her twins were mono-mono twins. This is a rare occurrence when the twins share not only the same placenta, but also the same amniotic sac. In addition to being at a greater risk for having twin-to-twin transfusion syndrome there is a large risk of cord compression or cord entanglement which can cut off nutrition and blood flow to one or both twins. At 16 weeks they learned that the girls had developed twin-to-twin transfusion and their cords were twisted together.

Callista and her husband were terrified and felt helpless as there was little they could do to help the girls. The plan was to go in for ultrasounds every two weeks to check on the girls cord flow and growth disparity. She would then be admitted for hospital bed rest and constant monitoring at 28 weeks and as long as the babies were doing well, there would be a planned delivery at 32 weeks. After 32 weeks the babies are so large, that the risk of one or more dying in utero because of restricted cord flow is so great that it is considered safer to deliver than allow the pregnancy to continue. Unfortunately, Callista never got to that point. At 24 weeks Callista got very ill. It was actually the weekend of her sister-in-law's wedding and Callista had to leave the rehearsal dinner because she felt so terrible. At home she started getting violently ill and felt stabbing pains in her back. She went to the labor and delivery unit and they found she had a kidney stone that was causing her pain and vomiting, but she was also having several Braxton Hicks contractions so she was admitted to the labor and delivery unit until her kidney stone passed. At first, the girls were doing well and were very active, but an ultrasound showed that the cord flow for one of the girls was blocked and Callista started to retain water and swell and in two days she gained 18 pounds.

The doctors gave Callista her first dose of the steroid shots to mature the babies' lungs and told her they needed to deliver her daughters. They called her husband as she was being prepped for surgery, and as they were wheeling her down the hall both she and her husband were crying knowing that it was far too early for their twins to be born. As she lay on the operating table during the surgery, Callista heard a cry and then one of the people in the OR said "there is baby B." She knew this meant that had already gotten baby A out and there had been no crying. Baby A was Cami and she came out not breathing and they had to do chest compression to revive her. Baby B was Maddi and although she came out breathing on her own, they quickly had to put her on a ventilator. When Callista and her husband were able to see the girls an hour later, they were unprepared for just how small the girls were weighing just 1 pound 3 ounces and 1 pound 7 ounces. Their skin was so thin that it was almost translucent, and their eyelids were still fused together.

Despite how early they had been born, the doctors were impressed with how well they were doing and quickly labeled the girls as fighters. They quickly moved off of the ventilators to C-PAP machines and Callista and her husband were able to do kangaroo care with the girls before they were a week old. When they were a week old, the girls had head ultrasounds and Callista and her husband were warned that grade 1 and 2 brain bleeds were to be expected. Later that night, they got a call from the hospital telling them that Maddi's scans did not look good and they were sending the films over to the local children's hospital to get a second opinion. When Callista and her husband got back to the hospital they were told that the scan had detected bilateral grade 4 bleeds and in the last hour, Maddi had started having seizures as a result of the brain damage and had been put back on the ventilator. A care conference was called where doctors presented the prognosis for Maddi which was not good. Due to the extent of the brain bleeds doctors predicted that if Maddi lived she would have quadrilateral cerebral palsy which impacts all four of the limbs. Doctors warned that there was a possibility that Maddi would never walk or talk. One option was to have surgery to place a shunt to drain some of the fluid off her brain, but her odds of surviving the surgery were low, and even if she did survive, doctors believed she would still have major physical and cognitive impairments. Following the conference and a repeat head ultrasound that showed the same results, Callista and her husband made the heartbreaking decision to let her go. Maddi's aunt who had gotten married the weekend before was still on her honeymoon, so they asked the doctors to keep Maddi alive until her aunt could get back so that Maddi could meet all of her family before she passed. In the meantime, their parents and siblings came to the hospital to meet Maddi and to say good-bye. A priest came to baptize both girls and a photographer came and took family pictures. Callista was given the opportunity to hold both girls at the same time, something she is thankful for as this was the only time she was able to have her girls together with her as twins.

As she sat in the NICU with her daughter, Callista had the realization that her daughter would pass away without ever being outside. Callista and her husband are both avid runners and it seemed so wrong to them that their daughter would never get to experience the outdoors and they would never be able to share that part of their lives with her. They spoke with some of the nurses on the floor who went to the hospital administration to see if there was any possible way to allow Maddi to go outside while she was still living. Maddi's aunt made it to the hospital, and shortly after her aunt was able to spend some time with her Maddi's heart rate started to plummet. The doctors' unhooked the ventilator and hospital administrators let Callista and her husband take Maddi out onto an outdoor pavilion that was being constructed in the respite unit. They were certainly not ready to say good-bye, but Callista says that the situation was as good as it possibly could have been. It was a beautiful sunny day, butterflies were flying around, and she was able to hold Maddi as she took her final breaths and together they said good-bye to their daughter. The loss was devastating, but Callista and her husband had to go on because they still had their other baby Cami in the NICU. Immediately following Maddi's passing, Callista went home to rest and it was very difficult for her to gather up the emotional strength to go back to the NICU unit. She wanted to lie in bed and mourn for her daughter and she did not want to go back to the place where she had just seen Maddi take her last breaths, but she knew it was what Cami needed. So the next day she got up and went back to the hospital to continue, which would end up in an almost six-month NICU journey with her surviving daughter.

Morgan and her husband were another couple who experienced the loss of one of their twins. Shortly after Morgan and her husband found out they were expecting twins, they learned that her sons shared a placenta, but each had their own amniotic sac. This put them at a greater risk for complications such as twin-to-twin transfusion and premature birth, but for the first trimester things were going really well. When she was around 20 weeks, an ultrasound showed Morgan's cervix was shortening slightly so her doctor suggested that she start to take things a little bit easier and to decrease her activity level, but did not place her on complete bed rest or start her on any medications. At 24 weeks and 3 days, Morgan was completely shocked then, when her water broke. She was admitted to the hospital and put on a magnesium drip to slow her contractions. At that point the plan was for her to stay in the hospital until the twins were born and optimistically doctors felt they could hold her off for until at least 28 weeks and if she could go even further, that would be great. This was not the case though, and Morgan's pregnancy lasted just 36 more hours. Her sons Jonah and Austin were born at almost 25 weeks weighing 1 pound 9 ounces and 1 pound 12 ounces, a very good size for their gestation, but still far too small and way too premature.

The first few weeks were rough as Morgan was still healing from her surgery and the boys struggled with basic preemie problems such as breathing and eating. When they were two weeks old, head ultrasounds showed that Jonah had a grade 2 brain bleed and Austin had a grade 4. Austin's brain bleed caused periventricular leukomalacia which is damage to the white matter in the brain. Repeat ultrasounds showed that he had a lost a significant amount of brain tissue from the initial bleed and more tissue was continuing to die. Quality of life was very important to Morgan and her husband and based on the extent of damage in his brain, it was very unlikely that Austin would ever be able to walk or talk. As his general health continued to deteriorate, they made the decision to withdraw life support when he was two months old. Morgan said that although they were incredibly sad to lose their son and still mourn all that they were never able to do with him, at the time she and her husband also knew they were making the right decision and had a sense of peace about what was happening. She is very thankful to the medical staff who were completely supportive of their decision and some even went out of their way to applaud them for their decision to let their son go so that he would not continue being subjected to a lifetime of invasive medical procedures. Like Callista, Morgan and her husband had to mourn their son, but they also had to keep going so they could care for their surviving son Jonah. This meant going back to the NICIU each day where they had held Austin as he passed away and celebrating each of Jonah's successes even though they grieved all of the milestones his brother would never have.

Tonia also lost one of her twins shortly after they were born. She and her husband used in vitro fertilization to conceive her twins and she was overjoyed when she learned that the procedure had worked. She was cautious though as she knew that having twins and her age, which was 38, put her pregnancy at a greater risk for something going wrong. From the beginning of her pregnancy, one of the embryos measured larger than the other which doctors said most likely indicated that one of the embryos had implanted before the other. At 24 weeks Tonia was not feeling well and started to have abdominal cramps every three minutes. Her husband was out of town so she drove herself to the hospital and the pain began to intensify. She recalls walking down the corridor to the check-in area and thinking that there was no way she was going to make it. As soon as she was sent up to the labor and delivery unit they started to do everything they could to stop her labor including putting her on an IV of magnesium sulfate and putting in a catheter. Her husband was trying to get to the hospital from his business trip and the entire experience was painful and stressful. Her contractions continued and she delivered baby A, a boy, that night shortly after her husband arrived. At that point her labor stopped so the doctor on call made the decision to deliver baby B via C-section. Looking back, other doctors have questioned why the second baby was delivered that night as theoretically Tonia could have stayed pregnant for several more weeks. The decision was made though, and an hour later baby B, a girl, was born.

Tonia and her husband had the feeling that no one who was there that night, including the medical staff thought that the babies would make it. After her son was born, making no noise at all, something inside told Tonia that she did not want to even look at him. When her daughter was delivered, everyone in the OR was shocked as she came out screaming. This time Tonia asked to see her baby and she says that in that moment she knew that her daughter who they named Presley would be okay. After the surgery she was very out of it as a result of the medications as well as the trauma of their births and it was barely registering in her mind that her twins had been born. Throughout the night, the nurses would wake her up and urge her to go to the NICU to see her son who was not doing well, but she refused. Finally her husband told her that she had to go up to see him and that she needed to be a mother to her son, so she did have her husband wheel her up to the NICU unit so that she could spend some time with her baby. He was in such critical condition that she was unable to hold or touch him, so she sat by his incubator and sang to him. After about 16 hours, one of the nurses came and spoke with Tonia and her husband and told them that she felt that she needed to be honest with them, and the fact was that this little boy was really struggling and if he would somehow survive, he would almost certainly be facing a lifetime of medical issues. She told them that every baby deserves to be held at least once, so they made decision to withdraw life support and she held her son as he passed away.

These stories of loss were heartbreaking to feel and as much as I tried to be professional and neutral while interviewing and gathering these stories, it was impossible to listen to these mothers describe watching their babies die without tears coming to eyes, and even now as I write their stories down I start to well up. These women lived out the worst possible ending to their stories, but the things that amazed and continues to amaze me is their ability to continue on and honor the memory of their child who passed away while still being a parent to their other children or in many of their cases the surviving twin. Research on death and dying in the NICU has documented the challenges of parents who lose one baby while the other survives and the tension parents feel between joy and hope for their surviving child and grief and despair for the child they lost (Anscombe 2008). Other research has focused on best practices for supporting parents during these difficult times. One key finding is that parents who are involved in making end-of-life decisions such as withdrawing life support fair better than parents who do not participate in the decision-making or make the decision without input and support from the medical team (Caeymaex et al. 2011; Brinchmann, Førde, and Nortvedt 2002). After parents have made a decision to let a child go or it becomes obvious to the medical team that a baby is not going to survive, the support and actions of the medical team during this time can impact parent's experiences and coping with the loss. Allowing and encouraging parents to hold and have skin-to-skin contact with their babies as they are dying has been shown to be a source of comfort for parents and help parents to have a sense of closure (Kymre and Bondas 2013). The mothers I spoke with all appreciated that they were able to hold their child as they passed away and those who made the decision to withdraw treatment all reported feeling a sense of peace with their decisions.

COPING STRATEGIES

Given how stressful the NICU experience is, parents develop a variety of coping strategies. According to Lazarus and Folkman's (1984) Theory of Stress and Coping, a person who encounters stress engages in two distinct processes; cognitive appraisal (evaluation of the stress) and coping (way of handling the stress). In this model, coping is situation specific and an individual may employ a variety of coping techniques over an array of stressful situations. Coping methods generally can be broken down into three categories, problem-focused, meaning-based, and emotion-focused techniques (Folkman 1997; Lazarus and Folkman 1984). Problem-focused coping attempts to solve the problem and control the situation through activities such as gathering more information, gathering resources, and aggressive interpersonal efforts. Meaning-based coping involves trying to see the situation through a more positive light or reassessing the situation. Mothers of premature infants frequently reminded themselves that their situation could be worse (i.e., the infant could have been born even sooner), as a way to reassess the situation. Emotion-based coping includes strategies that aim to minimize the distress caused by a stressful situation. This includes both avoidance strategies such as denial or escaping and emotional acceptance strategies which are attempts to express and understand emotions in a healthy way such as seeking social support.

For some women, the thing they needed most from their social network was understanding and space. Dealing with the emotions and needs of friends and family who were both upset about the premature birth and wanting to see the new baby was a challenge for some women. For many parents, once their child is born, their NICU becomes their entire world and they have neither the time nor energy to keep up with friends, family, and social engagements outside of the hospital. This can be difficult for family and friends who want to stay informed and connected and may feel as if they are being ignored, but as some women explained, they simply were unable to keep up with everyone and sometimes talking about all of their child's medical issues itself was stressful and upsetting. When I asked one woman if there was anything that could have possibly made her NICU experience less stressful she responded that she wished the people around her would have given her the time and space to just be at the NICU as much as she could. She explained,

> When people would offer to come visit I would say no and people would get upset when I did not return texts and phone calls. I had a cowoker who was really mad because I did not call personally to update her. I wish I had a point person to send out information. I did develop a database and I would send out a blast email every couple of days to update everyone. I needed the space to do what I needed to do and not make me feel like I needed to allow people to visit. We were just so afraid of germs.

The issue of having visitors in the NICU was not just problematic for this family. Typically when one has a baby, the hospital is flooded with visitors and the parents are eager to show off the new baby who is often passed around so visitors can ooh and ahh over how cute the newborn is. When the baby is in the NICU, the experience of having visitors is quite different. Depending on the time of year, visitation to the NICU is sometimes restricted to prevent the spread of infections such as the flu or RSV. Different NICUs had different policies, but often the only people allowed to hold the baby are parents and grandparents, and this is only when the baby is stable and healthy enough. NICUs often limit the amount of visitors allowed in at one time, meaning that large family groups are unable to go in together. Additionally, for visitors who have never been in an NICU or are not prepared for what a preemie looks like, a trip into the unit can be very upsetting. For all of these reasons, some of the families I spoke with opted to limit who they allowed to visit to the NICU, a decision that sometimes created tension between NICU parents and their family and friends. After Ashley had her twins at 29 weeks, she and her husband did not allow anyone into the NICU to visit, even their immediate family. Ashley explained that that their family resisted their decision, but the way she and her husband saw it was that they had worked so hard for these babies, and they were not going to risk letting anyone come in and expose the twins to something and causing a major setback. In a way she says she was also too selfish to have vistors. She and her husband did not know if their children would surive, and she was not willing to share what time they had with anyone else.

Helping friends and feel cope with their own grief, anxiety, and emotions also took its toll. There were many situations where mothers found themselves comforting others and feeling like they had to hold themselves together emotionally and be strong for those around them, when the reality was that they were the ones who need to be taken care of. DeeAnn said that dealing with her family's stress and axiety over her daughter Kendra who was born at 25 weeks became almost too much to handle. She explained, "once Kendra was born, everyday somebody wanted an update. My dad is a complete worry wart, I finally stopped telling him the real details. She was only 1 pound 4 ounces and 12 inches long. At the beginning she really was day to day and he would text me and ask me how she was doing and I would answer and he would call me all freaked out. That was really hard to deal with." To keep her father calm she started to shield him from some of the problems and issues Kendra was having and in the process lost a potential source of support for herself.

Tonia also found herself needing to support and comfort her family rather than being the one who was being comforted. Some of Tonia's in-laws worked in the medical profession, but not in the NICU. When they would come to visit, they would ask a lot of questions and criticize some of the care and interventions Presley was receiving. Tonia felt like she had to spend a lot of time defending the NICU staff and her daughter's treatment so that her family would calm down. Her step-children who were teenagers at the time started to act out and Tonia and her husband received calls daily from her husband's ex-wife relating to the children's latest issues and requesting that Tonia speak to them and explain how the baby was going to be ok. When her step-daughter came to visit her new sister, she often fell apart and had to leave because she could not control her crying. Tonia felt for her, but at the same time, as a woman who could barely take care of herself, dealing with others' stress and anxiety was just too much.

No matter how women tried to cope with their circumstances, how early their children were born, or how long they were in the NICU, having a child in the NICU was a stressful and emotional experience. As this chapter has illustrated, a roller coaster ride really is an apt metaphor for describing the NICU journey as parents experienced some of the lowest lows, bouts of absolute terror, and some of the highest highs. Even the long tedious days can be compared to the long lines one must stand and wait in before getting on the ride. What almost every NICU parent will tell you though is that the ride was something they were not prepared for. No matter how much they had read, or heard, or had tried to prepare themselves for the early birth, as soon as they stepped into the NICU it was as if they were in an entirely new world. Each woman and family differs in how they attempt to cope with the stress, anxiety, and tedium, and what women said they needed most was for the people around them to respect and understand their ways of dealing with the situation.

Chapter 10

Life after the NICU

Not a day goes by that Cindy's life is not impacted by her daughter's premature birth. When Cindy got pregnant with her daughter Zoey she was considered high risk and was closely monitored as she had lost a previous pregnancy at 18 weeks. Everything was going fine with her current pregnancy until she was 20 weeks along and started to feel some painful cramping. She went to her doctor who did an ultrasound which showed that the baby was fine, but her cervix was already dilated to one centimeter. She was rushed to the hospital to have an emergency cerclage and remained on hospital bed rest until she was 27 weeks and 1 day pregnant. That day some friends came and threw a baby shower for her in her hospital room and throughout the shower Cindy just felt that something was not right. She was feeling nauseated so she got up to use the bathroom and when she got there she threw up. When she sat down to go to the bathroom she noticed a lot of blood. Her cerclage had started to tear and the next thing she knew, the baby's head was coming out. There was no time for a C-section as is the typical mode of delivery when a woman has had a cerclage and by the time the doctor got there, Cindy's cerclage had completely torn out, and after pushing just twice, Zoey was born weighing 2 pounds 4 ounces and measuring just 13 inches long. After a long and difficult NICU stay, Zoey came home on oxygen and with a G-tube for feedings. At age three Zoey is still not walking but with the help of early intervention service she can pull herself up and walk with the assistance of a walker. She has a speech delay and shows some signs that she may have a learning disability. Cindy is a single mom as she and her husband have divorced since Zoey was born and she spends her days taking care of Zoey and managing all of her medical and therapy appointments. Cindy is unable to work because she cannot find a childcare center she can afford that is willing to take a child with Zoey's medical needs, which means that Cindy relies on government assistance and struggles to make ends meet each month. Zoey does qualify from some home nursing and respite care each week and it is during those hours that Cindy is able to run errands and do what she needs to do to get by. As I spoke to Cindy it was obvious that despite the daughter's ongoing issues, she loves her fiercely and will do anything to give her daughter every opportunity and every advantage. Cindy's story also is an excellent example of the long-term impacts of prematurity on both children and their parents.

When people learn that I have triplets the first question they almost always ask after how early were they born is how long were they in the NICU? Occasionally someone will ask if they have any long-term health issues, but in general the questions focus on my pregnancy and the girls' time in the hospital. This is very telling as it demonstrates the focus that many people have on the critical period around the birth and the prevailing belief that once an infant is discharged to go home, the hardest part is over. For many NICU families though, although discharge is an exciting and happy day, there are still months if not years ahead of health issues, developmental delays, doctors' appointments, and anxiety. Even if infants are doing relatively well, most preemie parents will tell you that bringing home a preemie from the hospital is much different than bringing home a typical newborn. It is already stressful to bring home a new baby, but that stress sometimes multiplied for NICU parents, They often have had an extremely high level of anxiety after watching their child struggle to perform basic tasks such as eating and breathing, and that heightened state of fear and watchfulness takes time to subside. Additionally, there is often a fear that without all of the monitors and medical staff that something will go seriously wrong and parents worry that their child may stop breathing or be unable to eat once they are not under the constant care of the medical team.

Many preemie moms reported feeling unprepared for what life would be like once they brought home a premature infant. Several mothers commented that they wished they had heard more stories about what happened after their pregnancies and about raising premature infants. Often women were so focused on coping with a high-risk pregnancy, staying pregnant for as long as possible, and after the birth on their child growing and surviving in the NICU, that they did not have a lot of time to contemplate the future. Women mentioned wanting to know about specific issues such as how to feed multiple infants or how to get their infants on a schedule. The types of stories they wished they had heard or read contained details about the birth, the first days of their infants' lives, and their NICU stay, as well as the time after women brought their infants home from the hospital. Some had even been too afraid that their baby or babies would not survive, so they would not let themselves think about life after for fear that it would never come. Once they began to face the challenges of raising their infants, they wished they had heard or read more stories to help them know better how to navigate this new phase of their lives.

For some parents the day their children "graduate" from the NICU, the term used to designate an infant who has successful learned all he or she needs to learn to survive outside of the hospital and is ready to be discharged, is one filled with mixed emotions. On one hand there is joy and excitement that the baby or babies has made it and is going to come home. For children who spent months in the NICU, there was often a sense of disbelief that this day had actually come after so many hurdles and setbacks. On the other hand though, graduation day could result in anxiety and even sadness as parents often had grown close to NICU staff members and even though they were glad to be leaving, they were sad to say good-bye to the people who had come to feel like family in some cases. Often parents felt a sense of fear as they wondered how they would be able to care for their child who previously needed round the clock medical care. Many of the women I spoke to described wanting to take all of the monitors and a nurse or two home with them because they were unsure that they would be able to do it on their own. After spending days, weeks, or months not feeling like the primary caregiver, the transition to home can be very difficult. Jolee, whose son Noah who was born just prior to 24 weeks, talked about how things were almost worse for her emotionally when her son Noah finally came home. As she got settled in and found a routine for caring for her son who had various medical needs, the reality of her situation hit her and this is when she began to notice her postpartum depression. While in the NICU, it was always day to day, and there was so much to be done between taking care of her home, her older children, and her baby in the hospital, and once she was home she was able to be a little more still, which gave her the time to process just how serious and frightening their situation had been. She felt like things happened in the NICU so fast, so it took all of her energy just to keep up with the latest test results or crisis, and once life slowed down she had more time to think and allow herself to feel all of the emotions she had been ignoring for the past few months.

Even though Jolee felt like things slowed down somewhat when Noah came home, there was still a lot of issues that she had to deal with on a daily basis. When Noah was released from the NICU he came home on supplemental oxygen and remained on it for a year. He also came home on a heart monitor and due to some ongoing kidney issues he had frequent visits to see a urologist during his first year. Because of his oxygen and feeding issues he had daily home nursing care. After he was two that care was reduced to a weekly visit. He had ROP when he came home which meant bi-weekly visits to the eye doctor. Luckily the ROP went away on its own without surgery, so one problem was checked off the list. In addition to PT to help him with reaching his developmental milestones such as reaching for objects and sitting up, he was also in speech therapy to help with his speech delay. Reading this list might make any parent feel overwhelmed, but Jolee has an amazingly positive attitude. At one point she sat down with Noah's team of specialists and they talked about all of the issues he could have had due to his prematurity which Jolee said made her thankful that all of her son's issues were manageable and considering what the list might have included she felt like her son's list was pretty good.

One of Noah's huge struggles was with eating and gaining weight. After the first year of being at home, he was still very physically delayed so at eighteen months he had a feeding tube put in. Even with the feeding tube he continues to remain small and has a hard time gaining weight which has raised a lot of concern from his doctors who at one point thought that maybe Jolee and her husband were not feeding him enough. Jolee explained that he gets 100 percent of his nutritional needs from his G-tube, but due to his high energy level and constant activity he uses everything he consumes. Eventually Jolee switched to a new pediatrician because she said the old doctor was always focused on what was wrong with Noah and what he could not do versus what he could do. She explained that Noah eventually would meet his milestones, but he just preferred to do them on his own time, or Noah time as she called it. She also said that Noah has his own normal and while that may be different than that of typical full-term kids, he was a micropreemie and his body had not yet caught up.

Some of the mothers told me that they and those around them had been so focused on the early birth and getting out of the NICU, but they had never really taken the time to think and learn about what life after the NICU might be like and found themselves at a loss for how to manage the logistics of caring for their babies once they were home. This was especially true of mothers of multiples. The stories their friends told of taking care of one infant did not explain how to feed or care for two, three, or more infants simultaneously, or how to keep track of who was doing what and when they were doing it. Denise, mother of triplets, felt like she had gotten the information she had wanted about her pregnancy, but had no idea what to do when her infants came home. She described the stories she wished she would have heard,

> I think it would have been more like the scheduling. I think all of the pregnancy stuff and the, I think that would have just freaked me out. I just look back and I really don't think I could have done anything different than I did. I don't think that anything I could have done would have changed the outcome. I would have had 28-weekers. But I think as far as just the scheduling and the making the bottles, easy ways to do that. I think that would have been helpful.

For so many preemie parents taking a premature baby home from the hospital is different than taking home a full-term baby. Many preemies come home needing additional medications, may be on apnea or heart monitors, have multiple follow-up physicians appointments, can still have trouble eating leading to extended feedings times, they may need to be woken up through the night for feedings, and in general have an immune system even more compromised than a full-term infant. Because of these difference parents need to hear stories from people who have navigated similar roads because the typical stories they have heard of caring for newborns are not always completely applicable.

Denise was not alone in wishing that she had access to more stories about how to simplify life with young infants. Women provided two explanations for why they did not read or hear more stories about these topics. As described previously, the first reason was women were so concerned about the outcomes of their pregnancies that they were unable to think past their infants' health and survival to the basics of day-to-day living at home. The second reason was that women lacked access to others who were facing similar situations in the number of infants or the health situation of their infants. They had plenty of friends to ask for advice on how to take care of a full-term infant, but did not have friends who knew what it was like to have a baby on a heart monitor or how to use a G-tube.

Another thing that makes it difficult when their babies finally come home from the hospital is that for many women, the fear that something could go wrong or that they could still lose their child takes a long time to go away. Many preemies are more medically fragile than your average child and their immune systems and lungs take a long time to develop their full strength, making preemies more vulnerable to common childhood infections. Parents who have spent weeks and sometimes even months watching their child struggle to breathe and have grown used to the sound of alarms going off constantly lived in a state of high alert and it can be difficult to let go of that intensity. We met Stephanie in chapter 5. Her first son was stillborn, and her second son David was born at 29 weeks. When he was ready to be discharged from the NICU Stephanie was terrified. Nothing felt safe to her. She explained that even the standard baby equipment like bathtubs and car seats seemed way too big for her tiny baby who weighed only 5 pounds. Even though he came home with only a few minor issues, she said she still worried about losing him every day and even now worries that something will happen to him. Anytime he was sick as a baby she was worried that he would end up back in the hospital again. David did come home on an apnea monitor and Stephanie was very reluctant to stop using it. Even after the pediatrician said he no longer needed it she asked to keep him on it because it gave her the security of knowing that if he ever did stop breathing that the alarm would go off and she or her husband would be able to assist him. When they finally did stop using the monitor she was terrified and woke several times a night to go and check on him to make sure he was still breathing. Even though he is now eleven, Stephanie admits that she stills stops in his room each night before she goes to bed to check and make sure he is okay, and there is always a small bit of fear that she walk in and her son will be in some kind of distress.

Heather was another mom who struggled with anxiety over her daughter's health once she was home from the hospital. Her daughter was born at 28 weeks and spent 6 weeks in the NICU. Heather's first child, a son passed away from SIDS when she was just 17. The official cause of his death was unknown and knowing that her daughter was early made Heather even more afraid that her daughter would also pass away in her sleep. To help ease her mind she requested that her daughter come home on an apnea monitor and her daughter's doctor agreed even though he did not think it was medically necessary, but the doctor understood that Heather needed to be able to sleep and have some sort of peace in order to care for her daughter.

Another thing that many preemie moms felt that other people did not understand is that many preemies have ongoing issues and parents are still very much involved in the medical and therapy world after their children are discharged. Over and over women told me that it isn't over just because you get to leave the hospital. Coming home is a huge milestone, so big in fact that some families celebrate both their child's birthday and their coming home day every year, but coming home rarely means the end of a preemie parent's worries and involvement in the medical care or their child. The first few years are generally the most intense as this is when preemies are the most medically vulnerable as their immature immune systems struggle to catch up. The first three years are also an important time for early intervention services which means that premature infants often spend the first three years of life being shuttled from appointment to appointment in order to get the medical care and therapy they need to be as healthy and developmentally on track as possible. Managing the medical and therapy appointments can be overwhelming and at times seem like a full-time job in itself. Jessica's daughter Quinn was born at 25 weeks and after she came home her life was full of a variety of doctors' appointments to manage her respiratory and digestive issues. She also had a feeding therapist who came each week to work with her on her eating. Eventually, she did learn to eat, but is still not a huge eater and there is an ongoing concern about her getting enough calories and staying on her growth curve. She qualified for speech therapy just before she turned three to help with a minor speech delay and also had ROP in both eyes. Quinn's issues have required a large amount of intervention services and routine doctor's visits.

As Jessica is quick to tell anyone though, it is miracle that these are the extent of Quinn's problems, and while it has not always been easy, she is constantly amazed by how strong her daughter is.

Elaine is another mother whose life after the NICU was still very much consumed with caring for her twin daughters and meeting their medical needs. Elaine, is the mother of twin girls Carol and Lydia who had a lengthy stay in the NICU. After the girls were home, they still had serious medical issues that required frequent follow-up visits to various doctors and almost round the clock medical care. Lydia was in the hospital for almost ten months. Due to the loss of much of her large and small intestines because of NEC, Lydia came home with a G-tube on continuous feeds and also has cerebral palsy on her right side due to a brain bleed. Her sister Carol was born with an atrial ductal defect. She came home earlier than her sister Lydia, but due to her heart condition she struggles a lot with her breathing and will need to have a heart surgery before she turns four to fix it. Despite all of their medical issues, Elaine remains in high spirits and every day is grateful for her daughters. As she told me, she never has the time to fall apart or dwell in her sadness because she is just always running and always doing something for her girls.

When Ashley brought her twins home from the hospital she felt like she basically transformed her home into an NICU so that she could care for them and keep them healthy which meant keeping everything sanitized and making sure that any visitors to her home "scrubbed in." Ashley felt like it was almost a full-time job to protect the twins from germs and viruses that could set them back. The twins were discharged from the hospital taking all of their feeds by mouth, but once at home they started to struggle with eating and were not gaining enough weight, so they had to go back on NG tubes. It was hard for Ashley to see her twins having setbacks and the tubes required a lot of extra care. The tubes needed to be changed every four days, but Ashley could not bring herself to fish the narrow plastic tube through her babies' noses down to their stomachs. Luckily, one of their primary nurses from the NICU lived just five minutes away and she offered to come over and change the tubes for Ashley, something she is still incredibly grateful for. It was only after the first year that Ashley felt like their life, though still full of challenges, started to take on a semblance of normalcy.

Melissa also felt like life was far from normal and routine after her son Elijah came home from the hospital. She explained that with a normal birth, after you come home from the hospital you are flooded with friends and family who are eager to drop off a warm meal and meet the new baby, but in their case they kept visitors out and Elijah in, as like many preemie parents they were terrified of germs and possible infections. The only time they left the house was for medical appointments which were fairly frequent, and weekly trips to the pediatrician to have his weight checked. One of the major issues he had was bad reflux which made his eating difficult. When he was ten months old his reflux caused him to aspirate and he was readmitted to the hospital and then a few weeks later he aspirated again and this time had to be taken to the hospital by an ambulance. This resulted in Elijah needing to be held upright for an hour after every feeding and needing to sleep on an incline. In addition to his eating issues, he had several developmental delays and received services through their state's early intervention program including speech and occupation therapy and he saw a developmental therapist to work on fine and gross motor skills.

Initially Melissa had returned to work full time eight weeks after Elijah was born. When he was discharged from the hospital she went to part time and family members came to their house to babysit. After a few months Melissa's boss informed her that she would need to resume working full time and Melissa made the difficult decision to quit her job. Her son's needs were just too great and she could not be away from him for 40 hours a week and provide the care for him that she wanted to. It has been a stretch for them financially, but she explained that they make it work and it has been well worth it. By being home she can play an active role in all of his therapy and medical appointments and can work with him throughout the week whereas while she was working some of the appointments took place while she was gone.

Another thing that can be frustrating for NICU moms is that a child's gestational age is not always a good indicator of the type of long-term issues he or she will deal with. A child born at 25 weeks might grow up to have relatively few medical issues whereas another baby born at 31 weeks might have a multitude of ongoing problems and delays. Heather's first child, a daughter, was born at 27 weeks and her second child, a son was born at 31 weeks. Although her daughter was in the NICU longer and had to be on supplemental oxygen for the first six months she was home, she overcame her respiratory issues and with the help of early intervention services was able to catch up in areas where she had developmental delays. Heather's son who was healthier at birth and spent less time in the NICU and never needed supplemental oxygen has actually gone on to have more health and developmental issues than his older sister. As a baby he had a febrile seizure and now that he is three he continues to have respiratory issues. His immune system is still weak and he catches things very easily and often sick. He has a speech delay and a sensory processing disorder and had a paraprofessional aide who works with him at preschool. She is confident that many of issues he will eventually outgrow with the help on continuing interventions, but she often tells people that you can never predict how a preemie will do by gestational age alone.

ISOLATION

Another thing that many preemie parents faced was continued isolation after their children came home from the NICU in both the physical and emotional senses. Debra Discenza, author of *The Preemie Parent's Survival Guide to the NICU,* explains that the way a preemie's life starts out is far different than a typical infant and parent face different challenges and different worries. She writes, "the public, not understanding this scenario, is left to devise assumptions about the family's actions regarding the child. This further isolates the parents, breeding a sense of mistrust and ongoing isolation which has severe consequences on the health of the parents that is both physical and mental" (Inspire, Support, and Special 2011). Physically, many preemie families are isolated as the fear of their medically fragile coming into contact with germs is so great that families go into self-imposed lock down. As one mom told me, "you can't even be normal when you come home." Many preemie families limited guests from coming to visit and insisted that anyone with any signs of illness such as a cough or a cold stay away. Guests who were allowed in were often required to scrub their hands or use hand sanitizer, a ritual reminiscent of scrubbing into the NICU. Not only did families keep people out of the home, but they also kept their babies inside and rarely ventured out in public except for trips to doctors. Women could not even venture out for a quick trip to the grocery store to pick up milk or diapers for fear that their baby or babies would pick up an infection and end up back in the hospital. Many mothers expressed some regret over yet another unmet expectation, which was taking their baby out in public and having strangers stop to admire their son and daughter and tell the mom how cute the new baby was. Having a stranger poke their head into a car seat and possibly breathe on or touch their baby became many women's worst nightmare. Women who did venture out often covered the car seat with a blanket or hung a small sign on the car seat that asked people not touch or identified the baby as medically fragile. Sarah, whose second child was born early, described taking her toddler out to the store and leaving her preemie at home. When people commented on how cute her son was she had an overwhelming urge to tell them that she actually had two children and her baby was at home.

Jen, whose twins were born at 28 weeks, described how little they left the house the first year they were home due to fears over them getting sick, especially with RSV. If they did ever go to the grocery store or to Target Jen made sure it was an off time and never took them on the weekends as there were just too many people. Jen and her husband's reluctance to take their twins out was hard for some people to understand. For example, some family members lived about two hours away and a few times suggested that they meet halfway for dinner so they could see the twins and were angry when Jen and her husband declined. Restaurants were too crowded and Jen feared that other customers would want to check out the twins and put them at risk. She explained that other people could not understand how susceptible her twins were to illness, especially respiratory infections and even though they thought she was just being overprotective, her greatest fear was one of them landing back in the hospital, so she was not going to take any chances. The few time they did take the twins out it was a local restaurant where they knew the slow times and they always sat at a booth in the back where there was little foot traffic. When friends and family did come to visit they were greeted with a hello, a bottle of hand sanitizer, and strict instructions to wash their hands frequently.

Carrie's daughter Tarin was born at 31 weeks. Her time in the NICU was very difficult for Carrie as she had an older daughter at home and she and her husband were struggling to make ends meet financially which meant that her husband was working extra shifts whenever possible. Carrie was constantly torn between being with her daughter at the hospital and taking care of things at home. When Tarin was discharged, Carrie was surprised by how difficult things still were. She was no longer torn between the home and the hospital, but life did not just resume as usual. She explained that she was still very isolated and exhausted as she tried to meet all of her daughter's needs. She described the first few months, "I was still homebound. I was not ready to let other children come into the house. She had breathing issues so I was doing all of these respiratory appointments. She had a bad suck swallow reflux. She could not breastfeed so I was pumping exclusively." Because caring for her daughter took so much of her time and energy she felt that many of her relationships including her one with her husband were strained. She felt like she was stuck in her house day after day and there was no way for her to get out to see friends and when she and her husband were together there was always the stress and exhaustion from taking care for their daughter.

The isolation after being discharged from the NICU was one of the things that really surprised Jessica whose daughter Quinn was born at 25 weeks. When they were finally able to bring Quinn from the hospital they were excited to start living life as a normal family, but quickly found that their life was still not typical. In addition to the constant appointments that dictated how they spent a lot of their time, there was an overall concern for Quinn's health. Because she was born so early, both her lungs and immune system were weak and to make matters worse, she was discharged from the hospital at the beginning of RSV season. Jessica and her husband were so worried about Quinn getting sick and having to go back to the hospital they spent almost all of her first year on what she described as lock down. One of the hardest things during that year was missing out on holidays and family celebrations. If anyone else in the family was sick they opted to just stay home and Jessica remembers Quinn's first Thanksgiving which was just the three of them at home which felt a little sad and lonely, but it was not worth exposing Quinn to something, so they made the best of it. Even if they did want to venture out, the fact that Quinn was on full oxygen and a feeding tube when she came home made it difficult as they had to take her tank and all of her equipment with her. Unlike a typical baby who requires a bottle or jar of baby food when on the go, Quinn's feeding regimen required careful measuring and timing as well as careful clean up and sterilization making it a complex and time-consuming process.

In addition to be physically isolated, many preemie moms continued to feel emotionally and socially isolated. Part of this was due to the physical isolation, but even after women felt more comfortable venturing out with their children, they still felt isolated because they felt so different from the other women and moms they knew. Some women described still living in a constant state of stress and anxiety as they cared for the baby while those around them had moved on and could not understand why they were still so worried and upset all the time. Friends and family members would encourage them to lighten up or stop being so overprotective which lead many women to withdrawal. When talking with other moms, the sense that their lives and experiences were very different from other mothers heightened feelings of isolation. It was hard to be the mom that was explaining what adjusted age meant and was familiar with a wide variety of health and developmental issues in a group where other mothers had full term and seemingly healthy children.

Another factor that contributed to both physical and social isolation for some women was a change in their working status or childcare after their child was born or came home from the NICU. Due to fears of overexposure to germs in childcare settings as well as the difficulties of getting a child to various medical and therapy appointments some women who had planned on going back to work after the baby was born decided to stay home. After Shelly's daughter Riley was born at 28 weeks and spent 78 days in the NICU, Shelly who had planned on going back to work made the decision to quit her job so she could stay home with Riley. While she is glad that she has been able to protect her daughter's health and play an active role in her various therapies including occupational therapy, speech therapy, and physical therapy, she has found that staying home has been more difficult that she thought it would be. She really misses her former job and the interaction she had with other adults.

NAVIGATING EARLY INTERVENTION

One thing that the majority of premature parents become familiar with is early intervention services. Early intervention is a system of services such as speech, physical, and occupational therapy for children from birth to age three managed by the state government. Each state is required by the Individuals with Disabilities Education Act to have an early intervention program. The act which became law in 1986 mandates that extra services be made available to individuals with education and learning challenges. One of the large benefits of these programs is that services are provided regardless of a family's ability to pay, and in many states, the service providers will come to a family's home or childcare center. Mothers who were leery of taking their children out, especially to crowded waiting rooms where germ exposure is almost inevitable were thankful that therapists would come to them. Despite the benefits, these programs can also be stressful for parents as there is a lot of paperwork that needs to be filed and there are often strict eligibility criteria and children in the program need to go through annual assessments in order to requalify for services, leading to a tension between wanting a child to develop and also wanting to be sure that the child still qualifies for the services she or he needs.

When Jamie's daughter Aubrey was discharged from the NICU she started working with early intervention right away to help her continue to develop and meet her physical and cognitive milestones. One of her big issues was that her hip joints were tight and she did not have full range of motion in her legs. Her early therapy and intervention services worked, and when she went for her NICU follow-up appointment at age two she was actually discharged from the follow-up program because she no longer had any significant delays and shortly after graduated from early intervention services. Jamie explained that her daughter lagged behind for quite some time, but then something clicked and she started to gain skills quickly. Now at age two the only lingering thing they notice from her prematurity is that she still has a fairly weak immune system and as Jamie put it, "gets sick at the drop of a hat." Every day Jamie is incredibly thankful at how well her daughter is doing and how she had access to quality intervention services that helped her to catch up to her peers.

In addition to the stress of dealing with the logistics of attending therapy appointments, there can also be an emotional toll. Even when their children begin to overcome their physical challenges and start to catch up on their developmental milestones, many parents continue to worry about the long-term impact of prematurity. Partly this is because there is still a lot that is unknown as far as what exactly the long-term impacts are as far as preemie's physical, intellectual and social health, and overall well-being are concerned. Many studies have focused on shorter-term impacts of prematurity such as the first two or three years. Longitudinal studies are much harder to conduct and with so many intervening factors such as home environment, socioeconomic status, and genetics, it is hard to provide direct causation between prematurity and health problems that develop later in life. Some problems such as learning disabilities and social difficulties are not identified until a child is older and in school, so even when a three-year-old appears to be developing normally there is a still a fear that school will reveal additional problems or delays. Parental anxiety about the future can easily be increased when researchers report findings such as the fact that premature infants have a greater risk of early mortality. A 2011 article published in the *Journal of American Medical Association* reported that infants born at less than 37 weeks were 38 percent more likely to die in early adulthood than infants born full term. This makes for a splashy headline and can drive fear into a preemie parent's heart, but further reading of the details of the article show that the overall risk is still very low, with it being only 1 in 1000. There is still a concern that the risk is higher and the researchers indicated that even when a preemie has grown up and appears healthy, they should still be more closely monitored by their physicians as there might be health conditions that develop later in life.

Jennifer, mother of twin boys who were five when I spoke with her, told me that she has had to stop reading reports like this because each time she did, she had a new set of worries about her boys. They were doing wonderfully and had fully caught up to their peers, but there was always a nagging feeling that something could still go wrong. There was also a sense of guilt when any problems did arise that it was because they were born early when in reality there might not have been a direct correlation. "When can I stop worrying," she asked. "When they are married?" Cora, mother of Lily, a 29 weeker also deals with ongoing anxiety about her daughter's future. When Lily turned one and was doing very well as far as her health and meeting her developmental milestones were concerned, Cora started to have nightmares about her birth and time in the NICU. "At what age can we stop worry about her getting Alzheimer's or other brain-related things? It happens every year. It never goes away." Every six months Lily has an appointment with the neonatologist to assess her progress, and this causes a great deal of anxiety as Cora is always worried about a new diagnosis or the identification of a new delay.

Something that women found difficult once leaving the NICU and that often contributed to their anxiety and feelings of isolation was the lack of a formal support system. Women with multiples were sometimes able to tap into a local multiples club, but for mothers with single preterm babies or living in smaller towns with no multiples groups there is not often a support group for preemie parents. Leslie delivered her twins Kadri and Xavier at 25 weeks after she went into premature labor that doctors could not stop. Once her twins were discharged from the NICU after 104 and 105 days she felt a little lost and alone. Her NICU staff had provided a strong support community and the local March of Dimes had offered assistance and support, but once she was home there was nowhere to turn. Some days she just wanted to call up the NICU and talk to a nurse, because they had been her support for so long and she knew that they would be able to relate to what she was going through and offer some encouragement. After her boys were older she learned about the parent mentor program provided by Hand to Hold, a nonprofit organization where preemie parents can request to talk to other preemie parents who have been there. She told me something like that would have made a lot of difference to her as she was struggling to figure out how to parent two premature and medically fragile babies. When she was feeling lonely, scared, or had a parenting question it would have been great for her to have a preemie parent who was further along in the journey who should quickly call or send an email.

WHAT NOT TO SAY TO A FORMER NICU MOM

In almost every interview I conducted and in a lot of conversations that I have had with preemie moms, the subject of the insensitive and offensive things people said to them almost always came up. I vividly remember talking with another mom at a playgroup who was pregnant with her second child. She was about seven months pregnant and feeling quite uncomfortable and was complaining about severe heartburn. In an effort to commiserate with her I mentioned that I had terrible heartburn with the triplets, way worse than my pregnancy with Anna. "Yeah," she said to me, "but at least you were only pregnant for seven months." I chose not to respond because nothing that would have come out of my mouth would have been polite or appropriate, but inside I was seething. I now see that this mom did not truly understand what a having a high-risk pregnancy was like or how much guilt I carried for the fact that the girls were born 8 weeks early. I wanted to start lecturing her about how important every day in the womb is for a child and a part of me also wanted to start listing everything I had been through physically and emotionally during those seven months, but it did not seem like the time or place so I let it go and chalked it up to a general lack of knowledge of what a high-risk pregnancy is like. Ironically, several years after she made this comment she was pregnant with twins and delivered them early. I ran into her when her boys were about five months old and she apologized for any insensitive comments she ever made about what it was like to have multiples as she had no idea until she had her own.

Unfortunately, I am not alone in having an experience of dealing with unwanted and even rude comments as almost every woman I talked to could recall at least one time when either a friend, family members, or stranger said something insensitive and hurtful. Insensitive and negative comments are so common, that numerous blog posts have been written and shared detailing what people should not say to a preemie mom. A popular post on the Preemie101 website, a site dedicated to providing parents information about raising preemies from birth into childhood, details a list of things not to say to a parent while his or her child is in the NICU including things like, well at least you can get some sleep at night, or asking if he or she going to be normal. Based on the number of comments and times the article was shared on social media, it is clear that the article struck a chord with preemie parents. Upsetting remarks are so common, that Inspire, an online support community for preemie parents published a report in 2011 entitled Insensitive Comments and Their Impact on Preemie Mothers. The organization surveyed 630 preemie mothers about their conversations with others about their preterm birth or the premature child. Over half of the respondents reported that insensitive comments made by friends, family members, or strangers caused them additional stress. The comments made by people women knew caused the most stress and in some cases comments lead to the end of a relationship a fact that is troubling as women need a strong social support network to deal with the emotional and physical stress of caring for a preemie.

The most bothersome comments to women were those that implied directly or indirectly that she had done something to cause the premature birth such as directly asking what she did wrong or more indirectly asking questions about her prenatal care and activity levels while pregnant. The Inspire report explains that the common belief that premature birth is due to the behavior of the mother is an indication of the misinformation and misunderstanding there is in the general public about premature birth and its causes. One of the reasons that comments like these may be particularly hurtful to women is that so many preemie moms already harbor feelings of guilt and blame themselves for their premature delivery. When someone suggests that she is potentially at fault for going into early labor, it reconfirms her beliefs in her own culpability. It is natural for people to want to know the reason for the early delivery, and most women did not mind sharing this information. The problem arose when the questions were asked in an accusatory or offensive manner Women did not appreciate being asked if they had done anything wrong to cause their early labor. Stephanie, whose son David was born at 29 weeks, had the terrible experience of being in a store when a stranger came over and inquired about David's age. After Stephanie explained why he was so small, the woman point blank asked her if she had done drugs, because that was the only reason she knew of for babies being born so early. Needless to say, Stephanie was speechless and had to just turn and walk away rather than get into altercation in the middle of the store.

The most commonly reported types of comments were those that implied that a preemie mother was in some way lucky because her pregnancy ended early and she was able to avoid some of the discomforts associated with pregnancy. Nicole, whose twin sons were born at 24 weeks and 6 days when doctors could not stop her premature labor, shared some of the bothersome things that strangers have said to her. Because her sons are identical twins a lot of people will come up and ask her questions about her pregnancy and their birth as Nicole has noticed that people tend to be particularly fascinated with twins. After learning how early they were born, she has had people actually ask her in front of the boys if they are ok mentally which she finds highly offensive. One time she was talking to a woman who told her how lucky she was that the boys came so early because she did not have any post-pregnancy "pudge." Nicole could hardly believe that someone would ever think someone was lucky to have micropreemies who might not have survived and she simply stood up and walked away, as she did not trust herself to not either start crying or yelling. Nicole knew that this women was not thinking when she said this, but at the same time all she could think of was everything she missed out on as a new mother and how much her boys had gone through. She would have gladly gained and kept on pounds of baby weight if it had meant that her sons would have been born full term and healthy.

In a similar vein, women also resented comments that implied that she was somehow fortunate to have her baby or babies in the NICU rather than being at home with a newborn. Julie's triplet sons were born just after 26 weeks and spent three months in the hospital dealing with a series of medical issues. Julie spent almost 12 hours a day at the NICU and when she was home she was up throughout the night pumping to provide her sons with breast milk. She was exhausted and constantly worried about her sons and their progress and could not believe it when a friend told her that she was pretty lucky because having them in the NICU was sort of like having a built-in babysitter for three months. Her friends comment implied that she was able to do what she pleased and go out whenever she wanted without having to worry about who would be taking care of her sons, when in reality, Julie's life was anything but care or stress free. Kellie, whose son was born at 25 weeks had a friend tell her that even though it must be very hard to have her son in the hospital, at least she would be well rested when he was discharged. For a mother who was spending 15 hours a day at the hospital and waking up every three hours during the night to pump breast milk for her son, she was more exhausted than she had ever been. For her, there was nothing restful about having a preemie.

Another category of comments that 40 percent of the women reported as bothersome were those that implied that parents were being too overprotective or going too far in their efforts to protect the health of their children. Again, there seems to be a general lack of knowledge among the general public about the complications that arise from prematurity. The report explains that there is a "consistent myth that once the baby is discharged from the NICU that everything is suddenly "OK" (Inspire, Support, and

Special 2011). Infants born even three to four weeks early still have a weaker immune system than full-term babies and any breathing or lung issues makes them more susceptible to respiratory infections. Mothers felt ridiculed when people made comments about their refusal to send their toddler to daycare or preschool or continued to insist that visitors use hand sanitizer before they were allowed to touch the baby. One woman I talked with, Haley, talked about how her mother-in-law is a pediatrician. Rather than making her more sympathetic to the anxiety her daughter-in-law felt, she approached the situation from a more clinical perspective. Haley was frustrated by what she felt was lack of support,

> I was trying to talk to her about, but she told me the baby was going to be ok. I knew he was going to be going to be okay, this is not what it was going to be about. I felt like people were saying, if your baby is not going to die than you must be ok with it. The experience itself is really awful and the loss and the time and everything. Even pregnancy books and child rearing backs and are all about early bonding is so important and hold them and breastfeeding.

Because her child had lived and no long-term health issues, Haley felt as if she did not have a place to complain and be sad because those around her were so focused on what had gone well for her.

Many women were bothered by comments about their children's size. Women knew their children were smaller than other children their same age, and comments just reminded women that their children had been born too early. Tonia, mother of Presley, a 24-weeker described her frustration with the remarks people would make about her daughter who at 11 months old weighed only 15 pounds. "People have no regard with what they say and do not think at all. They think it is ok to comment on her size. I don't need ten people to tell me she is small." Presley's twin brother did not survive, so in addition to trying to cope with Presley's health issues, Tonia was also grieving for her son. She recalled the most insensitive thing that she remembered someone saying to her. "I had a friend, and I use that term loosely, who came to see me while Presley was still in the NICU. She had a toddler and a baby, and she said to me, 'hey can I have that twin stroller?'" Tonia was so taken aback by the request that she did not even know how to respond, and could not believe that her visitor had the nerve to ask for such a thing. Along the same lines, some people made comments about preemie's appearance. Due to their early birth, many preemies, heads appear to be proportionally larger than is normal and spending a lot of time lying flat while the skull bones are still so soft and malleable can lead to preemie heads being misshapen. One mother recalled a woman in the grocery store asking in a very concerned voice if her son would ever look normal.

Another thing that many preemie moms resented was when other people would try to compare their preemies with full-term babies and children. Once again, women felt that those around them had a hard time understanding that just because their child had lived for a year, did not mean they were developmentally or physically on par with a typical one-year-old. Moncia's son was born at 28 weeks due to her elevated blood pressure. In addition to typical preemie issues, he also got an *E. coli* infection while in the NICU which set him back some more and he was in the NICU for four months. After coming home, he did fairly well, but did have some slight physical delays and was in physical therapy to work on his gross motor skills. Monica's sister had been pregnant at the same time and had her baby was boy 3 weeks before Monica delivered. If Monica had gone full term her nephew would have been almost four months older, but given the circumstances of her son's birth, the boys were close in age. Even though Monica repeatedly tried to explain to her family about what it meant to have an adjusted age and how her son's early health problems contributed to his delays she found that people were constantly comparing the two boys in terms or size and meeting different milestones such as rolling over, sitting up, or walking. This was hard for Monica as her son was behind and even though she knew he should be behind, the constant reminders or what he could not do still bothered her.

Sometimes the comments people made did not fit into a certain category, but were just plain rude and incredibly thoughtless. Yvette, whose twins were born early and continue to have developmental issues spoke at length about how the average person just does not understand what it is like to have and raise a preemie. She talked about some of the things people have said to her,

> You get the most insensitive comments. A woman told me should me would rather have a miscarriage than have a kid with a lot of medical issues. She knows my history and this the comment that came out of her mouth and I just looked at her. I said I don't think a woman gets pregnant and wants a kids with special needs. You can see they do not get it. I want to say to them, go to the grocery stores and buy a pound of ground beef. Get 5 sticks of butter and that is how much my daughter weighed.

Another mother with twins told me that a woman in a grocery stores once stopped her and told her that she would shoot herself if she ever found out she was having twins.

Heather, mother of two premature children had a similar conversation that still bothers her. She was talking to a woman she did not know about her children and this woman mentioned that she had a friend who had a daughter born very early. She then went on to say that her friend was pregnant again and she could not believe that this woman would put a child at risk again to be born early and that she thought it was terrible what her friend was doing. Heather was so angry that she wanted to scream at the woman, but instead she calmly told her that many women who have preemies go on to have more children and have perfectly healthy pregnancies, and many other women have preemies and also have complications with their second pregnancies, but there is no reason that once a woman gives birth early that she should no longer be allowed to have children.

Forever Changed

Many NICU moms will tell you that experience of having a child in the NICU will forever change you and forever change your perspective on the world and life. Sometimes that change can be negative as it can lead to sadness and ongoing anxiety, but so many women I have met have told me about the positive changes their pregnancies and their children's prematurity brought to their lives. Over and over women talked about how their experiences taught them to have a greater appreciation for the value of life and the small moments and milestones. After coming close to losing a child, or seeing other children pass away in the NICU, and in some cases even losing a child, preemie parents know all too well how fragile life actually is and how miraculous it is to have a healthy full-term baby. After a parent has celebrated that his or her child has gained an ounce or is able to breathe room air, they often expressed having a deeper appreciation for all of the little milestones that had their child not been born early, they could have easily overlooked or taken for granted. Callista whose twin daughter Maddi passed away in the NICU after living for a week talked about how much she has grown and learned from both losing her daughter and raising her surviving twin, Cami. She has been given a deeper appreciation for the importance of the small things in life as well as a deeper bond with both her husband and her daughter.

Stephanie, the mother who started a foundation after one of her twin sons had NEC and almost died, talked about how her experiences after her sons were born taught her to be grateful even when circumstances were difficult. She told me, "prematurity has taught me that there is always someone worse off than you. We got that perspective when the woman who was next to us in the NICU lost her baby. Our son had NEC, but he survived. We are better off than the woman next to us. No matter how bad my day is there always someone who is worse off than me." Many people might look at Stephanie and what she and her husband went through, premature twins, emergency surgery, having their twins stay in NICUs at two different hospitals, and think that they have it pretty bad, but Stephanie says that when she saw the worst in the NICU it made her own problems seem so much smaller. Her experiences with prematurity also spurred her and her husband to start the foundation to raise awareness of NEC and to provide support for families going through similar situations. Prematurity has pushed her to get more involved and to become an advocate to raise awareness of NEC and money for research, something she would have never even thought to do had her sons not been born early.

Yvette had this to say about how the entire experience of her pregnancy and her twins' time in the NICU impacted her.

> It forever alters you. You see your children through a different lens. You talk differently. When you get together with moms with children who have delays you hear things like, those are some great gross motor skills. In a lot of good ways you see life through a different lens. When you do find another preemie mom it is like there is another mom who understands me and understands my story. You have walked in those shoes. It is not that other people lack the ability to have empathy, but to actually walk in those shoes is different.

Even though much of her twins' pregnancy and life has been difficult and full of challenges, Yvette recognizes that all obstacles and hurdles have given her a deeper understanding about life and what truly matters. Her experiences also allowed her to connect on a deeper level with fellow preemie moms who understood each in a way that other moms without a similar experience could not.

Like Yvette, Kari also talked about how losing her triplets and then giving birth to her twins being and then her singleton early completely changed the way she and her husband approached life and the way they parented as well as her career path. Kari who is a nurse switched her area of specialty to neonatal nursing after her triplets were born. Having been through life and loss in the NICU, she feels that she has greater compassion and understanding for the parents she works with. On a personal level, one of the biggest ways she and her husband were changed was in giving them perspective about what was really important. The day we met for me to interview her, her three kids all had strep and she had just come from taking them to the doctor. Rather than being stressed or upset about it Kari told me that it is just a part of life and she would much rather be the mother of three kids who get sick than to not be a parent at all. She explained,

> I get to go through you know the bumps and the stitches and the strep throat. And you know I get to go through that. But that's all I have to do. You know, I'm not hanging tube feeds every night, and not having to have a visiting nurse come every night to relive me from my child that has a trachea. And, you know those kinds of things. I think it has changed me a lot being a nurse and a lot being a mom.

She has also found that her experiences strengthened her relationship with her husband. While many marriages face a lot of strain and sometimes even fail when presented with a stressor like a premature infant, in Kari's case she and her husband do not let too many things bother them. At the end of the day common things that couples argue about such as money, sex, or division of labor around the house are minor to them as they have literally faced life and death together as a couple and that has made them stronger.

Samantha's experience with both loss and the NICU also gave her a greater appreciation for the smaller things in life. During her first pregnancy with her son Landon, her water unexpectedly broke when she was 16-and-half weeks pregnant. Because it was so early the doctors said there was little they could do and because there was so little amniotic fluid left in Landon's sac they said he would soon pass so they recommended that they induce labor. She and her husband opted against this believing that if her body had not gone into labor yet there was still a chance. She went home on strict bed rest and after a week they learned that her fluid had tripled and they thought that possibly the amniotic sac had resealed. They went home feeling hopeful until the next day when she started to have fast and painful contractions. By the time they got to the hospital her son had passed. She went ahead and delivered her son vaginally that day and went home from the hospital that night. She was understandably heartbroken, but is thankful at how well the hospital where she delivered handled things. They let her hold her son and they took pictures which they placed in a memory box along with his birth certificate and footprints.

A few months later Samantha learned that she was pregnant again, but this time it was with twins. She was obviously concerned given the outcome of her first pregnancy, so she was closely monitored by a high-risk doctor and got weekly progesterone shots with the hope that this would help to strengthen her cervix. She carried her girls to almost 26 weeks, but even though they were very early and had to endure very long NICU stays with a lot of complications, both of her girls survived. Samantha says that ever since losing her son, she takes nothing for granted. When she sees her daughters walking and hears them talking she knows that it is somewhat miraculous that her daughters are here and doing so well. She knows what can go wrong, and because of that she feels that she has a greater appreciation than most people for the things that go right. She told me, "people who have these perfect amazing pregnancies with no complications have no idea how lucky they are." When one of her twins hits a milestone or has a good checkup she and her husband truly celebrate because they know that there was a very real chance that these accomplishments might not have happened.

For Nicole, the experience for having her twin sons in the NICU taught her some important lessons about patience and letting go. She told me, "before

I was pregnant before this happened I was very much a type-A control freak. After I went through this and spent a lot of time in a hospital bed learned I am in a control of nothing. I am a recovering control freak." As much as she wanted to speed up the time her boys were in the hospital and wanted to ensure that they met all of their milestones, the reality was that there was very little she could do so she learned to focus on the things that she could do such as providing breast milk while they were in the NICU or doing their therapy exercises when they were home. For the things that she could not control she had to simply relax and not spend too much of her mental energy getting upset about it because it was just a waste of her time.

Monica also learned some important lessons about patience when her son was born at 28 weeks. She had heard from others that babies were usually released around their due date, but her son's due date came and passed and he was still there and still having issues with his breathing and eating. This made her incredibly anxious and frustrated because in her mind he had been there long enough and once his due date came he was supposed to be home. She eventually had to accept that her son would do things on his time and being impatient was not going to get him home any faster. Deanne told a similar story to Monica. She talked about the lessons she learned from her daughter Kendra's time in the NICU. "Up until I had my daughter, I was very impatient and when she was born I was force fed patience. You can't worry about what tomorrow is going to bring. You just have to wait and see, what is and what is. That was really hard to let go of that. Now I am probably one of the patient people I know."

Sometimes women are forever changed by the preemie experience because even though they were able to bring their child home from the NICU, the ongoing health issues were so severe that their child passed away after coming home. Again this points to the very real fact that the preemie journey does not end when a baby gets to come home from the hospital. I spoke with Kiera after I had already been reading her blog for several months. The mother of triplet daughters born at 25 weeks, I found Kiera's story when I was Googling for triplet stories and was immediately captivated by her story which was both inspiring and heartbreaking. While all of Kiera's daughters struggled as they were born so early, her daughter Zoe, who was actually the largest at birth weighing 1 pound 10 ounces struggled the most. Due to serious respiratory and feeding issues, Zoe spent 291 days in the NICU and was almost ten months old when she was finally discharged and able to come to join her sisters. She came home on oxygen and a feeding tube and needed home nursing care, and she also had moderate to severe hearing loss due to some of the treatments she received to save her life when she was born. Thrilled to have her home with her sisters, Kiera and her husband took on the daily challenges of caring for three infants with various medical needs.

Everything was going extremely well until Zoe caught a cold when she was fourteen-months-old. Kiera took Zoe to the doctor to check for an infection and her pediatrician sent them to the ER when he detected an elevated heart rate. At the ER she underwent several tests, but X-rays showed her lungs were clear so we she was discharged. After a few days of increased coughing, a high heart rate, and the inability to tolerate any feeds, they took Zoe back to the ER where she was diagnosed with the flu and pneumonia and was admitted to the hospital for IV fluids and after two days when her oxygen needs stabilized she was again sent home. Just two days later after giving her round the clock breathing treatments and upping her supplemental oxygen levels it became evident to Kiera and her husband that Zoe had taken a turn for the worse and took her back to the hospital. X-rays revealed that her pneumonia had gotten much worse and her lungs were barely functioning. Zoe had to be placed on a ventilator and was given medication to partially sedate her both to try and lower her heart rate which was hovering around 200 beats per minute and to keep her from fighting the ventilator. Zoe's stats continued to worsen and when her heart stopped beating and team of doctors and nurses had to perform manual CPR to resuscitate her. When she crashed again, the team asked Kiera and her husband if they wanted them to try to save her again or if they wanted to just hold her and let her go. Not wanting Zoe to be in any more pain, they opted to let her go and Kiera held her as she took her last breath. Needless to say their family was devastated and could not believe that their little girl had fought so hard and had overcome so much and was now gone.

Donna was another mother who lost her son after he had come home from the hospital. Donna's first pregnancy was with twin boys Joey and Danny who were born at 30 weeks and 5 days after her water broke and doctors could not stop her labor. Up until that point her pregnancy had been going perfectly smoothly, so Donna was in shock and completely unprepared to deliver her sons so early. In addition to being born more than 9 weeks early, her son Danny was born with a rare syndrome that caused several genetic anomalies including the lack of an anus to eliminate waste, and a malformed esophagus. When he was just ten hours old he was transferred to the local Children's Hospital so he could have a surgery to have an ileostomy placed. He spent the next five months in the NICU where doctors worked on getting him to grow and he also had several other surgeries in attempts to repair some of his other physical abnormalities. He never was able to eat by mouth as he aspirated any liquid he tried to ingest and he came home on IV medications and fluids, a 24-hour feeding pump and still had his ileostomy. Donna worried about his future and wondered if he would ever be able to eat on his own, but focused each day on taking care of her twins and keeping them healthy and growing.

When he was seven months old, two months after he had come home from the hospital, Donna's husband was on his way home from a business trip. He called from the airport and she asked him to stop at the pharmacy on the way home to deal with a problem with a prescription. She went to change Daniel's IV and noticed that he was choking on his saliva. This was a common occurrence, but this time he was not recovering. She quickly called 911. When the ambulance got there, the paramedics rushed in and neighbors came out to see what has happening. Donna yelled to a neighbor to call her husband and warn him so that he knew what he was coming home to. When her husband did get home he was there just in time to see his son being transported to the helicopter ambulance which arrived to transport Daniel to the hospital more quickly and Donna and her husband were actually allowed to ride in the helicopter with him. Despite the best efforts of the paramedics on the scene and in the air, they were unable to revive him, and he passed away that day. They knew their son had major medical issues that he would be dealing with for his entire life, but they never imagined they would lose him when he was so young.

Tracey and her husband also lost their son after he came home from the hospital. When Tracey was in her early 30s, she had a surgery to remove some uterine fibroids which sent her into early menopause. Because of this she and her husband sought treatment with a fertility specialist. At her first ultrasound after a successful treatment the ultrasound showed two tiny beating hearts and she and her husband were excited to be expecting twins. When she went for a follow-up ultrasound they found that the third baby had been hiding behind one of his siblings. Tracey said they came around to the idea of having triplets pretty quickly, excited that she was pregnant and they would instantly have a large family. Her pregnancy was progressing well until 21 weeks when her cervix started to funnel so she went in for an emergency cerclage which triggered contractions. The doctors determined that the cerclage was irritating her cervix so at 24 weeks they removed the cerclage and told her she would be in the hospital for the remainder of her pregnancy. In addition to having contractions, monitoring showed that baby A, who was their son Conner, had a heart rate that was repeatedly decelerating. At 25 weeks and 6 days, Conner's heart rate dropped into the 30s and was not recovering. Doctors told them they could either continue with the pregnancy and baby A would pass away, or they could deliver and hope for the best. Tracey and her husband chose to deliver, as they wanted to give all of their children the chance to survive. The triplets did survive and all came home from the hospital after long NICU stays.

Her daughter Cheyenne was the biggest at birth and came home on oxygen and has some vision issues, but otherwise did very well. Her son Caden spent the longest time on the ventilator of the three and also came home on supplemental oxygen. Conner who had the most health issues came home on oxygen, had a G-tube, and needed frequent suctioning due to his respiratory issues. At one point there had been concern that Conner would never be able to come home as his oxygen needs were so high and they had talked about the possibility of him being transferred to a long-term care facility, so Tracey and her husband were beyond excited when he was well enough to come home. He had a shunt placed in his skull to help drain some of the fluid off of his brain while he was in the NICU, and when he was home the shunt malfunctioned and he had to be life-flighted to the hospital in Omaha where his shunt was repaired. When he was eleven months old he was having seizures and he had a bad reaction to the valium they gave him at the hospital to sedate him and he coded and had to be revived. While he was in the hospital recovering he caught pneumonia and when he was eleven months and seven days old during a breathing treatment a mucus plug got trapped in his airway and he choked and passed away. Tracey commented that after all he had been through and all he had survived, it seemed so crazy that it was something as common as pneumonia that took his life.

REACHING OUT

Throughout this book, a common thread to women's stories was the feeling of being alone and isolated and feeling like they were one of the only people in the world who had gone through what they had gone through. These feeling prompted many women to reach out to other preemie moms to offer support and to share their stories. Josie struggled with PTSD after her daughter Elin was born at 31 weeks. One of the ways she found healing was by volunteering with her local March of Dimes chapter and helping to put together and deliver care packages for NICU families. Another thing she has been working on is helping parents to get to the hospital to visit as easily as possible. Josie is from a large city with a lot of traffic. There is a toll road she could have taken that would have drastically reduced her drive time to the hospital, but over time the toll road became very expensive and she had to stop using this route. Knowing that many other parents were in similar situations, she applied for a grant to pay for NICU parents, use of the toll road. It is often those little things that can make a huge difference for NICU families as it gives them one less thing to worry and think about. When her daughter was in the NICU there was a large bulletin board over the sink where parents had to scrub in. It was covered with Christmas cards and pictures of NICU graduates. She would look at the pictures of the smiling and happy babies, but she had a hard time imagining that they would ever get to that point. In her work as a volunteer she wants to share her story with parents and let them know that it does get better with time that most of the time they will too have a smiling happy baby at home with them.

Heather also took the sadness, trauma, and fear of her two high-risk pregnancies and early deliveries and used it to reach out and help others. In addition to getting involved with the local chapter of the March Dimes because of the encouragement of a friend, she also started a local support group for parents of preemies. One of the things that is unique about her group is that it is not just for parents who currently have children in the NICU, but also for parents who are raising preemies and coping with the day to day challenges that so often come along with this. Not only has she made some wonderful friends through the group, but being able to support and encourage other mothers and families has helped her to make sense of her experiences and to find something positive out of the negative.

For Leslie whose twins Kadri and Xander were born at 25 weeks, getting involved with the March of Dimes was an important way that she was able to reach out and also start to heal from that trauma of their birth and their long months in the NICU. She is very passionate about sharing her story, providing education about premature birth, and providing support to other preemie parents and families. Through her volunteer work with the March of Dimes she is able to go into the NICU where her twins were and talk to some of the parents there and offer encouragement. She was also asked join the research and training committee at the hospital to provide a parent's perspective on safety in the NICU. This gave her away to go back to the hospital and into the NICU which held so many negative memories and start to make more positive ones. As she works to improve the quality of care and the quality of life for NICU patients and their parents she feels a deeper sense of purpose and helps her to feel as if she was able to take the many challenges her family faced and create good out of them. In addition to her formal volunteer work, Leslie is also committed to actively trying to share her story and get it out there. When she started to go into labor prior to 24 weeks and when her twins were in the NICU she struggled to know what to expect and to understand her experiences because she had never encountered a story like hers. Her hope is that if another mother goes through the same thing, they will at least have the knowledge and comfort that there have been others who have walked the same path.

Kiera was another mom who took her incredibly difficult and trying circumstances and tried to create something good out of them. After her triplet daughter Zoe passed away from complications directly related to her prematurity she and her husband created the Zoe Rose Memorial Foundation in her honor. The mission statement of the foundation is to "provide emotional support, educational resources, and awareness focused events, which inspire hope in parents of preemies while in the NICU, post discharge and for those who have suffered a pregnancy or infant loss." Kiera recognized that many other preemie parents feel alone, scared, and uneducated when it comes to all aspects of having and raising a premature infant or infants and her hope is that the foundation can fill in some of the gaps for parents and be a source of support that she and her husband did not have. Creating the foundation was an important way for her and her husband to memorialize Zoe and ensure that the joy that their daughter brought them and her sisters was spread to others. The foundation was also an important way for Kiera to heal as the work and reaching out to others gave her a sense of purpose and allowed her to remember and talk about Zoe with others.

Like Kiera, Kellie's experience with prematurity inspired her to start an organization to help other preemie parents and families. After her first son was born unexpectedly at 24 weeks, Kellie and her husband decided to have another child, and two years later their daughter was born at 34 weeks because of a rare blood disorder and also had to spend the first weeks of her life in the NICU. In some ways around the second time around was even more difficult, even though her daughter was so much older and bigger than her son had been, it brought back so many terrible memories. Kellie was desperate to find some support from other women with similar experiences, but as much as she went on-line and searched, she really could not find what she was looking for. Even once both of her children were home from the NICU she continued to struggle as she spent her days dealing with insurance companies, managing her children's multiple therapy appointments, and researching different treatment options. Again, she felt alone as she knew no one else who was dealing with similar issues. When her younger daughter went to kindergarten she was emotionally and mentally ready and now had the time to start doing something to help others. After informally polling other preemie parents about what the types of information and support they wished they had she conceived the idea for what is now Hand to Hold. Hand to Hold is a non-profit foundation whose mission is to, "enable a network of families to offer support, comfort and understanding to one another, and to provide them with knowledge, information and resources to reduce the impact of prematurity and ensure the best outcome for their children and family."

The organization started out small and the primary purpose was for it to be a peer-to-peer support network where parents could easily connect with other parents who were further down the road of the preemie journey to get information and support. The organization took about three years to get off the ground and running and now has a variety of support services including support groups in Texas NICUs where the organization is based, a website with resources for parents, families, and medical personnel, a blog featuring posts by preemie parents, a Facebook support group, and a parent mentor program where parents can request a parent mentor and be pair up with a mentor who they can communicate with privately. One of the important components of the support is that it exists for all stages of the preemie process including pregnancy, the NICU, life after NICU. Kellie was amazed at how quickly the organization grew as the blog and website got more and more views and followers and more and more people commented on the Facebook page. The growth of the organization is simply proof to Kelli of how much this type of resources and support is needed and she continues to work daily to get parents the support and information and support they need so that they are not alone in coping with their experiences and navigating the often difficult world of parenting a preemie.

One way that some NICU parents I met have reached out is to share their story with others. Some did this in a formal way by becoming a parent mentor either through their NICU, in a local mom's group for preemies or multiples, or through a national organization such as Graham's Foundation or Hand to Hold. Others reached out to others more informally by talking with friends and family and friends or friends and family or commenting on online forums. Monica's son was born at 28 weeks due to her consistently high blood pressure. When she had her son she did not know anyone else who had ever had a preemie or a baby in the NICU and she felt incredibly alone as no one could share stories with her or understood what it was like to have a two pound baby. Now whenever she learns of someone in her town who has a preemie or of someone's friend or family member she makes a point to reach out to them and send an email or call them just so they can know that there is someone out there who has had a similar experience and they have someone who can answer questions or even just listen to what a fellow mom is going through without passing judgment.

In both large and small ways, the women and families who have been impacted by prematurity found ways to help others and to create good out of what were oftentimes extremely hard and painful experiences. No matter how a woman reacts to her high-risk pregnancy or premature birth experience she is rarely the same person when it is over, whether it changes her perspective, the way she parents, how she looks at her child, or even just her awareness of pregnancy complications. It was a desire to share with others how they were changed that motivated many of the women who agreed to speak with me. They wanted the public to understand how their experiences changed them in both positive and negative ways and also to recognize that the impacts of high-risk pregnancy and premature birth are often ongoing. By educating others, their hope was that people would be a little more sympathetic to others in similar situations and be better able to provide the emotional, relational, and tangible support they need.

Chapter 11

The Emotional Journey

Jana, mother of twins born at 32 weeks, talked about how unprepared she was for the emotional strain of having a high-risk pregnancy. Prior to her pregnancy she had not heard too many stories that focused on the different complications women could experience or of babies born too early. She knew that it could happen and she knew what an NICU was, but she had never considered what it was like for a woman who went into early labor or what it would be like to spend your first weeks of motherhood in the NICU. Jana actually never thought she herself would be pregnant. Jana has Crone's Disease and autoimmune disease that attacks the digestive system. As a result of several surgeries and the removal of parts of her intestines she had a lot of internal scarring and doctors had told her she would be unable to get pregnant. She and her husband were completely shocked then when not only did she have a positive pregnancy test, but was pregnant with twins. At this point she started to seek out more information and look for stories of women like her. She described the stories she read, "I heard that you are on bed rest. That was one of the stories for me. You hear about the typical exhaustion you are going to experience when you are pregnant and you kind of get a feel for that in your first trimester." She then went on to describe what was not included in these stories, "No one really tells you about the mental exhaustion. I was not prepared for at 20 weeks my brain to stop working. Really I could just sit on the couch for seven hours and just stare and I was fine to just stare." Not only were the days long and repetitive, but she lived in a state of almost constant fear and no one had warned her about this. She described the fear, "All of your concerns are magnified because you're just sitting there and I remember the narrative of, sort of the one day in equals one day out. You sit there and try to focus on keeping them in just day by day and hour by hour, and in doing so, you have nothing else to focus on, every pain is magnified, every contraction, you just sort of live in this one ball of anxiety." The stories Jana read prepared her somewhat for the physical challenges of a twin pregnancy, but not for the emotional and mental strain.

It is not surprising or earth shattering to learn that having a high-risk pregnancy or a premature baby is an intensely emotional experience. While the emotions tend toward the negative side of the emotional spectrum, many preemie parents also experienced intense positive emotions in response to their children's progress. Anytime one's health or the health of one's child is in jeopardy, it is a basic human response to feel fear and sadness. What was interesting as I spoke with mothers and experienced my own premature delivery was the range of emotions I and these other women felt. Not only was there a high level of anxiety but also that of anger, envy, grief, and a deep sense of isolation. It was also interesting to me how willing women were to talk about the negative emotions they experienced. Many told me that it felt good to talk so openly about their struggles as they felt that people they knew who had not experienced a high-risk pregnancy or early delivery were not as comfortable in discussing the full range of emotions that accompanied a high-risk pregnancy. Also, because they had rarely heard or read these types of stories, they felt unprepared for the emotional roller coaster they experienced. Because their emotions did not match the stories they heard there were also several moments when women wondered if something was seriously wrong with them, because their emotions did not feel as if they were in the realm of normal based on what they had heard. This also led some women to keep quiet about some of their more negative and intense emotions as they did not want others to judge them.

When I asked women what they wished they had known prior to their pregnancies and births, many told me that they wish someone had told them just how difficult the emotional ups and downs would be. Women also wished they had known that their feelings were typical for a preemie mom and they were not the first mom in the world to have a complete breakdown, to fear calling the hospital for an update, or to dread going to spend another long day in the NICU. They also wish they had known that sometimes they would not want to be in the NICU, or that it might be difficult to feel connected to a baby that you are not allowed to hold. Even though women acknowledged that knowing about the emotions ahead of time would not have changed the emotions they felt, it would have at least given the reassurance that the emotions they were feeling were okay and normal for the situations they were in.

Along the same lines, when I asked women what they wished others knew about what it was like to have a high-risk pregnancy or a preemie, the most common answer was that they wanted other people to know how emotionally difficult it is for mothers. Over and over women said they felt those around them did not understand what they were going through and because of their inability to experience true empathy, they were unable to provide the social support the women needed. Many women hoped that by sharing their stories they would not only help other women, but also educate those who know and support these women so that they were better equipped to respond to and help women through these difficult times.

Anxiety

The most commonly mentioned emotion was anxiety which women also referred to as fear and worry. Like Jana, many mothers echoed the idea that they almost were consumed by the constant anxiety they felt from the time they were diagnosed with a high-risk pregnancy until delivery and then if their babies were born early for weeks, months, and sometimes even years. Women felt as if the outcomes of their pregnancies were out of their control, and they constantly worried about the health and lives of their unborn children. This anxiety was so different than the emotions women routinely heard described in pregnancy stories such as joy, excitement, and anticipation. Many women do experience some level of anxiety while pregnant, even if it is not a high-risk pregnancy, as they worry about the health of their unborn child, have concerns about the delivery, and frequently have worries about their ability to parent the new child. However, the level of anxiety experienced by women during a high-risk pregnancy, in the NICU, and while raising a preemie is at an entirely different level and often consumed women to the point that they had a difficult time coping. This anxiety was the type that never went away and ruled every thought and action women took. Women often wished they had been exposed to others who had the same emotions both to prepare them as well as to provide reassurance that emotions women were experiencing were within normal range and were justified and acceptable.

For Amy, mother of twins, her anxiety and fear came from the unknowns about being pregnant with multiples. Her first pregnancy with her son had been a typical pregnancy and she felt as if she experienced all of the typical things she read about and heard about. When it came to her pregnancy with her twins, she was struck by how little she knew, and how difficult it was to find information that would help her understand her situation which led to constant feelings of anxiety. She explained,

> I just wish I would have stopped working sooner and would have relaxed and taken it easy. . .It was stressful not knowing. For me during my pregnancy, I was constantly like, how is this supposed to go? Like constantly thinking about, you know, what, what's going to happen. You know, just the unknown was very stressful. You know, with the regular pregnancy I had experienced it before, but with a regular pregnancy, like my first pregnancy. You are all caught up in the

> excitement of having a baby. You know, it is fantastic. You read the books on like step by step what to expect. . .You know, after I got through my couple of months of sickness with my son it was like great you know. You do the whole baby showers, you get the nursery ready. So, when you become pregnant with your second, it was sort of like old hat. But then when you find out you are having multiples, you're just like, you know, what's supposed to happen? What is? You know, and I read the books and you try to find out as much information, but you are still like, the unknown is out there.

She went on to talk about how she wished it had been easier to access stories like her own. She found the experience of carrying twins so vastly different both emotionally and physically than carrying her singleton, and wished more stories had been readily available to help her deal with these differences.

Laura was another mother whose first pregnancy had been a typical pregnancy with no medical complications. When she learned she was pregnant with twin girls during her second pregnancy and that the twins shared just one placenta, she felt as if her first pregnancy had not really prepared her for what this high-risk pregnancy would be like. I met with Laura over lunch one day when her older son was five and her twin daughters were twenty months old. She explained that the fear started the minute she found out it was twins. She told me,

> And when they found out I was having twins they gave me what seemed like a novel about having a healthy pregnancy. And I basically read it all that whole weekend, and I was like scared half to death. You know it scared me because, like with my first pregnancy I was freaked out about every little thing. And then, I was like with this second pregnancy, I am going to enjoy it. I am going to lay down and relax. And then of course, I find out I am having twins. And then, you learned about all the ways you can die, all the ways the baby can die. So it was like I can do what I can do. And I was just trying to take care of myself as best I could.

Laura was closely monitored throughout her pregnancy and was incredibly fortunate that she carried her girls for 38 weeks and brought them home from the hospital with her. Even though she had a successful outcome and is not a preemie mom, there was no way of predicting the future during her pregnancy, so her anxiety over what could happen was still a constant presence and drastically altered the way she experienced her pregnancy. She eventually was able to adopt a healthy mantra to help cope with the anxiety of her pregnancy. Whenever she started to feel anxious she would repeat to herself, "I can do what I can do." The mantra did not make the fear disappear, but it did serve as a reminder that some circumstances were out of her control and her role was to take care of herself and follow her physician's orders and otherwise she just had to hope for the best.

One possible contributor to the high level of anxiety women experienced beyond the fact that very real risks were involved, was the fact that many women were placed on some form of bed rest during the pregnancy and once a baby was born prematurely, women spent many long days sitting in the NICU. This gave them a lot of time to think and consider all of the potentially negative possibilities as they had limited ways to distract themselves from their own anxious thoughts. Women who were on bed rest also had more time to get on the internet and seek out information, statistics, and stories which contributed to increased amounts of stress as they were able to find every possible thing that could go wrong. Women in the NICU were also privy to the stories of the babies and families around them, giving them additional complications and conditions to worry about.

The anxiety women felt did not always abate after their children were born or when they came home from the NICU. Karen, mother of twin boys, would be considered a success story by most. She delivered her twins at 35 weeks and each weighed over 5 pounds and did not have to spend any time in the NICU. The anxiety she felt during her pregnancy that something could go wrong just intensified though when she left the hospital three days after her sons were born. She remembers feeling overwhelmed as she left the hospital with the tiny babies in her hands. She was constantly worried that one of them would get sick or suddenly stop breathing. Not only was she worried about their health, but she also felt overwhelmed with the task of raising two babies at once. When I met her, her boys were four, and she admitted that she still went into their bedroom every night after they were asleep to check and make sure they were still breathing. After watching their children deal with medical issues on a daily basis, it was difficult for many women to turn off the constant worry that something could be wrong.

Guilt

After fear and anxiety, the most commonly mentioned emotion was guilt. Women referred to feeling guilty about the health conditions of their infants and/or guilt over not being able to carry their infants longer. Guilt requires a sense of responsibility for what occurred and a belief that one has done something wrong or harmed another. Even if women rationally knew that it was not their fault, they still blamed themselves for the outcomes of their pregnancies and the struggles and pain their children sometimes endured. In trying to find a reason for their early delivery a lot of women spent a lot of time going over their pregnancies and regretted actions they had or had not taken which they believed contributed to their early deliveries. Many women had goals of reaching a certain gestation based on what their physicians had told them and what they read. When they failed to reach that gestation, or when they saw their children struggling to perform basic bodily functions like breathing or eating, they often struggled with feelings of guilt and failure. Even in situations where others repeatedly assured them that there was no one to blame, they still harbored feelings of guilt over what they saw as their failure to have a positive outcome.

Much like the anxiety that women continued to feel, even after their children were older and healthy, feelings of guilt often continued years after their children were born. Tonia described the guilt she carried with her after her twins were born at 24 weeks and only her daughter Presley survived. Although she has come to accept what happened and takes comfort in the fact that Presley has few lingering issues due to her prematurity, she still was unable to let go of the guilt. "The only regret I have obviously is not being able to take care of them and keep them safe." Tonia blamed herself that her twins were born so early that her son could not survive. Even though Presley did survive, Tonia felt guilt over all that her tiny little baby had to endure. "I do carry guilt. For many, many months, every time I looked at her I had a tremendous sense of guilt. She had to have surgery in her right eye before she left. She will probably have glasses when she is older." Tonia could not help but think that had she been able to carry her twins longer, even just a few more weeks things would have been completely different.

Ashley is another woman that blamed herself for her twins' early delivery, and because of that she carried a tremendous amount of guilt with her. After struggling to conceive, Ashely and her husband had used IVF to get pregnant. Their first cycles had all been unsuccessful so she and her husband had decided that this would be the last time they would try because it was so draining both financially and emotionally. Based on her blood and hormone levels, her doctor had recommended that they wait a cycle and freeze the existing embryos, but Ashley and her husband opted to go ahead with the transfer because they were emotionally at the end of their rope. Much to their surprise, the transfer was not only successful, but they were pregnant with twins. She told me, "since we did IVF I blame myself a lot. I still blame myself a lot. Maybe we should have frozen. I was the one who pushed it. I blamed my body for not being able to get pregnant and not being able to keep them in longer. I had no control. I really felt like, is my husband going to blame me? Normal people do not go through this. What did I do?"

In addition to feeling guilty that they were born early, Ashley also struggled with guilt as she tried to divide her time and attention between her twins in the NICU. Her son James weighed 3 pounds 5 ounces and was much bigger than his sister Quinn who weighed just 2 pound 9 ounces and did much better after birth. Quinn had very low fluid levels in the womb. Without the protective fluids around her she was squeezed in utero which lead to her having clubbed feet and a misshapen skull. During the delivery she inhaled a large amount of blood and had to be put immediately on an oscillator. Her first days were very touch and go and she was so sensitive that even touching her hand was so overstimulating to her that she would go into respiratory distress. Because James was doing better, Ashley was able to participate in his care and do kangaroo care with him very early on, while Quinn had to lie undisturbed in her isolette. She explained, "I always felt so guilty. I would be holding James or doing kangaroo care and here I am holding one and she is stuck in the isolette." Even though there was nothing more that she could be doing for Quinn, she could not let go of the guilt.

For many women, their belief was that as a mother, it was their responsibly to care for and protect their children. When they delivered early and their children were exposed daily to tests, procedures, equipment, and pain, women could not help but feel guilt over the fact that their babies had not entered the world healthy and full term. Maggie described the overwhelming sense of guilt she felt when her triplets were born prior to 30 weeks, "What I wasn't prepared for in addition to all of the stress in the NICU was the onset of PPD (postpartum depression) or what I was calling survivor's guilt. Even though I had all survivors, the guilt that I could breathe and they couldn't without help, that I could eat, but didn't want to because they were having difficulty, the fact that I couldn't hold my one daughter for three weeks and she promptly de-satted [had low oxygen levels] after about 30 seconds of our first encounter, not producing enough breast milk then getting mastitis." Even though most of these circumstances were out of her control such as developing mastitis, an infection of a milk duct, she blamed herself and harbored guilt for her young infants' struggles early on. She felt even worse that she could not provide some of the basic things her children needed such as breast milk and comfort, and in her mind because she could not do these things she had failed as a mother. She still carries this guilt with her, and even though her triplets are doing well now, she still regrets the circumstances of their early birth and subsequent time in the NICU.

Kari had an interesting perspective to share with me about prematurity and guilt. Kari is the NICU nurse who is the mom of triplets who did not survive, and twin daughters and a son who were all born prematurely. When we spoke, nine years had passed since her triplets had passed away, and she still sometimes felt the pangs of guilt over them being born too early to survive. She explained to me,

> But it's normal to have mommy guilt. I mean that's normal. It is. I mean you talk to anybody who has had a preemie and it is normal for you to blame yourself. Like you did something. Or you could have done something different. With the

> triplets I had the emergency cerclage at 21 weeks and then I was on bed rest for a couple of weeks. And by like the second week I was getting antsy and I was only supposed to get up to go to the bathroom. I remember thinking, there's bananas on that counter, so if I went up to the bathroom and I just happened to go through the kitchen and get a banana. And I wasn't doing stairs or anything. And I kept talking myself into doing a little bit more. And one time I think I checked the clothes in the dryer and they weren't dry, so I just restarted the dryer on the way to the bathroom. Then I was convinced it was my fault. It was my fault. I think you want to explain it. You just want a reason why. And there's really not any reason why. And I think that that's just your normal instinct as a mom.

Although the majority of the women needed no prompting to feel guilt when their infants were born early, the stories of others who had better outcomes often sparked increased feelings of guilt. In the earlier discussion of social comparison, it was evident that many women compared themselves and their infants to others. After hearing or reading the stories of other women who had similar complications but who carried their infants for a longer time, some mothers felt guilty. When I asked why those stories sparked pangs guilt some replied that those stories made them feel as if they had could have done more. Had they been mentally stronger of if their bodies had been stronger then they would have been able to carry their infants as long as other women. There seemed to be a prevailing belief among a lot of the women I spoke with that if another woman could carry triplets to 36 weeks, then it was possible for any woman if she tried hard enough to do the same, and if a woman with an incompetent cervix was able to make it full term then again and woman with a similar problem could as well.

When women made comparisons to others and fell short they often assumed that it was something they had done or not done that contributed to their poor performance. Amy, mother of twins born at 34 weeks, described how hearing stories about other mothers of multiples who had carried their twins or triplets closer to full term made her question why her body had such a difficult time carrying her twins.

> I know a mother in town who has triplets who, you know, just carried them to full-term somehow. And there are, they were, you know, I don't know if there's no issues, but I think it was really nice that she was able to do that. And it's like, why couldn't I do that, what did I do wrong? You know, even looking back, I had eating disorders when I was young and I think, oh, did I somehow mess my body up? And there's nothing you can do about it, and I try not to go down that road, but yeah, there's, there's a lot of guilt.

Women also felt guilty about their emotions toward their children, especially if they did not have the rush of maternal feelings they had anticipated.

Bonding with a baby can be a very difficult thing for parents in the NICU as a large part of the bonding process is spending time together, having physical contact, and providing for the baby's needs. Women often assumed that feelings of connection and love were instinctual and when it took longer for those feelings to develop women assumed they were doing something wrong. Carrie, mother of triplets shared how difficult it was to feel a bond with her babies, "I was definitely not prepared for the lack of connection. First, the amount of drugs pumped into me following my C-section was crazy. I was out of it for a while, and then I did not even see them for about 16 to18 hours after the birth. It is also hard when you have to ask permission to hold your own baby or told you can or can't come hold your baby." Carrie knew how she was supposed to feel, and felt guilty that her emotions did not meet expectations. She felt like she was not the mother she should have been. Even though she was there every day for her triplets she felt that she had in some way given them less than what they needed as if they could somehow sense her initial sense of disconnect.

Journalist Jessica Valenti documented her premature birth experience in *The Guardian* after she delivered her daughter Layla at 28 weeks because she developed HELLP syndrome. The birth was traumatic and unexpected and Valenti spent almost all of the next 56 days in the NICU fearing that her daughter who had several medical setbacks would not survive to go home. One of the things that made the experience even more difficult for her was the all-consuming guilt she felt over not feeling bonded to her daughter. She wrote, "The guilt of looking at my baby with fondness, not an overflow of emotion is overwhelming. What kind of mother doesn't go ga-ga over her infant?" In her piece she explains that she loved her daughter and did not want to see her hurt, but she did not experience the rush of love that she had heard so many others describe. Given the gift of time she is able to look back on her experience and see that a lot of her struggling in bonding was partly due to her being limited in her ability to physically care for her daughter and it was also a form of self-protection. She wrote in her brutally honest way,

> When your entrance into parenthood isn't marked with flowers and congratulations, but a deadly disease and a baby that is 2lb of sagging skin hanging from fragile bones, your brain simply doesn't let the possibility of a happy ending enter the picture. Better not get attached, it tells you. This does not look promising (Valenti 2011).

The desire to protect herself from potential loss was not unique to Valenti. Studies of parental attachment in the NICU have repeatedly found that some parents have trouble bonding with their baby due to the overwhelming fear that the baby will not make it. The thought of completely falling in love with a child only to have them not ever get to leave the hospital is too much to handle (Johnson 2008; Hoffenkamp et al. 2012).

Throughout the interviews, women seemed almost relieved to be able to share this part of their story with me and when I shared a little of my story with them they were often glad to hear that another mother had similar emotions. Women were sometimes ashamed of their feelings and they worried that their feelings of disconnect were an indication of a lack of maternal instinct. Had the women known that the feelings of disconnection did not make them bad mothers, but were in fact an expected reaction to the extreme stress and trauma they had endured, they could have possibly felt less guilty.

Sometimes hearing others' negative stories about the consequences of prematurity provoked feelings of guilt as women felt bad about the ongoing challenges their children faced or would face due to their early births. Jennifer, a mother of twins, described how reading stories about premature infants as they grew made her feel guilty,

> I am always reading stories of babycenter.com, about research they have done and you know, it is always negative about premature babies. You know, it's like they don't have this, and they don't have this, that, and the other, and then I am getting to the point where I just can't even read it. So I'm like, it's bad and I know they are. You know, so why am I reading this? You know? But I have some guilt sometimes, you know, because I exercised, and sometimes I think that is why they came early. Because I didn't you know. . .I went to a baby shower when I was on modified bed rest. I asked the doctor what I could do and he just said take it easy, and now I wish I hadn't gone because that's you know when I was at 27 weeks.

Reading stories about the negative outcomes for premature infants made Jennifer feel guilty and soon after reading these types of stories online she would begin to question her actions during her pregnancy as she placed blame on herself for her early delivery. Because of this guilt she began to avoid reading these kinds of stories knowing it would only lead to feelings of self-blame and regret.

Jennifer was not alone in questioning her activity level. Amy, whose twin daughters were born at 35 weeks, often questions how long she kept working. Although she was following her doctor's orders, she still wonders if she could have rested more and perhaps prevented her daughters from needing to spend time in the NICU. "I felt a lot of guilt, and I still feel some guilt. Like I say, and I look back and I sort of wish I would have done things differently." Over and over women held themselves responsible for the outcomes of their pregnancies, convinced that something they did or thought caused preterm labor and early delivery. At this point it is important to address this key component of a high-risk pregnancy which is the pressure and responsibility many women felt for the health and well-being of their children. Again, pregnant women in general feel this responsibility as they are the ones who are growing and nourishing the baby and are the ones making choices about what to or not to consume and what to expose their unborn children to in terms of drugs, alcohol, and chemicals. There are certainly situations, especially those that involve drug use or refusal to follow doctors' orders, where women directly contribute to the premature birth of their child, but in the vast majority of cases premature labor and birth are caused by physical factors out of a woman's control.

Loneliness

Another thing that many women I met spoke about was the sense of isolation and loneliness they felt during their pregnancy and while their children were in the NICU and sometimes even after. Their isolation was both physical and emotional. Isolation during pregnancy often occurred because of medial restrictions. Many of the mothers were on some form of bed rest which limited how often they were able to leave the house which in turn served to seriously limit their face-to-face interaction with others. Isolation occurred because others in women's social and support networks had not had similar experiences and had difficulty relating to what women were going through. Women also felt that even when they had a strong support network, they were ultimately the one responsible for the pregnancy and their baby's health.

For example, Cynthia, mother of twins, found that her unique situation made it difficult to find other stories like hers. What made Cynthia's situation unique was that she was originally pregnant with quadruplets as a result of fertility treatments. Her doctors recommended selective reduction to reduce the risk of premature delivery. While making the difficult decision about whether or not to reduce to twins, she found that she had no one to go to for stories or advice other than medical professionals. She did contact the organization, MOST, mothers of super twins, to ask some questions about quadruplet pregnancies as well as the reduction procedure. The woman she spoke with recommended that Cynthia contact a woman from her hometown with quadruplets. Cynthia, who was seriously considering reduction, felt uncomfortable calling this mother. She explained, "I'm not going to call her to say, well I know you have quads, and I do too, but I think I am going to get rid of them. I mean I just don't feel comfortable with all that. I mean, that just seems sort of rude. I mean I just don't feel comfortable approaching anyone." The extreme nature of her situation, made Cynthia feel isolated as she was reluctant to share her story and she had no other stories to turn to for comparison. She believes she could not find any stories because most of the women who made similar choices also were uncomfortable sharing their stories.

She went on to describe a situation after her twins were born when she was at a business function and met a woman who was pregnant and had recently reduced from quadruplets to twins. She did talk with this woman at the party and felt so relieved to find someone like herself. The women did not continue their relationship though as the topic was just too painful to discuss at length. Interestingly, when I sat down for coffee at a Panera to talk with Cynthia she led with the disclaimer that she was going to share a part of her story few people knew. It was an important part of her story, and one she felt should be shared in order to assist other women who had to make similar decisions, but she still did not feel like she could tell friends or family members about the reduction for fear they would judge her for her choice. The anonymity of the interview made her feel more comfortable sharing a part of the story that even friends and family members did not know.

Michelle, mother of triplets, was another woman who felt like her situation was just too different from most of the people she knew for her to be able to relate with other moms. Often people who were eager to talk to her about her triplets shared stories with her to convey that they somehow could relate to or understand what she had been through, but very rarely were their stories really that similar to her experiences and because of this, Michelle had trouble connecting with them. She acknowledged that there were some general pregnancy and parenting issues that went across the board, regardless of whether one had multiples or not, but there were many issues surrounding a triplet pregnancy and raising triplets that were unique, and her friends with singletons had different situations and their stories did not relate to hers. "But when they start to get all generalized and start talking about the hospital it is like, you don't even know what they are talking about. And like, I mean you can't be judgeful about that." Her friends did not know and could not understand what her situation really was like because their situations were too different from hers. She tried to be understanding and not to condemn them for their lack of knowledge, but at the same time it was hard for her. Sharing birth and baby stories is a way that women can find common ground and connect, but when a mother's story starts with being knocked out for an emergency C-section and having three critical babies in the NICU, it can be hard for that preemie mom to relate to women sharing typical birth experiences.

Once a woman's high-risk pregnancy was over, many of their babies spent time in the NICU which meant they did as well, which contributed to feelings of isolation and loneliness. The majority of NICUs had strict regulations regarding visitors including who was allowed into the NICU and who was allowed to touch or hold the infants. Due to these regulations as well as the precarious health of their infants, many women had very few visitors come to the NICU. Marie, mother of triplets, explained how they limited who they invited to come to the NICU to visit her girls, "The only people who visited us were my mom and dad. I didn't let anyone hold them." The reasons for limiting visitors included rules and regulations from the hospital, limited space, feeling that visitors would be too upset when seeing such small and sick babies, and fears of spreading infection. One mother told me that she was so paranoid about her twins getting sick that she would not even let the priest come to baptize her sons as she was not convinced that the holy water was sterile enough to be introduced into the NICU.

After their infants came home from the hospital, some women still found themselves very isolated. Due to their premature status, many of the infants remained at a higher risk for contracting respiratory infections and other illnesses. Especially during the winter months, many women kept their infants isolated at home and allowed very few visitors to minimize the amount of germs their infants were exposed to. In addition to being protective in the NICU, Marie also was protective once her daughters came home. Her daughters were born in March and Marie was still worried about exposing them to germs. "Yeah, I was kind of crazy about the beginning. You know, they were only born in March, but I didn't let anyone come see them until May or June." This self-isolation during the cold, flu, and RSV season was not only common, but was often medically recommended to protect premature babies from illnesses that their still immature immune and respiratory systems could not handle. After spending too many days in the NICU, the last thing parents wanted was another hospital stay so they endured the social isolation and barred even family and friends with any signs of an illness in order to protect their children.

Kiera, mother of triplets, described how she isolated herself from most of her friends after her daughters were born at 25 weeks. "Yeah, I definitely retreated from most of the people that I knew because we didn't let anyone come to the hospital except for our parents and our sisters until towards the end of their NICU stays and then a very close friend was allowed to come and see them for 30 minutes." Her daughters were very ill, and it was difficult for Kiera to handle the situation and socializing with friends was not high on her priority list, but in isolating herself from friends she lost some of the support and connection she craved.

Anger

Women were not just sad about their situations, but many times they were angry because what was happening to them or what was happening to their babies was just not fair and was just too painful and too hard. This was one of the emotions that women had the hardest time discussing and acknowledging as this was not an emotion traditionally associated with pregnancy and birth. It was also an emotion that they felt was not necessarily productive or one that others would be comfortable with. Some felt that they did not have the right to be mad or express that anger because it made them look ungrateful or negative and they were constantly being told to look at the positives of their situations or reminded that things could be worse.

Stephanie was one of the women who felt a lot of anger when she started to have serious pregnancy complications. To give you a little background, Stephanie is a twenty-nine year old from South Carolina whose son David was born at 29 weeks after her first son Payton was stillborn at 25 weeks. She was refreshingly honest during our interview and I appreciated her candor in discussing how hard both of her pregnancies were for her. When she was 25 weeks pregnant during her first pregnancy she started to have some major pains in her side. She suspected it was a kidney stone and went it into the doctor's office. She was 22 at the time and told me how young and naïve she was, never imagining anything was wrong with the baby. They performed an ultrasound in the office and explained to her that she had suffered from a placental abruption and the baby no longer had a heartbeat. She had not gone into labor so they needed to admit her to the hospital to induce labor so she could deliver the baby. She desperately wanted a C-section so she could just be knocked out and not have to know what was going on and suffer through a delivery, but they would not perform the surgery as they said a vaginal delivery was safer for her.

At this point she was crying hysterically and admits that she was mean and nasty to anyone who was with her. She knows she said terrible things, but she was just so mad. "I was like people have crack babies all of the time and why is my baby dead?" After the delivery she held her son but did not take any pictures. She was discharged from the hospital and went home to mourn and had a very difficult time being around people and she could not handle them asking how she was doing. She spent a lot of time isolating herself trying to figure out how to move on after her loss. When her doctor gave her the go ahead to have another baby she and her husband started trying right away. When she found out she was pregnant she was thrilled but simultaneously terrified. The doctors never could tell her why her first son had passed away in utero and she was so afraid that it would happen again.

Her pregnancy progressed normally until she was 26 weeks and 5 days and she had a kidney stone. She went into the hospital and while they had her hooked up to the fetal monitor they detected that the baby's heart rate dropped. It went back up so they continued to monitor and it happened again. At this point the doctor determined that his umbilical cord had compromised flow and Stephanie was given the steroid shots and placed on full bed rest. She was scared, but she was also so angry. She could not believe this was happening again. Even if the baby did survive she was convinced that he would be horribly disabled. She told me very bluntly, "I was a real bitch, they weren't letting me up and I was tired, and I was like even prisoners get to go outside for an hour." At one point a relative told her that she couldn't wait to see the baby's face and she snapped and yelled, "why would you say that? He is going to be blind, deaf, and stupid, and I am going to bring a child into the world who has no quality of life." She grew tired of how optimistic everyone around her was trying to be and felt like those around her were not facing up to the possibility that her son might not make it, and if he did live, he might face a very difficult life. Stephanie's son was born about 2 weeks later and although he was small and needed a lot of medical interventions, he did survive and is now a healthy child with no long-term delays or disabilities. She is thankful every day that David is thriving, but still easily recalls the anger she felt about her situation.

Another mom, Morgan shared how anger sometimes hit her when she least expected it. I do need to preface this by saying that Morgan was one of the most upbeat and positive women I have ever spoken with. Despite delivering her twin boys at 24 weeks and 5 days and losing one of her sons about two months after his birth, she made a conscious decision to be thankful for her son who survived and to be inspired by her sons' strength. When I commented to her how remarkable she sounded given that her son Austin was still in the NICU when we spoke she told me that she and her husband were generally positive people, but as positive they were, they still had their down days and moments. She said one of the most difficult things for her was seeing friends' pictures of healthy full-term babies on Facebook. She and her husband did not post any pictures of their son on Facebook until he had his ventilator removed because you could not really see his face, and they didn't know if other people would be alarmed by seeing photos of his tiny, frail body. Seeing the pictures of people holding their newborns and babies smiling made her angry, not at her friends, but at her situation and circumstances. She wanted two full-term, healthy twins, and she did not get that.

Jacque whose daughter was born at 26 weeks and given the misdiagnosis of a serious brain condition shortly after birth spent a lot of her daughter's time in the NICU being angry. She described how she felt,

> I was really pissed. I was mad at the doctor, I felt like if I had listened to that little voice on Friday night maybe I could have gone in and they would have been able to put me on bed rest for longer, then maybe the whole brain defect thing would have not even happen. I had just bought maternity clothes that I never got to wear. I cried constantly. My face hurt from crying. I was so pissed. I just wanted to rewind life. My life was perfect on Friday and by Monday my whole world had been turned upside down. And then people would say to me, 'I just know it's going to be ok' and I wanted to say, do you have a crystal ball, really? You don't know that really.

Envy

Another emotion many women struggled with and sometimes felt overwhelmed with was envy. As the previous chapter on social comparison explained, women frequently looked to others around them to assess their situation. When women came up short in their comparisons they not only felt discouraged and disappointed, but the comparisons also sparked feelings of envy. When others had the experiences and outcomes they had wanted, women could not help but crave what those other people had and question why others were able to have healthy, full-term children when they were not. Yvette, mother of twins described how hard it was for her not to constantly look to other women and wish she had had the pregnancies and births they did. She explained that she still finds herself thinking about how difficult things were for her in comparison to others. She explained,

> To have this day I have to catch myself. The combined weight of my twins was three pounds, and she has a nine pounder. You are always comparing. I don't know how to get away from that. I am jealous. I wish I had that, to carry a child, to able to feel them kicking in you. At least I didn't get any stretch marks, but I would take a road map in exchange for full term babies, to be quote on quote normal. That is not our reality.

She went on to explain that even though she had experienced a pregnancy, she missed out on so many of the typical pregnancy and delivery experiences that she had a hard time relating when other moms started swapping stories, because she never did the typical things.

Cora, mother of a 29-weeker explained how her envy of women who had full-term babies and got a normal experience turned into bitterness. Cora was a first-time mother and had been so excited to have a baby and was devastated when her daughter came so early and had to be admitted to the NICU. Cora stayed at the hospital for the first ten days, but after that decided that she need to go home because being at the hospital 24 hours a day was not good for her or her mental and physical health. At that point she started to envy women who got to take their baby home from the hospital and for the next few weeks did nothing but care for the baby. She explained, "I got bitter about not being able to cuddle with my baby like a normal mom and I was mad that I wasn't one of those women who did not have to get up and look presentable to go to the hospital to visit their baby. Most people who have a baby don't even have time to shower and they can just lay around watching TV and holding their baby."

PTSD

One thing that has changed since I gave birth to my girls in 2008 is the increased recognition by the medical community of the emotional trauma of having a high-risk pregnancy, traumatic birth, and infant in the NICU and the possibility of parents and particularly mothers developing post-traumatic stress disorder (PTSD) in reaction to traumatic deliveries and NICU stays. It has long been known that all women have a risk for developing postpartum depression (PPD) and women who experience a difficult or stressful pregnancy are at a higher risk, making preemie moms especially vulnerable. There are cases however, that rather than PPD, women are actually experiencing PTSD or both. PTSD was first identified as a psychiatric disorder in 1980. It was discovered by studying the emotional difficulties of soldiers who had returned from war. The initial diagnosis of PTSD required that an individual was exposed to a traumatic event outside what one would normally encounter in everyday life such as an explosion or witnessing people being shot and killed. In 1994, the American Psychological Association changed the definition to define trauma as experiencing or witnessing dire threat to the self or others and those threats could occur within normal life. This meant that women experiencing difficult births or watching their child struggle to breath in the NICU were now included as traumatic events under the DSM-II definition. Once the definition was changed, physicians began to recognize and diagnose more and more cases of PTSD in their patients. In 2009, researchers at Stanford University found that of eighteen parents whose children were admitted to the NICU, three were diagnosed with PTSD after four months and seven of the parents were considered high-risk for developing PTSD (Shaw et al. 2009). Another study done at Duke University found that African American mothers who experienced extreme emotional distress in the form of high anxiety were more likely to still be experiencing post-traumatic symptoms a year after the birth of their child than similar women who had lower levels of initial distress (Holditch-Davis et al. 2009). Studies have found that any pregnant woman can suffer from PTSD if the circumstance surrounding the birth are traumatic such as having an emergency C-section, but when the results of the birth are having a child spend time in the NICU, studies have found that parents are 26 to 41 percent more likely to have PTSD symptoms than parents whose infants do not spend time in the NICU (Holditch-Davis et al. 2003).

One important thing to understand is the difference between PPD and PTSD because some of the symptoms overlap, and PTSD is often misdiagnosed as PPD. PTSD is characterized by three major categories of symptoms; avoidance of stimuli that trigger memories of the event, flashbacks or nightmares of the event, and a persistent state of arousal (Association 2013). Women who have PTSD may avoid sounds or smells that remind them of the hospital, have frequent flashbacks to the delivery or crisis situations in the NICU, and are often extremely agitated and prone to bouts of crying or anger. Noises similar to the alarms that so frequently go off in the NICU are often a large trigger for parents and many will go out of their way to avoid them.

Many women told me that the smell of disinfectant which was used liberally throughout the NICU was enough to put them right back next to their baby's bed side and bring back all of the feelings of fear and hopelessness.

Parents with PTSD do not just remember the difficult times, but almost relive the experience during their flashbacks including the physical sensations such as shortness of breath and sweating. One of the very difficult things for parents is that every time they see their child they are reminded of the birth and the NICU stay. One way that the persistent state of arousal manifests itself is in a high state of anxiety and hyper vigilance. Parents will become very overprotective in order to keep their preemies safe, going beyond what even their physician's recommend as far as protective measures. Each time their child gets ill they often relive the hospital experiences and can often have irrational fears that even a small cold will require hospitalization (Shaw et al. 2009; Feeley et al. 2011). On the opposite end of the spectrum from flashbacks are complete memory loss of certain aspects of the traumatic event as well as denial of problems resulting from the traumatic event.

One of the primary differences between PTSD and PPD is that PTSD develops as a result of experiencing a traumatic event whereas PPD develops as a result of a hormone imbalance following delivery. Postpartum depression is clinically defined as moderate to severe depression following childbirth. It differs from the baby blues, which is the common experience of mood swings and crying jags for the first two weeks following birth, due to its duration with symptoms lasting up to two years after birth. Common symptoms of PPD are difficulty sleeping, appetite loss, irritability, feelings of hopelessness, withdrawal, mood swings, and in the most severe cases thoughts of harming oneself or the baby (Kammerer et al. 2009). It is easy to see how PTSD might be mistaken for PPD. It is important to correctly diagnose a woman so that she can receive the proper treatment.

Josie was very open with me about the PTSD she experienced after her daughter Elin was born at 31 weeks. Throughout her entire pregnancy Josie had a lot of bleeding and constantly feared that she was losing the pregnancy. At about 24 weeks she started strict bed rest at home and was in and out of the hospital for the next 7 weeks. At 31 weeks, she started to have major hemorrhaging and they delivered Elin via emergency C-section. For being born 9 weeks early Elin did great. She was mostly a feeder and grower and was discharged after 4 weeks. Given the constant fear that she would come too early and the thoughts of what that would have meant made Josie feel somewhat prepared for the NICU, but even though she did well, the NICU experience was still traumatic. After Elin came home she did continue to struggle with her breathing and now that she is almost three has been hospitalized with RSV, pneumonia, and an upper respiratory infection. She says that the first time Elin was re-hospitalized with RSV she suffered from severe PTSD as being back in the hospital brought back so many traumatic memories. She was already on an antidepressant to deal with PPDand had to increase her dosage. One of the things that was really difficult for her was to drive the road back and forth to the hospital as it served as a trigger of the countless times she had to drive that road to visit Elin in the NICU. One of the ways that she was able to find some healing was getting involved with the local March of Dimes chapter to do some volunteer work. One of the things she did was deliver NICU kits for the families in the NICU. Each time she drove to the hospital to make a delivery she started to feel a sense of peace as now she was driving for a positive reason.

Dee Anne who had severe polycystic ovarian syndrome (PCOS) had been told by doctors that she would most likely never conceive on her own, so she was shocked and excited when she took a pregnancy test and it was positive. Dee Anne who is diabetic had anticipated issues with keeping her blood sugar under control, but she had not anticipated having high blood pressure and impaired kidney function. Around 20 weeks she started to have the symptoms of preeclampsia and was put on full bed rest at home. At 24 weeks her blood pressure was still running dangerously high so her doctor admitted her to the hospital and told her she would be there for the duration of her pregnancy. She started to mentally prepare herself to spend the next three months in the hospital, but continued to feel worse and worse despite the medications she was on. On Easter Sunday she was feeling particularly bad and due to her high blood pressure and she was having regular contractions. When the nurses brought the ultrasound machine in to check on the baby they found that with every contraction the baby's heart rate was decelerating. Dee Anne was rushed to an emergency C-section. Because she was so early, the walls of her uterus were still very thick, making it difficult for the surgeon to get the baby out. When the doctor pulled the baby, a girl named Kendra, out she was not breathing and had to be resuscitated in the OR. Dee Anne was moved to post-op and put on a 24 hour magnesium drop to help with her blood pressure and the next day was a complete blur for her.

Even though Kendra was incredibly small and had several health issues to overcome before she was able to come home, she eventually was able to come home with a feeding tube. Dee Anne who has since separated from Kendra's father spoke about how hard the entire experience was and how it changed her. She explained,

> Her father always says I was never the same after Kendra was born, he thinks I have PTSD. I haven't gone to talk to anyone about it. I am dealing with everything. He knows me better than anyone on the planet though. There was

> a nurse who had a particular scent a couple of days ago I smelled it and I kept looking around I couldn't quite place where I had smelled it. I felt apprehension and anxiety and fear and sadness and then I realized where the scent was from.

Nicole was another mother who found the birth of her twin sons, Thomas and Colin and their subsequent NICU stay to be very traumatic. Her sons were born at 24 weeks and 6 days after medications could not stop Nicole's labor. After they were born, Nicole had a difficult time handling the NICU and lived with a constant fear that one of her boys would die. She described their time in the NICU,

> By the second week I was a bit more aware of what was going on with them. They had to have PDA ligation surgery. I kept thinking, why is this happening to me, how did this happen? We didn't name them for weeks because I was afraid, if they die, I couldn't do it. We are Catholic and one of the priests asked to baptize them just in case, but I said no because I did not want anything not sterile that could cause infection. One of the nurses suggested I go see a therapist. After 15-20 minutes of sitting next to their beds I would just be close to a puddle on the floor. Little, little by it got better. They did put me on stuff. It was a roller coaster the boys would have good days and bad days.

With the assistance of medication and time Nicole was able to feel more like she was in control of her emotions, but she still looks back on that time with feelings of anxiety and sadness. Now that her boys are older she still is unable to go to baby showers and has a hard time listening to women talk about their pregnancies as it brings back so many negative memories.

Even though Tracey, mother of triplets and then another son who was also born prematurely, was never formally diagnosed with PTSD, she was very traumatized by her triplets birth at 25 weeks, the loss of one of her triplets when he was almost a year old, and then by her last sons' early birth and NICU stay. She described having many of the common symptoms, including flashbacks triggered by something that reminded her of the NICU. When her step-daughter had to go into the hospital to have her tonsils removed Tracey was overwhelmed by being in the hospital and while walking with her to the OR she became light headed, had difficulty breathing, and had to be escorted out by a nurse. When her second son was born early, even though he was older and larger than the triplets, she had a much harder time dealing with his NICU stay because it brought up to many bad and frightening memories of her triplets' and her son who passed away. She explained that even now she never knows what may trigger her emotions. She described brushing her daughter's hair and as she was parting it she caught a glimpse of a scar that was there from an IV in her head. It was small and faint, but it was enough to bring Tracey to tears as the memories of watching her tiny babies struggle to survive came back as vivid as ever.

COPING MECHANISMS

Having access to similar stories also could help women cope with and understand the wide range of emotions they experienced in conjunction with their high-risk pregnancies. Many of the emotions that women experienced such as extreme guilt, constant fear, or lack of connection to their infants are not emotions typically associated with motherhood. Many women commented that they were unable to enjoy or be excited about their pregnancies once they learned they were high risk. Instead of being excited and filled with joy, they lived with constant fear and anxiety about their unborn infants' survival and health. After enduring a stressful and emotional pregnancy, many mothers had to face the challenges of having infants who required time in the NICU. This was also a time of stress as women tried to physically heal and worried about their infants' health and progress. These overwhelming emotions combined with surges of hormones made the initial weeks after delivery emotionally challenging for many women. Some felt withdrawn, depressed, irritable, or angry and in turn did not feel the joy, love, and bonding they had expected.

Because these emotions did not match women's expectations of pregnancy and motherhood, many women felt isolated and ashamed to talk about their emotions. The feelings women described about needing to keep quiet about their negative emotions were similar to those of women who suffer from PPD. Feeling sad or depressed about the events surrounding a child's birth do not fit with the societal ideal of a "good mother." Feelings of depression and disconnection were a source of shame for many women as they believed that there was something wrong with them and their emotional reactions. Often women choose to hide or keep quiet about their feelings for fear they would be judged for having less than motherly instincts or feelings (Knudson-Martin and Silverstein 2009).

This silence creates a vicious cycle as women believe they are one of the only mothers who has ever felt so sad, anxious, or depressed about their situations because they had not heard or read stories in which women experienced similar feelings. They also were ashamed of their feelings and chose to keep quiet themselves so others cannot learn about their struggles, and in turn, their silence limited their ability to connect with others. The issue of struggling to feel connection with their infants actually came up often in the interviews, and women seemed eager to share their experiences and to be able to talk about what they had been through. Unfortunately, many of the women explained that their eagerness to share their stories in the interview situation was unique, and they rarely felt comfortable discussing their negative emotions in other settings. The feelings of isolation and guilt were perpetuated as women had nowhere to go to find stories that showed them that their feelings were not rare, but were quite natural.

A practical suggestion that could address concerns about the absent narratives of depression maternal disconnection is providing safe forums for women to both tell and hear these stories. Research has shown that talking about and sharing one's story with others is an important way that both mothers and fathers cope with the NICU experience. Mothers especially look to others outside of the family to share their stories with and in addition to nurses and doctors, other parents in the NICU are great sources for them to share their stories with (Coppola et al. 2013). The internet is another potential context for sharing what women view as less than desirable stories because women have the benefit of anonymity. Online forums and groups allow women to use a screen name and they are not required to share any identifying information. When women do feel comfortable enough to share their stories, it is crucial that those around them do not fault or condemn them. When these feelings are expressed in stories they need to be properly addressed and not dismissed as baby blues. The feelings women are experiencing are genuine, and in some cases might require medical interventions such as medication or counseling. Having access to other stories of PPD could make it easier for women to acknowledge their own feelings and ask for needed assistance.

One of the resources that several of the women mentioned as being very valuable were birthing and pregnancy classes specifically designed for their high-risk condition such as multiple infants or diabetes. The information was tailored specifically to their special needs and they were able to connect with other mothers dealing with the same issues and concerns. Marie, mother of triplet girls, talked very positively about a class that was offered at the hospital where she delivered for women pregnant with twins or more called Marvelous Multiples. In addition to learning valuable information about her pregnancy and how her delivery might differ from a non-high-risk delivery, Marie also was able to connect with other mothers and even made friends she kept in contact with after the class concluded. "Yeah, there were like three triplet moms and maybe like six or eight twin moms. Yeah there were quite a few people in there and now, my friend Alicia and our other friend Sarah, we all met in that class." Unfortunately, only women who lived in larger cities with larger hospitals had access to these types of classes. Based on the positive assessments of these classes, they should be made available at hospitals in all areas and women should be encouraged to participate. In situations where a woman is likely to be ordered on bed rest, she should be encouraged to take the classes early in her pregnancy or with current technology, it may be possible for hospitals to create online courses women could take from home.

Support groups are another context where women may feel safer sharing their stories as most likely other members had similar experiences and feelings. Several women mentioned support groups that were held within their NICU specifically for the parents. These groups often were facilitated by volunteers who were previous NICU parents. Having volunteers run the support groups is a great way to provide needed support to NICU parents without taxing hospital resources. Parents with infants in the NICU were welcome to attend and the meetings were spent sharing concerns as well as activities designed to alleviate stress and provide some enjoyment such as doing crafts or sharing a meal. Women appreciated the hour each week they were able to connect with other parents in the NICU as well as the insight they gained from women who had been through the NICU experience. Sam's daughter was born at 29 weeks and she really struggled emotionally to cope with the NICU experience. Her NICU had both a breastfeeding support group and a weekly lunch support group where the women would just talk and share their stories. Sam said it was so encouraging to hear that other people were going through similar things and both the other mothers and nurses were a great source of support and their stories and words were often the thing that kept her going. Beth, another preemie mom, also found that the support group in the unit not only provided an hour a week for her and other moms to talk about their situations, but it also helped them to connect and form friendships that sustained them throughout the week.

A support group gives parents in the NICU a formal way to connect and share their stories. This provides an excellent opportunity for women to connect when they feel uncomfortable approaching other women in the NICU as they want to respect their space and give them privacy. Newer hospitals are tending to build NICUs not as open units, but instead infants are given private rooms similar to those of other hospital patients. Although this design allows for more privacy, it can make it more difficult for mothers in the NICU to interact. Support group meetings should be held in a separate room to give mothers some time and space away from the NICU to relax and talk. Some of the things that women reported that they enjoyed most about the support groups they participated in was meeting other moms, having time to share stories and ask questions, and some groups even did a small craft or made scrapbook pages as a way to relax and take their minds off of all of the stress.

Some women also found support groups helpful while they were coping with their pregnancies. For example, Mandy, a mother with type I diabetes, talked a lot during her interview about a support group for diabetic mothers she belonged to during her pregnancy. Sponsored by her obstetrician's practice, the group met biweekly and the women, who were at all different points in their pregnancies, met to discuss different topics related to their diabetes and to ask and answer questions. Many of the members would return to the group with their infants after they gave birth to discuss questions about delivery and recovery. Mandy really enjoyed seeing all of the women with their healthy infants as it provided her with visual evidence of the positive outcomes women had which helped lessen her fears.

The need for support groups and connections with others does not end after infants are discharged from the hospital as was shown in the chapter Life After NICU. As women begin raising premature infants or multiple infants they continue to face challenges unique to their infants and their situations (Olshtain-Mann and Auslander 2008). For example, the first year of raising twins or higher-order multiples can be stressful and taxing as mothers reported feeling that their lives were put on hold during this time (Beck 2002; Glazebrook et al. 2004). Support groups for women dealing with similar issues such as raising multiples or infants with special needs or health concerns could provide a much needed form of support.

Some parents preferred and sought out more informal ways to connect. Anna, whose son was born at 30 weeks, talked about a weekly dinner the NICU held each week for the parents. During the meal parents were encouraged to talk and share their concerns. Not only was Anna able to connect with some of the other moms in the unit she also learned a lot of valuable information. For example, she did not know that parents could be involved in selecting a primary day and night nurse and after she asked for this her son received much more consistent care. The unit also had a more formal support group that was led by a social worker, but she felt uncomfortable attending the formal parent support group. She explained that her son did not have as many medical issues. He was a preemie and had major feeding issues that kept him in the NICU for a long time, but he had never been on a ventilator and was not a micropreemie. At the meeting she went to she felt very out of place as it seemed to her that all of the other parents had much more serious issues they were dealing with including breathing issues, brain bleeds, and surgeries, so she did not feel as if she had the right to complain about her son's problems. Other women I spoke with did not feel comfortable participating in face-to-face support groups, especially while they were in the NICU. Some women are by nature more private people and did not feel comfortable talking about their emotions in a group. One mom explained to me that she and her husband were not joiners by nature, so any type of group support made them very uncomfortable.

Another option for some women was to find support online from different forums and websites. Literature on internet support groups suggests that the ability to find others with similar problems is one of the advantages of online support groups, especially when their health conditions are rare or unique and people have difficulty finding similar others near their geographic locations (Rains and Young 2009; Taylor and Luce 2003). Women pregnant with higher-order multiples or who gave birth to micropreemies may be unable to find or contact others in the immediate area with similar experiences. Additionally, many of the women were on strict bed rest during their pregnancies and were unable to meet people or attend in-person support group meetings. The internet gave women access to others even when they could not leave home. With internet message forums such as Inspire, Triplet Connection, and preemie boards on BabyCenter women were able to connect with women from all over the world to discuss and swap stories about the unique challenges of a pregnancy with higher-order multiples and later the challenges of raising multiples. Women also were able to find the stories of other families with premature infants and could learn how those families coped with the many challenges they faced.

Access to these stories gave women ideas about what could be and allowed them to imagine various outcomes of their own stories. Many women could not personally conjure up a story about what life would be like with a premature infant or with multiples. Hearing or reading stories about people who had these experiences gave them the ability to create their own narratives. Other women were fixated on a certain narrative and hearing and reading others' stories provided them with alternative possibilities. For example, some women who learned they were carrying triplets or higher-order multiples were consumed with fears and doubts as they believed they would never be able to care for so many infants at once or that all of their infants would suffer from severe disabilities. Hearing or reading about triplets who were healthy and women who were raising thriving triplets created new possibilities and new potential storylines.

Not only did women need access to stories that provided help and information, but they also needed access to people who had similar stories. Even when they had a strong support network of family and friends, the existing support system was sometimes not adequate as their network members had not gone through similar experiences. For example, women found that it was difficult to relate to friends and family members who experienced typical pregnancies or singleton births. Having a fellow preemie mom as a friend and a source of support was one of the most helpful things for many women, and it was the thing that women most commonly wished they had. For example, Johanna, is the mother of two preemies. Her son Thomas was born at 30 weeks after her water broke and her daughter Theresa was also born at 30 weeks after her water broke early again. She explained that she had a huge support system thanks to a large group of friends, pastors at church, family, and coworkers, but one of the most important sources of support Johanna had come from an unexpected place. Johanna's sister had a friend who had given birth a preemie a few years earlier. Even though the two women had never met before, her sister's friend called her after Thomas was born and the two instantly connected. They would spend hours talking on the phone swapping preemie stories and for Johanna, having a friend who was further along down the road of the preemie journey was an invaluable source of answers to her questions and a source of encouragement when she became frightened or overwhelmed. "Being able to talk to that friend was totally helpful. You get what it's like to live the NICU and then go home every night without your baby. Even when you do bring your kid home, it is not like when you bring a full term baby home."

One of the reasons women seemed to desire relationships with those who could share similar stories was because they desired feelings of normalcy. Several of the mothers of multiples commented on how they quickly became tired of the endless comments by others of how difficult and unique it must be to raise twins or triplets. Although most likely intended to be an observation or compliment, these comments made women feel different and placed their experiences and stories into the category of unique or strange. When women participated in groups for mothers of multiples or made friends with other mothers with multiples they found that they no longer were the unique or different person in the group. Their stories were similar and women felt they could relate to each other and appreciated that the other women did not regard them or their families as oddities.

It is important to note though that the experiences of preemie moms were not all the same, and those differences sometimes made it difficult for women to relate and connect, even if they shared elements to their stories such as a high-risk pregnancy or premature birth. Just because two women had children in the NICU, did not mean that they would automatically be able to provide the support each needed. For some women, their children were born so early that they felt like their stories were too frightening for other NICU moms or it was too hard to relate to women whose babies were not as critical. Leslie, mother of Kadri and Xander, said that for the most part she felt very isolated from the other parents in the NICU. Because they were born so early and were so critical, her twins were in a pod that housed the micropreemies. In order to get to that pod, Leslie had to walk through a pod with the older and bigger babies who were just feeders and growers. She explained, "I hated walking through that room. My babies were the sickest in the unit. I didn't want to talk to the preemie parents that were there." For Cora, her concern was that her baby was so small and so sick that it scared the other parents. She described sitting in the pumping room talking with other parents and when she talked about her daughter or showed pictures to the other mothers who had four and 5-pound babies the other moms often had a hard time relating to her because their babies were so much healthier.

On the opposite side of the spectrum were mothers who felt like their children were too healthy to relate to other women whose children were dealing with much more serious and sometimes even life-threatening issues. Some women described as almost feeling guilty for how well their own children were doing and felt like their problems and issues paled in comparison to what others were dealing with. Kate articulated how even now when she thinks about her daughters who were born at 33 weeks she is sometimes hesitant to talk about them as preemies. I was somewhat surprised by this as they were born 7 weeks early and spent 11 and 18 days in the NICU, but Kate explained that even though they were preemies, they were almost 5 pounds at birth and their time in the NICU was relatively easy as they were both just feeders and growers. The truly hard part for Kate was her pregnancy, and once they were born and were for the most part healthy, things seemed so much easier. Compared to what other preemie moms went through in the NICU she felt like the NICU experience was about as easy and uncomplicated as it can get.

Another situation that made women feel abnormal or unique was when they heard or read stories about mothers or talked with mothers who gave birth to full-term infants. Mothers found that their concerns about their infants' health and development were often different than other mothers because premature infants often are more susceptible to illnesses, particularly respiratory infections, and frequently face some developmental delays. Mothers felt most comfortable with other mothers of premature infants as they did not feel judged or questioned about the actions they took that others sometimes labeled as overprotective or extreme. When they were with others who had similar stories, women felt they were understood and did not have to spend time explaining their situations.

Another frustration for women who experienced high-risk pregnancies, had preemies, were raising multiples or had medically fragile children was encountering other mothers who tried to compare what seemed to them to be incomparable experiences. For example, many women described others who complained of long and painful labors and equated this to women who had experienced contractions for weeks. A lot of women I have met talked about how their level of sympathy for others has in many ways gone down after their experiences. They of course did not want another person to having morning sickness or aches and pains, but they also saw the normal side effects of pregnancy as minor compared to some of the things they experienced. Other women talked about the anger they felt when a woman who was seven or eight months pregnant said that she was ready for the baby to come any day. Preemie moms know how important each day in the womb is and most would have given anything to carry their child just one day more, if not weeks more. Some women would tell mothers of twins or triplets they understood because they had two or three children of different ages. These attempts at connection by other mothers were generally alienating to the mothers interviewed as they felt that the comparisons were invalid and in many ways lessened their experiences.

In order to avoid being in situations like this, many mothers sought out other mothers whose stories more closely matched their own. Being with others whose stories were similar helped to validate and affirm women's experiences. Women felt more normal when they could talk with others who shared similar stories. The challenges women faced seemed less extreme when those around them experienced similar challenges. Women enjoyed talking with and sharing stories with those whose daily lives more closely resembled their own. This is not to say that women still were not frightened, frustrated, or stressed by their situations. However, when they found others with similar stories they felt understood and could consider their challenges more within the realm of possible experiences.

Another key factor in women being able to successfully cope with the NICU experience was having a strong support network outside of the hospital of family and friends. Research has found that having a strong social support system is a strong factor in protecting women against PPD and PTSD (Platt, Keyes, and Koenen 2014; Negron et al. 2013; Giurgescu et al. 2015). When I asked women how they survived their long days on bed rest or how they dealt with the ups and downs of the NICU one of the most common responses was support from our friends and family. Having close family and friends who were encouraging and willing to listen at any time were invaluable to women as they struggled to make sense of their circumstances and emotions. Even if friends and family could not always relate to what parents were going through, they could provide the tangible support parents needed by doing things such as providing meals, feeding pets at home, watching other children, and taking care of tasks that parents did not have the time or energy for.

Unfortunately for some women their social support was limited. Sometimes this was due to living far away from family and being new to an area. Other times women found that friends and family did not know how to effectively support them during this difficult time. Over and over women told me that other people just didn't know what to say and instead offered generic comments and platitudes that were meant to be helpful, but often had the opposite effect. One thing that really bothered some women was when others told them how lucky they were that their child or children were doing relatively well or that they were lucky that their child had survived his or her early birth. As I wrote in chapter 2, I had a hard time dealing with the stress and sadness I was feeling because so many people kept telling me how lucky and blessed we were that the girls were all here and doing well for their gestational age. I knew we were fortunate and blessed, but at the same time I also felt like there were a lot of not so great things about our situation, and I wanted to be able to acknowledge those without feeling guilty and I wanted to be able to complain and cry without someone trying to be sure that I was able to look on the positive side of things.

Cora, whose daughter Lily was born at 29 weeks weighing just 1 pound 10 ounces articulated how frustrating it was for her when people would rush in to console her with assurances that everything would be fine or to point out how things could be worse for Lily or that this was a part of God's plan. She explained, "I don't think people know what to say, think about how lucky you are when you have a sick baby? I avoided people. One time I snapped, are you telling me that people who have normal kids means they are personal friends or are closer to God? I wish someone would have said, I am sorry this is happening to you. The people who are very positive oriented, it is dismissive to people's feelings. She could have died." She knew that people's comments were coming from a good place, but their need to have her look on the bright side of things ignored the painful reality she was living. "You are entitled to have fear for your kid," she told me.

> I was sad for myself, and what about for her. Just recently we just had her follow up and they want to send her for hearing testing. I was upset I have to prepare myself for the fact she might have hearing loss, my dad said you know just focus on the positive. . .yes that is all very true, but I can be sad for her, I don't want her to have a disability. He focuses on the positive and I would rather just stare the bad news in the face and deal with it.

FAITH AND PRAYER

Another way that women coped with the stress and trauma of their experiences was by relying on their faith. In situations that where women felt like they had absolutely no control, the one thing they felt they could do was rely on their faith and prayer to get them through. Browsing on Pinterest one day I came across a picture with a baby in an isolette with the words, "The walls of NICUs have heard more prayers than most of the walls of churches." For many mothers, when they were in situations where they felt completely helpless and had no control, one of the only things they could do was pray and hope for the best. A few weeks after I interviewed Heather, whose third daughter was born at 27 weeks, she emailed that she had forgotten to tell me one of the ways that she managed to stay sane while she was on bed rest and during the long days in the NICU. Over and over she would recite the Serenity Prayer to herself, "God grant me the serenity to accept the things I can't change, the courage to change the things I can and the wisdom to know the difference. Living one day at a time; Enjoying one moment at a time; Accepting hardships as the pathway to peace." The familiar words brought her comfort and helped her to accept that she was in the situation she was in and for the most part it was out of her control so she had to trust that it was in God's hands. This was especially important to her as there were times when she found herself questioning why God was letting this happen to her. When she was admitted into the hospital with complications and while she was fearing that her daughter would not make it, she struggled to understand where God was in all of the struggles, but in the end she clung to her faith and was able to find a sense of peace and calm amidst the turmoil.

Several other mothers talked to me about how their faith and the support of their church communities was one of the only ways that they got through their difficult pregnancies and long NICU stays. Michelle's son Lincoln was born almost four months early after her water broke at 19 weeks. After 5 weeks of hospital bed rest he was born. Michelle said that despite him coming so early, she felt a sense of peace even as she was wheeled into the delivery room for an emergency C-section. She explained, "I have a lot of faith and I just knew it was going to be OK. Neonatology came and gave us all of the statistics and I was very peaceful." Her husband had a very hard time dealing with his son's birth and was very concerned that Lincoln would not survive, but Michelle said her faith kept her going every day and she always felt that in the end everything would be fine. This is not to say that her son's time in the NICU was not incredibly difficult and at times heartbreaking, but the one thing that she never did worry about was losing her son as she always had a sense that he was meant to live.

Dee Anne whose daughter Kendra was born early explained to me the complicated role her personal faith played during her pregnancy and while her daughter was in the NICU. When Dee Anne was nineteen her mother passed away which caused her to lose most of her faith as she could not understand why this had happened. She did not think about her faith very often until she was lying in her hospital room in the days leading up to her daughter's birth. A hospital chaplain came in a few times to talk and pray with her and she said this was a real turning point for her. When she was alone in her room she started talking to God for the first time in a long time and she was pretty blunt. "I said to him, OK big guy, show me what you got." She described how being so helpless as she waited for her daughter to be born and later to come home from the hospital led her to rely more on a greater power.

> I had done everything I was supposed to do. My placenta failed. It eats up all of the insulin I was crashing. They didn't tell me that then. There was nothing more I could have done right for this pregnancy and it just wasn't up to me anymore. That is the only way I got through it. Up until I had my daughter, I was force fed patience, you can't worry about what tomorrow is going to bring. You just have to wait and see, what is and what is. That was really hard to let go of that.

For Beth, her deep faith was the one thing that kept her going after both of her sons' premature deliveries. With her first pregnancy, she started to experience a lot of swelling around 18 weeks. At 24 weeks she had a bad headache that would not go away and when she went into her OB's office to be checked and her blood pressure was 160 over 110. Her doctor sent her to the hospital immediately and she was diagnosed with severe preeclampsia. An ultrasound revealed that her son's growth was restricted and physicians made the decision to deliver him immediately, so Tyler was born weighing just 1 pound 9 ounces. Beth spent a lot of Tyler's time in the NICU praying and leaning on her faith to get through this difficult time as the first months of Tyler's life were filled with constant ups and downs and frequent setbacks.

When Beth and her husband were ready to have another child they spoke extensively with their OB who explained that the odds of a woman having preeclampsia in a subsequent pregnancy were low. She got pregnant again and was having a great pregnancy and was feeling great. At 26 weeks even though she was still feeling good she told her doctor that it did not feel like her stomach had gotten any bigger in the past few weeks. An ultrasound showed that this boy was also showing growth restriction. They decided to give Beth the steroid shots in case they needed to deliver her son early, so she had to check into the hospital for monitoring and they went ahead and did a 24-hour urine catch which tested positive for protein and it was determined that she had borderline preeclampsia. She was discharged and when she followed up the next day with her doctor he told her that she would probably deliver early for sure and he would like her to stay at the hospital until her son was born as a precaution. She went back to the hospital mentally preparing herself for a long hospital stay. After she was checked in, the nurses hooked her up to the fetal monitor and they saw that the baby's heart rate kept dropping. This resulted in another ultrasound which showed that Beth had a 75 percent placental abruption. Had she not been checked into the hospital for borderline preeclampsia the likelihood is that she would have had a full placental abruption at home and would have lost her son as well as possibly her own life. Because they caught the abruption she was rushed to the ER where she was put under and her son Owen was delivered.

These two traumatic births would be enough to make anyone question why her pregnancies and births were so difficult, but instead of focusing on what went wrong Beth repeatedly told me how thankful she was that God saved her sons' lives and that she developed the symptoms she did when she did so that she was in the right place at the right time for her sons to be delivered. She explained, "I am a strong believer in Jesus. That got me through it. He gave us a peace, even with everything was going on with Owen, we had peace that people could not understand." One of the things that made both of her sons' NICU stays more difficult was that she and her husband lived two hours away from the hospital so Beth stayed at the Ronald McDonald House while her husband went home during the week to work and the during the second stay, to help care for their older son Tyler. The family did attend a local church by the hospital and through this Beth was able to connect with some women who became a strong source of support. Beth did spend a lot of time in the NICU alone though as none of their family lived close by and she spent a lot of her time praying and this helped her to stay strong and get through the long days.

As this chapter illustrated, women who experience a high-risk pregnancy or give birth prematurely experience a wide range of intense emotions both positive and negative. This is not a surprising finding, but what is noteworthy is the fact that so many preemie moms felt like they were alone in experiencing such intense emotions. Women felt as if this was not a common part of the stories they heard about pregnancy and birth and because of this many felt compelled to reach out and share their stories with others so other mothers would not feel so alone. It was also important that women found a source of emotional support at all points during their pregnancies and after their children were born whether that support came from face-to-face relationships or from the internet. Sometimes women's emotions were so overwhelming due to PPD or PTSD that they needed additional assistance to help deal with their intense sadness and anxiety.

Conclusion

When I embarked on this project I was in large part motivated by a desire to see if my experiences and feelings were normal as I like so many women who I met and spoke with had little access to stories about high-risk pregnancy, having premature babies, and having multiples. I wondered if other mothers were as upset as I was to find out their pregnancy was high-risk, if there were women who also struggled to feel like the babies they were visiting in the NICU were theirs and if the overwhelming feelings of guilt over their early births were par for the course. Was the rollercoaster of emotions I felt from the time I learned I was pregnant until the girls were almost three typical, or was it just me? As I met and talked with woman after woman I quickly realized that my experiences were in fact quite normal, but even more importantly, there were hundreds of stories that needed to be told and shared. Not only was telling her story cathartic for a woman, but it also provided an alternative narrative for the many women whose pregnancies and childbirth experiences do not match the prevailing stories they are surrounded by. When I was going through my pregnancy and then life in and after the NICU I felt very alone and struggled to navigate this new life without having the assistance of the stories of women who had walked this road before me. Knowing that feelings, reactions, and fears are common can go a long way in reducing some of the isolation and feelings of strangeness women feel.

Another goal in sharing these stories is that hearing some of these stories can also prepare women for some of the elements of a high-risk pregnancy or NICU stay that are not necessarily covered in a pamphlet or included in a pregnancy manual. As this book showed, women are full of expectations about pregnancy and motherhood and when those expectations are not met it can lead to feelings of anger, sadness, and confusion. Providing new expectations and finding creative ways to meet some of their other expectations could go a long way in easing some of the emotional pain and trauma women feel.

The stories in this book are not just beneficial to women and mothers with premature infants. Sharing these stories also offers insight and understanding to those who support these women whether medical professionals, social workers, friends, or family. For example, while it might be tempting to offer words of encouragement that ask women to gain a new perspective on their situations, these attempts might fall short as women may not be in a place mentally and emotionally where they are ready to compare their situations to others. Not every woman is comforted by stories of miracle preterm babies that survived or by reminders that their situations could be far worse than it is. Women had a variety of emotional and tangible support needs and when their support networks did not have direct experience with a high-risk pregnancy or having a preemie, it was often difficult for their support networks to know what to say or what to do. Each woman is different and has unique needs, but the one thing that women consistently shared with me is that they need is for the people around them to let them experience their emotions without judgment. Sometimes when a woman is sad she just wants to take the time to grieve and mourn what she has lost and when her child is grown and she has a nagging sense of anxiety in the back of her mind she needs people to accept that and not dismiss her concerns or make her feel like she is being ungrateful or dwelling too much on the negative. There is much evidence to support the benefits of positive thinking and the benefits of reframing a situation, but there are also times when someone needs to be able to complain or cry and hear nothing but I am so sorry this is happening to you.

Another important issue that is raised is finding the balance between ignorance and information overload when it comes to educating women about the premature birth and the risks, a task that is incredibly difficult as some women were self-professed information seekers while others avoided negative information at all costs. This led to many women being unnecessarily frightened while others were completely unprepared for the complications and situations they faced. While there is no specific answer to this question as each woman in unique in her informational needs, it is an issue that those working with and supporting women need to be aware of. Offering stacks of pamphlets of potential complications might not be the best strategy, but neither is completely ignoring the possibilities of preterm labor and birth. More research needs to be done to determine the best ways to educate and empower women when it comes high-risk pregnancies, preterm labor, and preterm birth in terms of the types of information and message channels.

As I sit and write these final pages, listening to my seven-year-old triplets laughing as they watch one of their favorite shows on the Disney Channel,

I am again struck by how fortunate my family is. In a situation where so many things could have gone wrong, there was so much that went right. At the time I did not have the knowledge of what the future would hold and I struggled to see how lucky we were. With each woman I spoke with I gained new perspective and a new appreciation for what it means to be a preemie mom. I learned that when it comes to high-risk pregnancies and premature birth there is always someone with what seems like they had a better outcome and there is always someone who seems to have had it worse. In the end though, the comparisons do not matter, as each individual is facing something that is difficult, challenging, and in some way will change them. The more I worked on writing this book them more I was reminded of the importance of sharing my story and using my experiences to help others whether it is by listening without judgment, offering advice, or using the platforms I have to share the stories of the incredible women and children that I have met and learned about. Additionally, as I spoke to more and more women and wrote and revised my chapters, my own story continued to change as well as I was able to better understand my own circumstances in light of what other women told me.

Just last week I spoke on the phone with a mother whose twins were born at 25 weeks. Her daughters are now almost two and doing quite well, but concern about developmental delays, weight gain, and overall health continue to permeate this family's life. During our nearly 40 minute conversation I did not do much talking other than to murmur things like, "I understand" or "me too." Later that day I received an email from her simply thanking me for listening and understanding what she felt. She told me that sometimes she just needed to hear someone tell her that her fears and anxieties were normal and she needed to know that other mothers had felt the same way. We have continued to talk and email since then and as new problems and issues arise and even though her worries and stress are very real and continue to be a large part of her life, she at least feels a little less alone.

In an ideal world there would no longer be premature births and scientists and doctors would discover ways to effectively stop labor, cure life threatening conditions that necessitate delivery, and assist women in having healthy full term pregnancies. While organizations like the March of Dimes are working to meet this goal, the reality is that even if the number of premature births is reduced, there will still be high-risk pregnancies and babies born too soon. What we can do then in addition to continuing to develop medical treatments for both pregnant women and premature infants is work to gather and share the stories of women who had these experiences and share those stories to raise awareness and understanding. We can also learn from those stories about what women want and need to help them cope with the often traumatic and life changing circumstances of their pregnancies and births. Even more importantly though, we can work to help shape the stories that women tell. As Fisher said, we must choose among the existing stories in order to live a good life. Even when two people are handed the exact same circumstance they can chose to tell vastly different stories about those events, which in turn shapes how they view and live in the world. One may focus on the negative aspects of the story, cast him or herself as the victim while another might chose to focus on the good that came out of trying circumstances and cast him or herself as the protagonist. How one chooses to tell his or her story is partly determined by personality, but it also determined by the stories that surround that person. As this book has shown, people pull from the stories they know and use those to make sense of their own situations and to craft their own explanations of their lives whether is it through comparison, emulation, or adoption of the language. It is my hope that my book as well as other books and stories told from the perspective of mothers will give women more possibilities to choose from as they construct their own stories to make sense of and understand what happened to them and their children and that with those possibilities women will be able to tell a story that is honest and accurate, but also is helpful to them as they work to cope and live with their experiences.

Bibliography

Abo-Yaqoub, S., A.-B. Mohammed, and H. Saleh. 2012. "The Effect of Second Trimester Emergency Cervical Cerclage on Perinatal Outcome." *The Journal of Maternal-Fetal & Neonatal Medicine: The Official Journal of the European Association of Perinatal Medicine, the Federation of Asia and Oceania Perinatal Societies, the International Society of Perinatal Obstetricians* 25 (9): 1746–49. doi: 10.3109/14767058.2012.663822.

Adval, R., and R. S. Wyer. 1998. "The Role of Narrative in Consumer Information Processing." *Journal of Consumer Psychology* 7 (3): 207–45.

Affonos, D. D. 1977. "'Missing Pieces'–A Study of Postpartum Feelings." *Birth* 4 (4): 159–64.

Alcalde, M. C. 2011. "'To Make It through Each Day Still Pregnant': Pregnancy Bed Rest and the Disciplining of the Maternal Body" *Journal of Gender Studies* 20 (3): 209 21.

Ali, L. 2003. "Muumuu No More." *Newsweek* 141 (17): 66.

Alijotas-Rcig, J., C. Palacio-Garcia, and M. Vilardell-Tarres. 2009. "Circulating Microparticles, Lupus Anticoagulant and Recurrent Miscarriages." *European Journal of Obstetrics, Gynecology, and Reproductive Biology* 145 (1): 22–26. doi:10.1016/j.ejogrb.2009.04.002.

Anderson, L. 2011. "Pregnant Women and Families Are Sharing More on Facebook, Web Sites." *The Washington Post*, June 10.

Anh, H.-Y. A., J. S. Park, and E. Haley. 2014. "Consumers' Optimism Bias and Responses to Risk Disclosures in Direct-to-Consumer (DTC) Prescription Drug Advertising: The Moderating Role of Subjective Health Literacy." *Journal of Consumer Affairs* 48 (1): 175–94. doi:10.1111/joca.12028.

Anscombe, E. 2008. "The Dichotomy of Containing Trauma amidst Joy: New Life and a Neonatal Death; the Experience of Working with the Parents of Twins on the NICU." *Infant Observation* 11 (2): 147–60. doi:10.1080/13698030802242849.

Ante, S. 2008. "Million Dollar Babies." *Business Week*, June.

Ardnt, B. 2006. "Role of the Media." *Australian & New Zealand Journal of Obstetrics & Gynaecology* 46 (Suppl. 1): 42.

Argus, B., J. Dawson, W. Connie, C. Morley, and P. Davis. 2009. "Financial Costs for Parents with a Baby in a Neontal Nursery." *Journal of Pediatric & Child Health* 45 (9): 514–17.

Association, American Psychiatric. 2013. *Diagnostic and Statistical Manual of Mental Disorders*. 5th ed. Washington, DC: American Psychiatric Association.

Baker, J. P. 2000. "Historical Perspective." 321–28.

Barshun, R. 1996. *Growing Sophia: The Story of a Premature Birth*. Saint Paul, MN: A Place to Remember.

Bates, B., S. Romina, R. Ahmed, and D. Hopson. 2006. "The Effect of Source Credibility on Consumers' Perceptions of the Quality of Health Information on the Internet." *Medical Informatics and the Internet in Medicine* 31 (1): 45–52.

Beck, C. 2006. "Pentadic Cartography: Mapping Birth Trauma Narratives." *Qualitative Health Research* 16 (4): 453–66.

———. 2002. "Releasing the Pause Button: Mothering Twins during the First Year of Life." *Qualitative Health Research* 12 (5): 593–608.

Belkin, L. 2012. "The Pregnancy Book That Made Me A Wreck Is Now A Movie | Lisa Belkin." *Huffington Post*. http://www.huffingtonpost.com/lisa-belkin/what-to-expect-when-youre-expecting_b_1520644.html.

Bener, M. 2005. "Stylish Mom-to-Be." *Working Mother*.

Berntrop, E. 2009. "Joint Outcomes in Patients with Haemophillia: The Importance of Adherence to Preventative Regimens." *Haemophillia* 15 (6): 1219–27.

Besser, A., and B. Priel. 2003. "Trait Vulnerability and Coping Strategies in the Tranistion to Motherhood." *Current Psychology* 15 (6): 57–72.

Betz, G. 2006. "Ambiguous Loss and the Family Grieving Process." *The Family Journal* 14 (4): 359–65. doi:10.1177/1066480706290052.

Bigelow, C., and J. Stone. 2011. "Bed Rest in Pregnancy." 291–302. doi:10.1002/MSJ.

Birth, P. 2007. Prevention Richard E Behrman, Adrienne Stith Butler, Understanding Premature Birth, Assuring Healthy, Outcomes Isbn, This Pdf, National Academies Press, and National Academy. *Preterm Birth: Causes, Consequences, and Prevention*.

Bochner, A. 2001. "Narratives Virtues." *Qualitative Inquiry* 7 (2): 131–57.

Boghossian, N. S. N. I. Hansen, E. F. Bell, B. J. Stoll, J. C. Murray, J. C. Carey, I. Adams-Chapman, et al. 2014. "Mortality and Morbidity of VLBW Infants with Trisomy 13 or Trisomy 18." *Pediatrics* 133 (2): 226–35. doi:10.1542/peds.2013-1702.

Bondas, T., and K. Eriksson. 2001. "Women's Lived Experiences of Pregnancy: A Tapestry of Joy and Suffering." *Qualitative Health Research* 11 (6): 824–40.

Bor, S. 2013. "Lucy's Two Babies: Framing the First Televised Depiction of Pregnancy." *Media History* 19 (4): 464–78.

Borschmann, R., K. Lines, and D. Cottrell. 2012. "Sun Protective Behaviour, Optimism Bias, and the Transtheoretical Model of Behaviour Change." *Australian Journal of Psychology* 64 (4): 181–88. doi:10.1111/j.1742-9536.2011.00049.x.

Boss, P. 2009. "The Trauma and Complicated Grief of Ambiguous Loss." *Pastoral Psychology* 59 (2): 137–45. doi:10.1007/s11089-009-0264-0.

Bränström, R., S. Kristjansson, and H. Ullén. 2006. "Risk Perception, Optimistic Bias, and Readiness to Change Sun Related Behaviour." *European Journal of Public Health* 16 (5): 492–97. doi:10.1093/eurpub/cki193.

Bravata, D., A. Rastegar, and R. Horowitz. 2002. "How Do Women Make Decisins about Hormore Replacement Therapy?" *The American Journal of Medicine* 113: 22–29.

Brick, M. 2005. "And Next to the Bearded Lady, Premature Babies." *The New York Times*, June 12. http://www.nytimes.com/2005/06/12/nyregion/12coney.html?n=Top%2FReference%2FTimes Topics%2FSubjects%2FB%2FBabies.

Brinchmann, B. S., R. Førde, and P. Nortvedt. 2002. "What Matters To the Parents? A Qualitative Study of Parents' Experiences With Life-and-Death Decisions Concerning Their Premature Infants" 9 (4): 17–19.

Brown, D. 2013. "Lady Sybil's Shocking Death." *Washington Post*, January 28.

Brubaker, S., and C. Wright. 2006. "Identity Transformation and Family and Family Caregiving: Narratives of African American Teen Mothers." *Journal of Marriage and Family* 5: 1214–28.

Bute, J. J. 2011. "When Public and Private Intermingle. . .Reflections on (re)production." *Health Communication* 26 (1): 104–6. doi:10.1080/10410236.2011.527627.

Caeymaex, L., M. Speranza, C. Vasilescu, C. Danan, M. Michèle Bourrat, M. Garel, and C. Jousselme. 2011. "Living with a Crucial Decision: A Qualitative Study of Parental Narratives Three Years after the Loss of Their Newborn in the NICU." *PLoS ONE* 6 (12). doi:10.1371/journal.pone.0028633.

Callister, L. C. 2004. "Making Meaning: Women's Birth Narratives." *Journal of Obstetric, Gynecologic, and Neonatal Nursing* 33 (4): 508–18. doi:10.1177/0884217504266898.

Callister, L. C., and I. Khalaf. 2010. "Spirituality in Childbearing Women." *The Journal of Perinatal Education* 19 (2): 16–24. doi:10.1624/105812410X495514.

Caponecchia, C. 2010. "It Won't Happen to Me: An Investigation of Optimism Bias in Occupational Health and Safety." *Journal of Applied Social Psychology* 40 (3): 601–17. doi:10.1111/j.1559-1816.2010.00589.x.

Carollo, K. 2001. "Preemies among World's Smallerst Surving Newborns Beating Odds." *Good Morning American*. http://abcnews.go.com/Health/follow-study-finds-worlds-smallest-surviving-newborns-fine/story?id=15121655.

Cassidy, T. 2006. *Birth*. New York, NY: Atlantic Monthly Press.

Cegala, D., and S. Broz. 2002. "Physician Communication Skills Training: A Review of Theoretical Backgrounds, Objectives, and Skills." *Medical Education* 36 (11): 1004–16.

———. 2003. "Provider and Patient Communication Skills Training." In *The Handbook of Health Communication*, edited by T. Thompson, A. Dorsey, K. Miller, and R. Parrott, 95–120. Mahwah, NJ.

Champagne, C. 1999. "Rattles and Ratings." *Advocate* 788: 107–8.

Charles, S., and T. Shivas. 2002. "Mothers in the Media: Blamed and Celebrted--and Examination of Drug Abuse and Multiple Births." *Pediatric Nursing* 28 (2): 142–45.

Chatwin, J. 2006. "Patient Narratives: A Micro-Interactional Analysis." *Communication & Medicine* 3 (2): 113–23.

Chism, D. 1997. *The High-Risk Pregnancy Sourcebook*. Los Angeles, CA: Lowell House.

Condor, B. 1995. "'ER' Episode Delivers More Drama Than Realism." *Chicago Tribune*.

Coppola, G., R. Cassibba, A. Bosco, and S. Papagna. 2013. "In Search of Social Support in the NICU: Features, Benefits and Antecedents of Parents' Tendency to Share with Others the Premature Birth of Their Baby." *The Journal of Maternal-Fetal & Neonatal Medicine: The Official Journal of the European Association of Perinatal Medicine, the Federation of Asia and Oceania Perinatal Societies, the International Society of Perinatal Obstetricians* 7058 (17): 1737–41. doi:10.3109/14767058.2013.798281.

Corry, M. P. 2013. "Listening to Mothers III Major Survey Findings," April.

Cottle, T. 2002. "On Narratives and the Sense of Self." *Qualitative Inquiry* 8 (5): 535–49.

Declercq, E. R., C. Sakala, M. P. Corry, S. Applebaum, and P. Risher. 2002. "Listening to Mothers: Women's Childbearing Experiences Listening to Mothers: Report of the," October.

Dias, L., and M. Lobel. 1997. "Social Comparison in Medically High-Risk Pregnant Women'," 1629–49.

DiMatteo, M. 1994. "Enhancing Patient Adherence to Medical Recommendations." *Journal of the American Medicla Association* 271 (1): 79.

DiMatteo, M. and H. Lepper. 1998. "Promoting Adherenc to Courses in Treatment: Mutual Collaboration in Physician-Patient Relationship." In *Health Communication Research: A Guide to Development and Directions*, edited by L. Jackson and B. Duffy, 75–86. Westport, CT: Greenwodd Press.

Doyle, L. 2004. "Neonatal Intensive Care at Borderline Viability: 'Is It Worth It?'" *Early Human Development* 80 (2): 103–13.

Durham, R. F. 1999. "Negotiating Activity Restriction: A Grounded Theory of Home Management of Preterm Labor." *Qualitative Health Research* 9 (4): 493–503. doi:10.1177/104973299129122027.

Eckerle, L. 2011. "Life in the NICU: A Few Ounces Away." *NPR*. www.npr.org/blogs/babyproject/2011.

Eggly, S. 2002. "Physician-Patient Co-Construction of Illness Narratives in the Medical Interview." *Health Communication* 14 (3): 339–60. doi:10.1207/S15327027HC1403_3.

Ellingson, L. L. 2006. "Embodied Knowledge: Writing Researchers' Bodies into Qualitative Health Research." *Qualitative Health Research* 16 (2): 298–310. doi:10.1177/1049732305281944.

Embler, P. 2006. "Midwifery and Conceptual Models of Nursing: A Comparison." *Midwifery Today with International Midwife*, no. 78 (January): 32–33. http://www.ncbi.nlm.nih.gov/pubmed/16841843.

"Ethics of Intensive Neonatal Care." 2000, 9198.

Evans, M., and B. O'Brien. 2005. "Gestational Diabetes: The Meaning of an at-Risk Pregnancy." *Qualitative Health Research* 15 (1): 66–81.

"Fathers in the Caribbean Have to Fight to See the Birth of Their Kids." 2014. *Public Radio International*. http://www.pri.org/stories/2014-03-12/midwives-take-action-no-dads-allowed-rules-trinidad-tobago.

Feeley, N., P. Zelkowitz, C. Cormier, L. Charbonneau, A. Lacroix, and A. Papageorgiou. 2011. "Posttraumatic Stress among Mothers of Very Low Birthweight Infants at 6 Months after Discharge from the Neonatal Intensive Care Unit." *Applied Nursing Research: ANR* 24 (2). Elsevier B.V.: 114–17. doi:10.1016/j.apnr.2009.04.004.

Festinger, L. 1954. "A Theory of Social Comparison Processes." *Human Relations* 7 (2): 117–40. doi:10.1177/001872675400700202.

Fioretti, B., M. Reiter, A. P. Betrán, and M. R. Torloni. 2015. "Googling Caesarean Section: A Survey on the Quality of the Information Available on the Internet." *BJOG: An International Journal of Obstetrics and Gynaecology* 122 (5): 731–39. doi:10.1111/1471-0528.13081.

Fisher, E., and B. Gainer. 1993. "Babyshowers: A Rite of Passage in Transition." *Advances in Consumer Research* 20: 320–24.

Fisher, W. 1984. "Narration as Human Communication Paradigm: The Case of Public Moral Argument." *Communication Monographs* 51: 1–22.

———. 1985. "The Narrative Paradigm: An Elaboration." *Communication Monographs* 52: 347–67.

———. 1989. "Carifying the Narrative Paradigm." *Communication Monographs* 56: 55–58.

Folkman, S. 1997. "Positive Pscychological States and Coping with Severe Stress." *Social Science & Medicine 1* 45 (8): 1207–21.

Frank, A. 1995. *The Wounded Storyteller*. Chicago, IL: The University of Chicago Press.

Friedman, B., K. Devers, C. Steiner, and S. Fox. 2002. "The Use of Expensive Health Technologies in the Era of Managed Care." *Journal of Health Politics, Policy & Law* 27 (3): 441–44.

Fuertes, J., L. Boylan, and J. Fontanella. 2009. "Behavioral Indices in Medical Care Outcome: The Working Alliance, Adherence, and Related Factors." *Journal of General Internal Medicine* 24 (1): 80–85.

Garten, L., L. Nazary, B. Metze, and C. Bührer. 2013. "Pilot Study of Experiences and Needs of 111 Fathers of Very Low Birth Weight Infants in a Neonatal Intensive Care Unit." *Journal of Perinatology: Official Journal of the California Perinatal Association* 33 (1): 65–69. doi:10.1038/jp.2012.32.

Gentile, K. 2011. "What About the Baby? The New Cult of Domesticity and Media Images of Pregnancy." *Studies in Gender and Sexuality* 12 (1): 38–58. doi:10.1080/15240657.2011.536056.

Gerbner, G. 1998. "Cultivation Analysis: An Overview." *Mass Communication & Society* 1 (3): 175–94.

Giurgescu, C., S. N. Zenk, T. N. Templin, C. G. Engeland, B. L. Dancy, C. Gi Park, K. Kavanaugh, W. Dieber, and D. P. Misra. 2015. "The Impact of Neighborhood Environment, Social Support, and Avoidance Coping on Depressive Symptoms of Pregnant African-American Women." *Women's Health Issues: Official Publication of the Jacobs Institute of Women's Health*, March. doi:10.1016/j.whi.2015.02.001.

Glazebrook, C., C. Sheard, S. Cox, M. Oates, and G. Ndukwe. 2004. "Parenting Stress in First-Time Mothers of Twins and Tripelts Conceived after in Vitro Fertilization." *Fertility & Sterility* 81 (3): 505–7.

Goldenberg, R., S. Cliver, J. Bronstein, G. Cutter, W. Andrews, and S. Mennemeyer. 1994. "Bed Rest in Pregnancy." *Obstetrics and Gynecoogy* 84 (1).

Golish, T. D., and K. A. Powell. 2003. "'Ambiguous Loss': Managing the Dialectics of Grief Associated with Premature Birth." *Journal of Social and Personal Relationships* 20 (3): 309–34. doi:10.1177/0265407503020003003.

Gray, J. E., C. Safran, R. B. Davis, G. Pompilio-Weitzner, J. E. Stewart, L. Zaccagnini, and D. Pursley. 2000. "Baby CareLink: Using the Internet and Telemedicine to Improve Care for High-Risk Infants." *Pediatrics* 106 (6): 1318–24. doi:10.1542/peds.106.6.1318.

Green, M. C., and T. C. Brock. 2000. "The Role of Transportation in the Persuasiveness of Public Narratives." *Journal of Personality and Social Psychology* 79 (5): 701–21. doi:10.1037//0022-3514.79.5.701.

Gubrium, J., and J. Holstein. 2009. *Analyzing Narrative Reality*. Thousand Oaks, CA: Sage.

Gupta, M., K. Emary, and L. Impey. 2010. "Emergency Cervical Cerclage: Predictors of Success." *The Journal of Maternal-Fetal & Neonatal Medicine: The Official Journal of the European Association of Perinatal Medicine, the Federation of Asia and Oceania Perinatal Societies, the International Society of Perinatal Obstetricians* 23 (7): 670–74. doi:10.3109/14767050903387011.

Gupta, S., and C. Gajilan. 2003. "Perils of Pregnancy." *Time*, November.

Hall, D, and G. Kirsten. 2008. "Kangaroo Mother Care--a Review." *Transfusion Medicine (Oxford, England)* 18 (2): 77–82. doi:10.1111/j.1365-3148.2007.00812.x.

Hamilton, J., and M. Lobel. 2008. "Types, Patterns, and Predictors of Copin with Stress during Pregnancy: Examiniation of the Revised Prenatal Coping Inventory in a Diverse Sample." *Journal of Psychosomatic Obstetrics & Gynecology* 29 (2): 97–104.

Han, S. 2013. *Pregnancy in Practice: Expectation and Experience in the Contemporary US*. Oxford, NY: Berghan Books.

Handfiled, B., S. Turnbull, and R. Bell. 2006. "What Do Obsetricians Think about Media Influences on Their Patients?" *Australian & New Zealand Journal of Obstetrics & Gynaecology* 46 (5): 379–83.

Harris, N.-E. 2013. "Full-Term Crisis." *Newsweek*, November.

Harvey, T. A., and L. Buckley. 2009. "Childbirth in China." In *Childbirth across Cultures Ideas and Practices of Pregnancy, Childbirth and the Postpartum*, edited by Helaine Selin, 5:55–69. Science Across Cultures: The History of Non-Western Science. Dordrecht: Springer Netherlands. doi:10.1007/978-90-481-2599-9.

Heermann, J., M. Wilson, and P. Wilhelm. 2005. "Mothers in the NICU: Outsider to Partner." *Pediatric Nursing* 31 (3): 176–81.

Helen, Julie, Jenny Hainsworth, and Stephen Thornton. 2008. "Women's Experiences of Hospitalisation with Hypertension during Pregnancy: Feeling a Fraud" 26 (3): 157–67. doi:10.1080/02646830701691384.

Hoffenkamp, H., A. Tooten, R. Hall, M. Croon, J. Braeken, F. Winkel, A. Vingerhoets, and H. van Bakel. 2012. "The Impact of Premature Childbirth on Parental Bonding." *Evolutionary Psychology* 10 (3): 542–61.

Holditch-Davis, D., R. Bartlett, A. Blickman, and M. Miles. 2003. "Posttraumatic Stress Symptoms in Mothers of Premature Infants." *Journal of Obstetric, Gynecologic, and Neonatal Nursing* 32: 161–71.

Holditch-Davis, D., M. Miles, M. Weaver, B. Black, L. Beeber, S. Thoyre, and S. Engelke. 2009. "Patterns of Distress in African American Mothers of Preterm Infants." *Journal of Developmental and Behavioral Pediatrics* 30 (3): 193–205.

Hughes, M., J. McCollum, D. Sheftel, and G. Sanchez. 1994. "How Parents Cope with the Experience of Neonatal Intensive Care." *Children's Health Care* 23 (1): 1–14.

Huynh, L., M. McCoy, A. Law, K. N. Tran, S. Knuth, P. Lefebvre, S. Sullivan, and M. Sheng Duh. 2013. "Systematic Literature Review of the Costs of Pregnancy in the US." *PharmacoEconomics* 31 (11): 1005–30. doi:10.1007/s40273-013-0096-8.

Hyden, L. 1997. "Illness and Narrative." *Sociology of Health and Illness* 19 (1): 48–69.

"'I Love Lucy,' 'Lucy Is Enceinte' More than 60 Years Later and More Talked about TV Pregnancies." 2013. *Huffington Post.* http://www.huffingtonpost.com/2013/07/25/i-love-lucy-lucy-is-enceinte.

Inspire, An, Preemie Support, and Community Special. 2011. "Insensitive Comments and Their Impact on Preemie Mothers," no. June.

Jesper, E. 2015. "Poor Quality Online Information for Pregnant Women Is a Global Problem: What Can We Do about It?" *BJOG : An International Journal of Obstetrics and Gynaecology* 122 (5): 740. doi:10.1111/1471-0528.13091.

Johnson, A. N. 2008. "Promoting Maternal Confidence in the NICU." *Journal of Pediatric Health Care* 22: 254–57. doi:10.1016/j.pedhc.2007.12.012.

Jones, L., D. Woodhouse, and J. Rowe. 2007. "Effective Nurse Parent Communication: A Study of Parents' Perceptions in the NICU Environment." *Patient Education & Counseling* 69 (1): 206–12.

Jorgensen, B. A. M. 2010. "Born in the USA–The History of Neonatology in the United States: A Century of Caring," no. June.

Kammerer, M., M. N. Marks, C. Pinard, A. Taylor, B. von Castelberg, H. Künzli, and V. Glover. 2009. "Symptoms Associated with the DSM IV Diagnosis of Depression in Pregnancy and Post Partum." *Archives of Women's Mental Health* 12 (3): 135–41. doi:10.1007/s00737-009-0062-9.

Kantor, J. 2005. "Expecting Trouble: The Book They Love to Hate." *The New York Times*, September 15.

Keane, E. 2009. "Evaluating Consumer Health Information: What Fails to Harm Us Makes Us Smarter." *Reference Librarian* 50 (2): 178–92.

Kline, K. 2007. "Midwife Attended Births in Prime-Time Television: Craziness, Controlling Bitches, and Ultimate Capitulations." *Women and Language* 30 (1): 20–29.

Knudson-Martin, C., and R. Silverstein. 2009. "Suffering in Silence: A Qualitative Meta-Data-Analysis of Postpartum Depression." *Journal of Marital and Family Therapy* 35 (2): 145–58.

Kruger, L.-M. 2003. "Narrating Motherhood: The Transformative Potential of Individual Stories." *South African Journl of Psychology* 33 (4): 198–204.

Kymre, I. G., and T. Bondas. 2013. "Skin-to-Skin Care for Dying Preterm Newborns and Their Parents-A Phenomenological Study from the Perspective of NICU Nurses." *Scandinavian Journal of Caring Sciences* 27 (3): 669–76. doi:10.1111/j.1471-6712.2012.01076.x.

Kyomuhendo, G. B. 2009. "Culture, Pregnancy and Childbirth in Uganda: Surviving the Women's Battle." In *Childbirth across Cultures Ideas and Practices of*

Pregnancy, Childbirth and the Postpartum, edited by Helaine Selin, 5: 229–34. Science Across Cultures: The History of Non-Western Science. Dordrecht: Springer Netherlands. doi:10.1007/978-90-481-2599-9.

Lagan, B. M., M. Sinclair, and W. George Kernohan. 2011. "What Is the Impact of the Internet on Decision-Making in Pregnancy? A Global Study." *Birth (Berkeley, Calif.)* 38 (4): 336–45. doi:10.1111/j.1523-536X.2011.00488.x.

Lazarus, R., and S. Folkman. 1984. *Stress, Appraisal, and Coping*. New York, NY: Springer Publishing.

Leichtentritt, R., N. Blumenthal, A. Elyassi, and S. Rotmensch. 2005. "High-Risk Pregnancy and Hospitalization: The Women's Voices." *Health & Social Work* 30 (1): 39–47.

Leigh, S. 2005. "When Preemies Reach 'Miracle' Status, Painful Truth Becomes a Footnote." *USA Today*, February 2.

Liamputtong, P. 2009. "Nyob Nruab Hlis: Thirty Days Confinement in Hmong Culture." In *Chil*, edited by Helaine Selin, 5: 161–73. Science Across Cultures: The History of Non-Western Science. Dordrecht: Springer Netherlands. doi:10.1007/978-90-481-2599-9.

Lowe, P., J. Powell, F. Griffiths, M. Thorogood, and L. Locock. 2009. "Making It All Normal: The Role of the Internet in Problematic Pregnancy." *Qualitative Health Research* 19 (10): 1476–84. doi:10.1177/1049732309348368.

Luke, B. 1994. "The Changing Pattern of Multiple Births in the United States: Maternal and Infant Characteristics." *Obstetrics and Gynecoogy* 84: 101–6.

Lupton, D. 2012. "'Precious Cargo': Foetal Subjects, Risk and Reproductive Citizenship." *Critical Public Health* 22 (3): 329–40. doi:10.1080/09581596.2012.657612.

MacDorman, M. F., T. J. Mathews, and E. Declercq. 2012. "Home Births in the United States, 1990-2009." *NCHS Data Brief*, no. 84 (January): 1–8. http://www.ncbi.nlm.nih.gov/pubmed/22617638.

Maher, J. 2003. "Rethinking Women's Birth Experiences: Medical Frameworks and Personal Narratives." *Hectate* 29 (2): 140–52.

Malik, S., and N. Coulson. 2008. "Computer-Mediated Infertility Support Groups: An Exploratory Study of Online Experiences." *Patient Education & Counseling* 73 (1): 105–13.

Mannering, L. 2009. "A Brief History of Maternity Clothes." *Huffington Post*. www.huffingtonpost.com.

"March of Dimes Peristats." 2014. www.marchofdimes.com/Peristats.

Marlow, N., D. Wolke, D. Ph, and M. A. Bracewell. 2005. "New England Journal," 9–19.

Martin, J. A., B. E. Hamilton, D. Ph, M. J. K. Osterman, S. C. Curtin, and T. J. Mathews. 2015. "National Vital Statistics Reports Births: Final Data for 2013" 64 (1).

Martin, J. A., B. E. Hamilton, D. Ph, M. J. K. Osterman, S. C. Curtin, T. J. Mathews, and V. Statistics. 2013. "Births: Final Data for 2012." 62 (9).

Matricardi, S., R. Agostino, C. Fedeli, and R. Montirosso. 2013. "Mothers Are Not Fathers: Differences between Parents in the Reduction of Stress Levels after a Parental Intervention in a NICU." *Acta Paediatrica (Oslo, Norway : 1992)* 102 (1): 8–14. doi:10.1111/apa.12058.

McCarty-Singleton, S., and A. C. Sciscione. 2014. "Maternal Activity Restriction in Pregnancy and the Prevention of Preterm Birth: An Evidence-Based

Review." *Clinical Obstetrics and Gynecology* 57 (3): 616–27. doi:10.1097/GRF.0000000000000048.

McDermott-Perez, L. 2007. *Preemie Parents: Recovering from Bab's Premature Birth*. Westport, CT: Praeger.

McIntosh, B., M. Stern, and K. Ferguson. 2004. "Optimism, Coping, and Psychological Distress: Maternal Reactions to NICU Hospitalization." *Children's Health Care* 33 (1): 59–76.

Mercer, R. T. 1995. *Becoming a Mother*. New York: NY: Springer Publishing.

Michinov, N. 2007. "Social Comparison and Affect: A Study among Elderly Women." *Journal of Social Psychology* 147 (2): 175–89.

Miller, K., J. Stiff, and B. Ellis. 1988. "Communication and Empathy as Precursors to Burnout Amon Human Service Workers." *Communication Monographs* 55 (2): 250–65.

Misra, D., D. Strobino, and B. Trabert. 2010. "Effects of Social and Psychosocial Factors on Risk of Preterm Birth in Black Women." *Paediatric and Perinatal Epidemiology* 24 (6): 546–54. doi:10.1111/j.1365-3016.2010.01148.x.

Morris, T., and K. McInerney. 2010. "Media Representations of Pregnancy and Childbirth: An Analysis of Reality Television Programs in the United States." *Birth (Berkeley, Calif.)* 37 (2): 134–40. doi:10.1111/j.1523-536X.2010.00393.x.

Negron, R., A. Martin, M. Almog, A. Balbierz, and E. A. Howell. 2013. "Social Support during the Postpartum Period: Mothers' Views on Needs, Expectations, and Mobilization of Support." *Maternal and Child Health Journal* 17 (4): 616–23. doi:10.1007/s10995-012-1037-4.

Neuman, W. R., and L. Guggenheim. 2011. "The Evolution of Media Effects Theory: A Six-Stage Model of Cumulative Research." *Communication Theory* 21 (2): 169–96. doi:10.1111/j.1468-2885.2011.01381.x.

Newman, A. A. 2009. "Once a Seldom-Heard Word, Pregnancy Is Now in the Spotlight." *New York Time*, April 9.

Noble, E., and L. Sorger. 2004. "Fetal Surveillance and the Nocebo Effect: Recommendations for a Normal Pregnancy, Vaginal Birth and Optimal Outcome-Session: Controversies on Obstetric Issues." *Twin Research and Human Genetics* 7 (4): 370.

Odd, D., D. Evans, and A. Emond. 2013. "Preterm Birth, Age at School Entry and Educational Performance." *PloS One* 8 (10): e76615. doi:10.1371/journal.pone.0076615.

Ogle, J. P., K. E. Tyner, and S. Schofield-Tomschin. 2013. "The Role of Maternity Dress Consumption in Shaping the Self and Identity during the Liminal Transition of Pregnancy." *Journal of Consumer Culture* 13 (2): 119–39. doi:10.1177/1469540513480161.

Olshtain-Mann, O., and G. Auslander. 2008. "Parents of Preterm Infants Two Months after Discharge from the Hospital: Are They Still at (parental) Risk?" *Health & Social Work* 33 (4): 299–308.

Osterman, M. J. K., and J. A. Martin. 2011. "Epidural and Spinal Anesthesia Use During Labor: 27-State Reporting Area, 2008." *National Vital Statistics Reports: From the Centers for Disease Control and Prevention, National Center for Health Statistics, National Vital Statistics System* 59 (5): 1–14.

———. 2014. "Primary Cesarean Delivery Rates, by State: Results From the Revised Birth Certificate, 2006–2012." *National Vital Statistics Reports: From the*

Centers for Disease Control and Prevention, National Center for Health Statistics, National Vital Statistics System 63 (1).

Padden, T., and S. Glen. 1997. "Maternal Experiences of Preterm Birth and Neonatal Intensive Care." *Journal of Reproductive and Infant Psychology* 15 (2): 121–39.

Pariera, K. L., H. J. Hether, S. T. Murphy, S. De Castro Buffington, and L. Baezconde-Garbanati. 2014. "Portrayals of Reproductive and Sexual Health on Prime-Time Television." *Health Communication* 29 (7): 698–706. doi:10.1080/10410236.2013.774653.

Paul, P. 2007. "What to Expect When Expecting? A Whole Lot of Loot." *New York Times*, June 24.

Pennebaker, J. W., and J. D. Seagal. 1999. "Forminy a Story: The Healtli Benefits Ol Narfative" 55 (10): 1243–54.

Peterson, E. 1987. "The Stories of Pregnancy: On Interpretation of Small-Group Cultures." *Communication Quarterly* 35 (1): 39–47.

Platt, J., K. M. Keyes, and K. C. Koenen. 2014. "Size of the Social Network versus Quality of Social Support: Which Is More Protective against PTSD?" *Social Psychiatry and Psychiatric Epidemiology* 49 (8): 1279–86. doi:10.1007/s00127-013-0798-4.

Potter, W. 1986. "Perceived Reality and the Cultivation Hypothesis." *Journal of Broadcasting & Electronic Media* 30 (2): 159–74.

Rains, S., and V. Young. 2009. "A Meta-Analysis of Research on Formal Computer-Mediated Support Groups: Examining Gruop Characterstics and Health Outcomes." *Human Communication Research* 35 (3): 309–36.

Reichman, S., A. Miller, R. Gordon, and K. Hendricks-Munoz. 2000. "Stress Appraisal and Coping in Mothers of NICU Infants." *Children's Health Care* 29 (4): 279–93.

Reid, T., R. Bramwell, N. Booth, and A. Weindling. 2007. "A New Stressor Scale for Parents Experiencing Neonatal Intensive Care: The NUPS (Neonatal Unit Parental Stress) Scale." *Journal of Reproductive and Infant Psychology* 25 (1): 66–82.

Resnik, D. 2005. "The Patient's Duty to to Adhere to Prescribed Treatment: An Ethical Analysis." *Journal of Medicine & Philosophy* 30 (2): 167–88.

Robinson, J., L. Callister, J. Berry, and K. Dearing. 2008. "Patient-Centered Care and Adherence: Definitions and Applications to Improve Outcomes." *Journal of the American Academy of Nurse Practitioners* 20 (12): 600–607.

Rooks, J. P. 1999. "The Midwifery Model of Care." *Journal of Nurse-Midwifery* 44 (4): 370–74. doi:10.1016/S0091-2182(99)00060-9.

Root, R., and C. Browner. 2001. "Practies of the Pregnant Self: Compliance with the Resistance to Prenatal Norms." *Culture, Medicine, and Psychiatry* 25: 195–223.

Rouck, S. D., and M. Leys. 2012. "Illness Trajectory and Internet as a Health Information and Communication Channel Used by Parents of Infants Admitted to a Neonatal Intensive Care Unit." doi:10.1111/jan.12007.

Sassi Matthias, M., and A. S. Babrow. 2007. "Problematic Integration of Uncertainty and Desire in Pregnancy." *Qualitative Health Research* 17 (6): 786–98. doi:10.1177/1049732307303241.

Saul, S. 2009. "The Twins Dilema." *New York Times*, October 11.

Scheufele, D. A., and D. Tewksbury. 2007. "Framing, Agenda Setting, and Priming: The Evolution of Three Media Effects Models." *Journal of Communication* 57 (1): 9–20. doi:10.1111/j.0021-9916.2007.00326.x.

Sears, C. A., and R. Godderis. 2011. "Roar Like a Tiger on TV?" *Feminist Media Studies* 11 (2): 181–95. doi:10.1080/14680777.2010.521626.

Seigel, M. 2013. *The Rhetoric of Pregnancy*. Chicago, IL: University of Chicago Press.

Shapiro, G., W. Fraser, M. Frasch, and J. Seguin. 2013. "Psychosocial Stress in Pregnancy and Preterm Birth: Associations and Mechanisms." *Journal of Perinatal Medicine* 41 (6): 631–45.

Sharf, B. 2005. "How I Fired My Surgeon and Embraced an Alternative Narrative." In *Narratives, Health, and Healing: CommunicationTheory, Reserearch, and Practice*, edited by L. M. Harter, P. M. Japp, and C. Beck, 325–42. Mahwah, NJ: Lawrence Earlbaum.

Sharf, B., and M. Vanderford. 2002. "Illness Narratives and the Social Construction of Health." In *Handbook of Health Communication*, edited by L. Harter, P. M. Japp, and C. Beck, 9–34. Mahwah, NJ: Lawrence Earlbaum.

Sharot, Tali. 2011. "The Optimism Bias." *Current Biology* 21 (23): R941–45. doi:10.1016/j.cub.2011.10.030.

Shaw, R. J., R. S. Bernard, T. Deblois, L. M. Ikuta, K. Ginzburg, and C. Koopman. 2009. "The Relationship between Acute Stress Disorder and Posttraumatic Stress Disorder in the Neonatal Intensive Care Unit." *Psychosomatics* 50 (2): 131–37. doi:10.1176/appi.psy.50.2.131.

Singh, G. K., and P. C. Van Dyck. 2010. "Infant Mortality in the United States, 1935–2007: Over Seven Decades of Progress and Disparities," 1–8.

Smith, T. 1999. *Miracle Birth Stories of Very Premature Infants*. Westport, CT: Bergin & Garvey.

Smith, V., B. DeVellis, A. Kalet, J. Roberts, and R. DeVeillis. 2005. "Encouraging Patient Adherence: Primary Care Physicians' Use of Verbal Compliance Gaining Strategies in Medical Interviews." *Patient Education & Counseling* 57 (1): 62–76.

Spock, B., and R. Needlman. 2004. *Dr. Spock's Baby and Child Care*. New York, NY: Pocket Books.

Spock, B. 1946. *The Common Sense Book of Baby and Child Care*. New York, NY: Pocket Books.

Stern, A., and H. Markel, eds. 2004. "Formative Years: Children's Health in the United States, 1880–2000." In , 66–90. University of Michigan Press.

Stevens, H. 2011. "Social Media Giving Birth to New Generation of Parents-to-Be." *Chicago Tribune*, December 28.

Taylor, C., and K. Luce. 2003. "Computer- and Internet-Based Psychotherapy Interventions." *Current Directions in Psychological Science* 12 (1): 18–22.

Thachuk, A. 2007. "Midwifery, Informed Choice, and Reproductive Autonomy: A Relational Approach." *Feminism & Psychology* 17 (1): 39–56. doi:10.1177/0959353507072911.

"US Maternity Apparel Market Size $4.8 Bn by 2015." 2010. *Commodity Online*. http://www.commodityonline.com/news/us-maternity-apparel-market-size-$48-bn-by-2015-25582-1-25583.html.

Valenti, J. 2011. "Learning to Love My Baby." *The Guardian*. http://www.theguardian.com/lifeandstyle/2011/aug/18/baby-pregnancy-premature-birth.

Vanderford, M., E. Jenks, and B. Sharf. 1997. "Exploring Patient's Experiences as a Primary Source of Meaning." *Health Communication* 9 (1): 13–26.

Vegni, E., S. Visioli, and E. Moja. 2005. "When Talking to the Patient Is Difficult: The Physician's Perspective." *Communication & Medicine* 2 (1): 69–76.

Ventura, S., J. Martin, S. Curtin, F. Menacker, and B Hamilton. 2001. *Births: Final Data for 1999.*

Vermeire, E., H. Hearnshaw, P. Van Royen, and J. Denekens. 2001. "Patient Adherence to Treatment: Three Decades of Research: A Comprehensive Review." *Journal of Clinical Pharmacy and Therapeutics* 26 (5): 331–42.

Von Gontard, A., S. Schwarte, A. Kribs, and B. Roth. 1999. "Neonatal Intensive Care and Premature Birth-Maternal Perceptions and Coping." *Archives of Women's Mental Health* 2 (1): 29.

Walczak, S. 2009. "Managing Personal Medical Knowledge: Agent-Based Knowledge Acquisition." *International Journal of Technology Management* 47 (1): 22–36.

Wall Street Journal. 2000. "Experimental Web Site Gives Parents a Link To Hospitalized Babies.," November 27.

Wegman, M. E. 2001. "Infant Mortality in the 20th Century, Dramatic but Uneven Progress." *J. Nutr.* 131 (2): 401S–408. http://jn.nutrition.org/content/131/2/401S.short#sec-2.

West, J. E. 2010. "Technology Knows Best: The Cultural Work of Hospital Birth in 21st Century Film." *Literature & Medicine* 29 (1): 104–26.

"What to Expect." 2004. *100 Years of Maternity Fashion*. www.whattoexpect.com/tools.

Wheatley, R., M. Kelley, N. Peacock, and J. Delgado. 2008. "Women's Narratives on Quality in Prenatal Care: A Multicultural Perspective." *Qualitative Health Research* 18 (11): 1586–98.

White, J. B., E. J. Langer, L. Yariv, and J. C. Welch. 2006. "Frequent Social Comparisons and Destructive Emotions and Behaviors: The Dark Side of Social Comparisons." *Journal of Adult Development* 13 (1): 36–44. doi:10.1007/s10804-006-9005-0.

White, M. J., L. C. Cunningham, and K. Titchener. 2011. "Young Drivers' Optimism Bias for Accident Risk and Driving Skill: Accountability and Insight Experience Manipulations." *Accident Analysis & Prevention* 43 (4): 1309–15. doi:10.1016/j.aap.2011.01.013.

Whitehead, N. S. 2012. "The Relationship of Socioeconomic Status to Preterm Contractions and Preterm Delivery." *Maternal and Child Health Journal* 16 (8): 1645–56. doi:10.1007/s10995-012-0948-4.

Williams, Z. 2012. "Why We Can't Get Enough of Childbirth on TV." *The Guardian*. http://www.theguardian.com/lifeandstyle/2012/jan/28/why-childbirth-on-tv-hit.

Wills, T. 1981. "Downward Comparison Principles in Social Psychology." *Psychology Bulletin* 90: 245–71.

Winterbottom, A., H. L. Bekker, M. Conner, and A. Mooney. 2008. "Does Narrative Information Bias Individual's Decision Making? A Systematic Review."

Social Science & Medicine (1982) 67 (12). Elsevier Ltd: 2079–88. doi:10.1016/j.socscimed.2008.09.037.

Worman-Ross, K., and T. L. Mix. 2013. "'I Wanted Empowerment, Healing, and Respect': Homebirth as Challenge to Medical Hegemony." *Sociological Spectrum* 33 (5): 453–81. doi:10.1080/02732173.2013.818509.

Yanagisawa, S. 2009. "Childbirth In Jpana." In *Childbirth across Cultures Ideas and Practices of Pregnancy, Childbirth and the Postpartum*, edited by Helaine Selin, 5: 85–94. Science Across Cultures: The History of Non-Western Science. Dordrecht: Springer Netherlands. doi:10.1007/978-90-481-2599-9.

Young, D. 2010. "Childbirth Education, the Internet, and Reality Television: Challenges Ahead." *Birth2* 37 (2): 87–89.

Zwelling, E. 2000. "The History of Lamaze Continues: An Interview with Elisabeth Bing." *The Journal of Perinatal Education* 9 (1): 15–21. doi:10.1624/105812400X87464.

Index

About the Author

Jennifer Hall teaches and serves as an Assistant Basic Course Director at Purdue University in the Communication Department, the same department where she earned her Masters and Doctoral degrees in Health Communication. She is also an adjunct faculty member at Southern New Hampshire University. Her previous publications include the coauthored health communication textbook *Health as a Communication Nexus* as well as journal articles about various health-related topics. In addition to teaching, she has a passion for nonprofits and loves the opportunity to take the concepts she researches and studies and apply them to assist different organizations in achieving their goals. She currently is on the board of directors for the Tippecanoe Child Abuse Prevention Council and Tippecanoe County Meals on Wheels, is a parent mentor for Graham's Foundation, an organization dedicated to providing support for preemie parents, and is a Girl Scout leader. She and her husband Brian reside in Lafayette, Indiana with their four daughters, nine-year-old Anna and seven-year-old triplets Sarah, Lucy, and Emily. The early birth of her triplets inspired her work on high-risk pregnancies and her goal is to provide a voice to the many women each year who experience difficult pregnancies and premature birth.

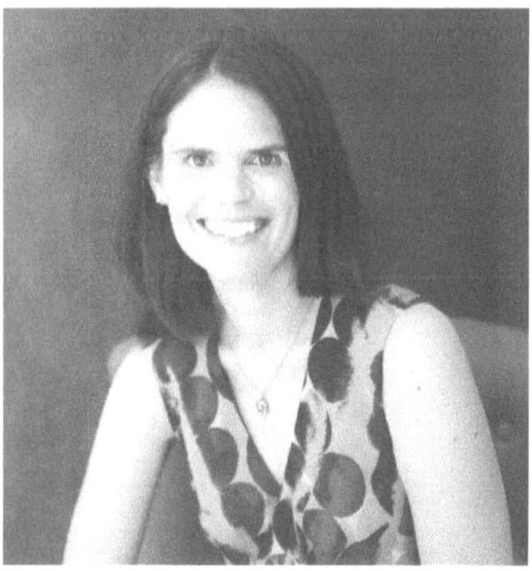

www.ingramcontent.com/pod-product-compliance
Ingram Content Group UK Ltd.
Pitfield, Milton Keynes, MK11 3LW, UK
UKHW041634031026
15587UKWH00001B/277

9 780739 195864